Fundamentals of Medical Imaging Systems

Fundamentals of Medical Imaging Systems

Cory Hibler

AMERICAN
MEDICAL PUBLISHERS
www.americanmedicalpublishers.com

AMERICAN
MEDICAL PUBLISHERS
www.americanmedicalpublishers.com

Cataloging-in-publication Data

Fundamentals of medical imaging systems / Cory Hibler.
p. cm.
Includes bibliographical references and index.
ISBN 979-8-88740-126-3
1. Imaging systems in medicine. 2. Diagnostic imaging. 3. Medical radiology. I. Hibler, Cory.
R857.O6 F86 2023
616.075 4--dc23

American Medical Publishers,
41 Flatbush Avenue,
1st Floor, New York,
NY 11217, USA

ISBN 979-8-88740-126-3 (Hardback)

Contents

Preface

The method and practice of functional and structural imaging of the interior of a body for the purpose of clinical examination and subsequent medical intervention is referred to as medical imaging. Medical imaging techniques help in creating visual representation of the structure and function of different body parts, organs or tissues. They have proved to be extremely beneficial in diagnosing and curing diseases. They also help in creating a normal anatomy and physiology database, allowing the detection of abnormalities. In medical imaging, two types of radiographic images are used: projection radiography and fluoroscopy. Fluoroscopy, like radiography, produces real-time images of internal body structures, but it uses a steady input of X-rays at a lower dose rate. X-rays, or projectional radiographs, are often used to diagnose the kind and extent of a fracture as well as to detect pathological changes in the lungs. X-rays can be used to visualize the structure of the stomach and intestines, which is helpful in diagnosing ulcers and some types of colon cancer. This book consists of contributions made by international experts. Also included herein is a detailed explanation of the various concepts and applications of medical imaging systems. For someone with an interest and eye for detailed research, this book covers the most significant topics in this field.

This book has been the outcome of endless efforts put in by authors and researchers on various issues and topics within the field. The book is a comprehensive collection of significant researches that are addressed in a variety of chapters. It will surely enhance the knowledge of the field among readers across the globe.

It gives us an immense pleasure to thank our researchers and authors for their efforts to submit their piece of writing before the deadlines. Finally in the end, I would like to thank my family and colleagues who have been a great source of inspiration and support.

Cory Hibler

1

Medical Imaging Systems: An Overview

Author: Andreas Maier

The design and manufacturing of modern medical devices requires knowledge of several disciplines, ranging from physics, over material science, to computer science. Thus, designing a single lecture as an introduction to medical engineering faces a lot of challenges. Nonetheless, the manuscript *Medical Imaging Systems – An Introductory Guide* aims at being a complete and comprehensive introduction to this field for students in the early semesters. Medical imaging devices are by now an integral part of modern medicine, and have probably already been encountered by all students in their personal life.

This book does not simply summarize the content of the lecture held in Erlangen. Instead, it should be understood as additional material to gain a better understanding of the theory that is covered in the lecture. To give a complete introduction, the lecture notes also cover basic math and physics that are required to understand the underlying principles of the imaging devices. However, we try to limit this to the very basics. Obviously, this is not sufficient to describe everything in the appropriate level of detail. For this reason, we introduced *geek boxes* (cf. Geek Box 1.1) that contain optional additional background information. This concept will be used in all chapters of the book which are summarised in the following sections.

Chap. 2 and 3 of this book cover an introduction to signal and image processing. Chap. 2 introduces the concepts of filtering, convolution, and Fourier transforms for 1-D signals, all of which are fundamental tools that are later on used across the entire book. We try to explain why these concepts are required and as most image processing is digital also emphasize the discrete algorithmic counter parts. At the beginning of Chap. 3, the transition to images is made, and therefore also the transition from 1-D to 2-D. The chapter

Geek Box 1.1: Geek Boxes

We designed the manuscript to be readable from the first semester on. However, we felt that we need to demonstrate that there is much more depth that we could go into. In order not to confuse a less experienced reader, we omitted most equations and math from the main text and relocated them to *geek boxes* that go into more detail and give references to further reading. In addition, we also refresh concepts that are already known to most readers. Nonetheless, the important concepts are already mentioned in the main text. This way, the reader can return to this book at a time when these concepts are introduced, e. g., in more advanced math courses seemingly unrelated to medical imaging. As such this book can be read twice: once omitting all geek boxes to get an overview on the field and a second time with a more throrough focus on the mathematical details.

covers the basics of image processing and explains how different image transformations such as edge detection and blurring are implemented as image filters using convolution.

The following chapters cover examples for imaging devices using standard optics. In this book, endoscopy and microscopy are discussed as typical modalities of this genre. Endoscopes, see Chap. 4, were among the first medical imaging devices that were used. Images can be acquired by using long and flexible optical fibers that are able to transport visible light through the body of a patient.

Microscopes also use visible light. However, tissue samples or cells have to be extracted from the body first, e. g., in a biopsy. Then the microscope's optics are used to acquire images at high magnifications that allow the imaging of individual cells and even smaller structures. Microscopes and the principles of optics are described in Chap. 5.

Magnetic resonance imaging (MRI), see Chap. 6 uses electromagnetic waves to excite water atoms inside the human body. Once the excitation is stopped, the atoms return to their normal state and by doing so emit the same electromagnetic radio wave that was used to excite them. This effect is called nuclear magnetic resonance. Using this effect, an MRI image is obtained. Fig. 1.1 shows a state-of-the-art MR scanner.

X-ray imaging devices, see Chap. 7, use light of very high energy. However, the light is no longer visible for the human eye. The higher energy of the light allows for a deeper penetration of the body. Due to different absorption rates of X-rays, different body tissues can be distinguished on X-ray images. Tissues with high X-ray absorption, e. g., bones, become visible as bright structures in X-ray projection images. Today, X-rays are among the most widely spread

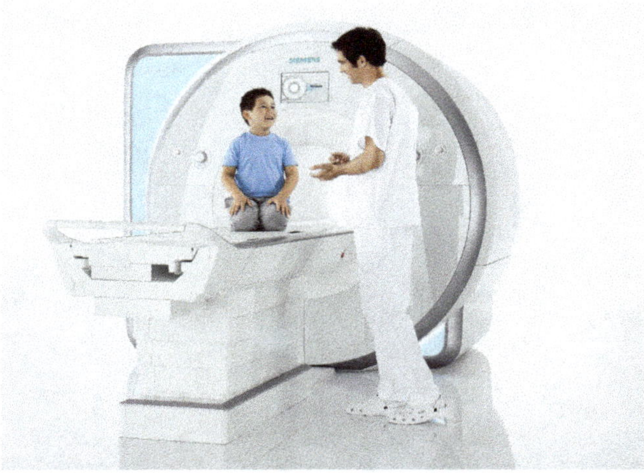

Figure 1.1: MRI is based on nuclear magnetic resonance which does not involve ionizing radiation. For this reason MRI is often used in pediatric applications. Image courtesy of Siemens Healthineers AG.

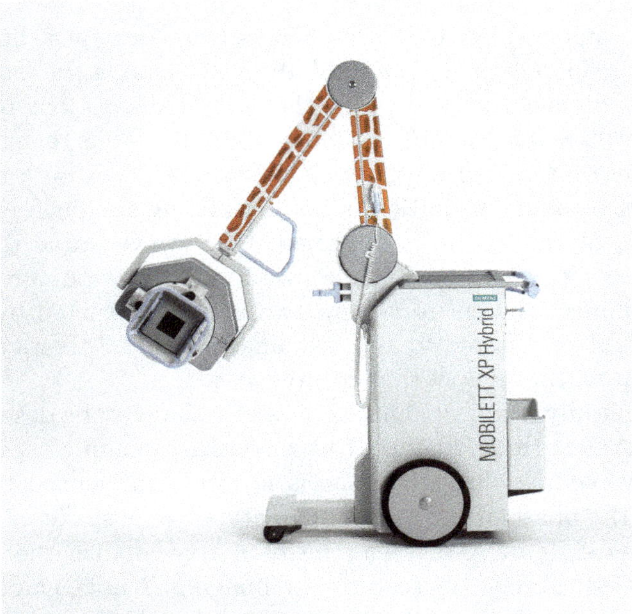

Figure 1.2: X-ray projection images are one of the most wide-spread imaging modalities. Image courtesy of Siemens Healthineers AG.

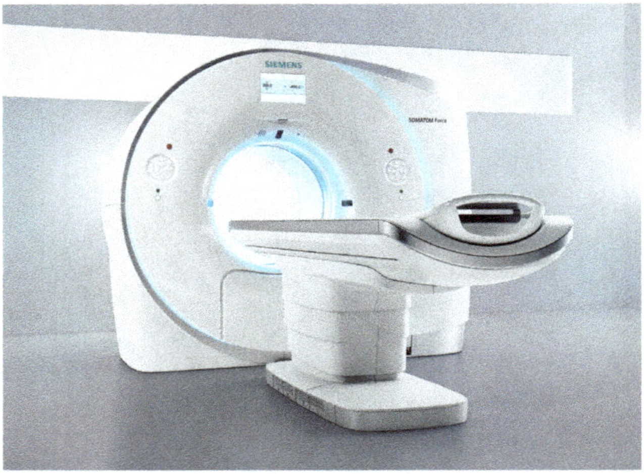

Figure 1.3: Modern CT systems allow even scanning of the beating heart. Image courtesy of Siemens Healthineers AG.

medical imaging technologies. An example for an X-ray imaging device is shown in Fig. 1.2.

Computed tomography (CT) uses X-rays to reconstruct slice and volume data as described in Chap. 8. The total absorption along the path of an X-ray through the body is actually given by the sum of absorptions by tissues with different absorption characteristics along its path. Thus, a measurement of the absorptions of X-rays from different directions allows for a reconstruction of slice images through the patient's body. In doing so, much better contrast between types of soft tissue is obtained. One is even able to differentiate between different tissue types such as brain and brain tumor. Once several slices are combined, the entire volume can be reconstructed by stacking the slices, which is then referred to as a 3-D image. Fig. 1.3 shows a state-of-the-art CT system with a gantry that rotates at 4 Hz.

X-rays essentially are electromagnetic waves that can be described by their amplitude, wavelength, and phase. Phase contrast imaging exploits the effect that an X-ray passing through tissue is not only influenced by absorption, but that also the phase of the electromagnetic wave is shifted. Chap. 9 shows that the phase shift of X-rays can be used to visualize the tissue the X-rays have passed. Today, phase contrast imaging is not yet used in clinical practice. In fact, due to the high requirements on the type of irradiation, such images often require a synchrotron as the source of the radiation. However, new developments in research now allow to generate phase contrast images using a normal clinical X-ray tube, which renders the application clinically feasible. At present, technical limitations allow only the scanning of small specimen such as peanuts and the mechanical design is still challenging. First image results indicate that the modality might be of high clinical relevance. Fig. 1.4 shows the reconstruction of peanut fibers that are in the range of

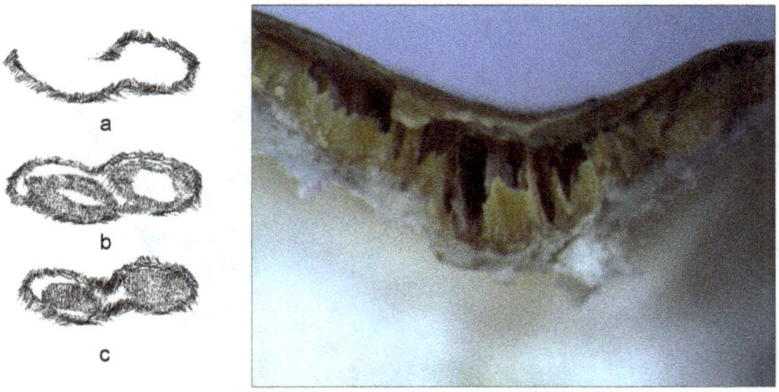

Figure 1.4: An X-ray dark-field setup can be used to reconstruct the orientation of fibers that are smaller than the detector resolution. The image on the left shows the reconstructed fiber orientation in different layers of a peanut. The image on the right shows a microscopic visualization of the waist of the peanut (picture courtesy of ECAP Erlangen).

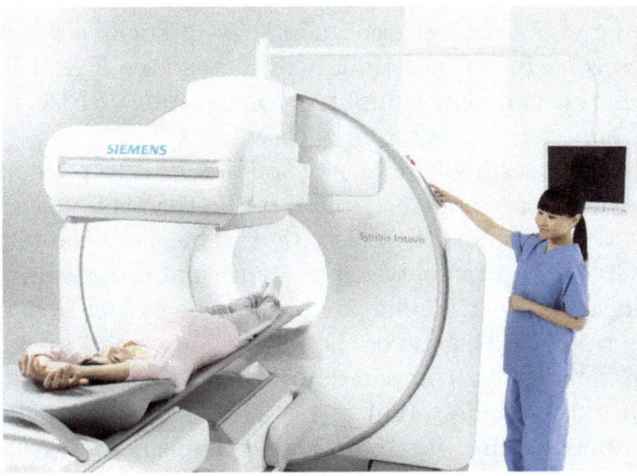

Figure 1.5: Modern SPECT/CT systems combine different modalities to achieve multi-modal imaging. Image courtesy of Siemens Healthineers AG.

several micrometers. Phase contrast allows for a reconstruction of these fibers, although the resolution of the used imaging device based on the absorption of X-rays was only 0.1 mm.

Emission tomography, described in Chap. 10, is used for imaging different bodily functions. It uses *tracers*, which are molecules that are marked with radioactive atoms. For example one can introduce a radioactive atom into a sugar molecule. When this tracer is consumed by the body it will follow the normal metabolism, and its path through the body can be followed. While sugar consumption is normal in certain parts of the body such as the muscles or the brain, tumors also require a lot of sugar for their growth. Thus, emis-

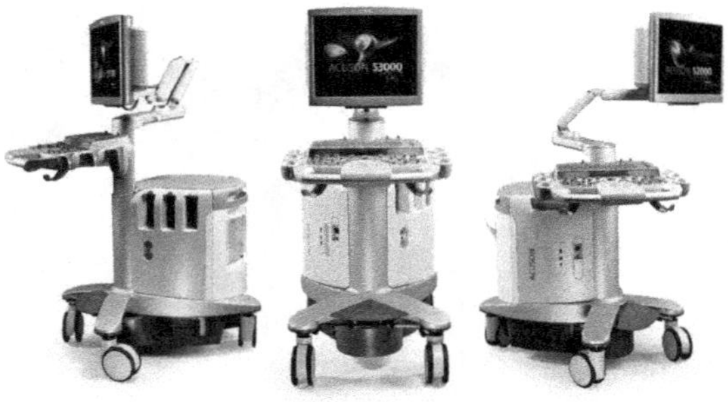

Figure 1.6: A typical ultrasound system as it can be found in clinics worldwide. Image courtesy of Siemens Healthineers AG.

sion tomography enables us to see anomalies in sugar consumption within the body which is useful to spot tumors or metastases. Fig. 1.5 shows a combined single-photon emission computed tomography (SPECT) / CT system that combines emission tomography with X-ray CT.

Ultrasound (US) uses high-frequency sound waves to penetrate bodily tissue. The sound waves are emitted from a probe that is in direct contact with the body. The same probe is then also used to measure the reflections of the sound waves. Given the time between the emission of the sound wave and the measurement of the reflection, one is able to reconstruct how deep the wave penetrated the tissue. US is one of the most wide-spread imaging modalities as it is rather inexpensive compared to other imaging modalities. Fig. 1.6 shows a clinical ultrasound system.

The measurement principle of optical coherence tomography (OCT) is quite similar to US. However, light waves are used instead of sound waves. Thus, the measurement process needs to be performed at much higher speed and penetration depth is much lower than in the case of US. Most applications are in eye imaging where 3-D images of the eye are generated.

2

Conversion from Continuous to Discrete Domain and the Role of Systems Theory

Authors: Peter Fischer, Klaus Sembritzki, and Andreas Maier

In the digital age, any medical image needs to be transformed from continuous domain to discrete domain (i. e. 1's and 0's) in order to be represented in a computer. To do so, we have to understand what a **continuous** and a **discrete signal** is. Both of them are handled by **systems** which will also be introduced in this chapter. Another fundamental concept is the Fourier transform as it allows us to represent any time domain signal in frequency space. In particular, we will find that both representations – time domain and frequency domain – are equivalent and can be converted into each other. Having found this important relationship, we can then determine conditions which will guarantee that also conversion from continuous to discrete domain and vice versa is possible without loss of information. On the way, we will introduce several other important concepts that will also find repeated use later in this book.

2.1 Signals and Systems

2.1.1 Signals

A signal is a function $f(t)$ that represents information. Often, the independent variable t is a physical dimension, like time or space. The output f of the signal is also called the dependent variable. Signals are everywhere in everyday life, although we are mostly not aware of them. A very prominent example is the speech signal, where the independent variable is time. The dependent variable is the electric signal that is created by measuring the changes of air pressure using a microphone. The description of the speech generation process enables to do efficient speech processing, e. g., radio transmission, speech coding, denoising, speech recognition, and many more. In general, many domains can be described using system theory, e. g., biology, society, economy. For our application, we are mainly interested in medical signals.

Both the dependent and the independent variable can be multidimensional. Multidimensional independent variables t are very common in images. In normal camera images, space is described using two spatial coordinates. However, medical images, e. g., CT volume scans, can also have three spatial dimensions. It is not necessary that all dimensions have the same meaning. Videos have two spatial coordinates and one time coordinate. In the medical domain, we can also find higher-dimensional examples like time-resolved 4-D MR and CT with three spatial dimensions and one time dimension. To represent multidimensional values, i. e., vectors, we use bold-face letters $\boldsymbol{t}$ or multiple scalar values, e. g., $\boldsymbol{t} = (x, y, z)^\mathsf{T}$. The medical field also contains examples of multidimensional dependent variables f. An example with many dimensions is the Electroencephalography (EEG). Electrodes are attached to the skull and measure electrical brain activity from multiple positions over time. To represent multidimensional dependent variables, we also use boldface letters $\boldsymbol{f}$.

The signals described above are all in continuous domain, e. g., time and space change continuously. Also, the dependent variables vary continuously in principle, like light intensity and electrical voltage. However, some signals exist naturally in discrete domains w. r. t. the independent variable or the dependent variable. An example for a discrete signal in dependent and independent variable is the number of first semester students in medical engineering. The independent variable time is discrete in this case. The starting semesters are WS 2009, WS 2010, WS 2011, and so on. Other points in time are considered to be constant in this interval. The number of students is restricted to natural numbers. In general, it is also possible that only the dependent or the independent variable is discrete and the other one continuous. In addition to signals that are discrete by nature, other signals must be represented discretely for processing with a digital computer, which means that the independent variable must be discretized before processing with a com-

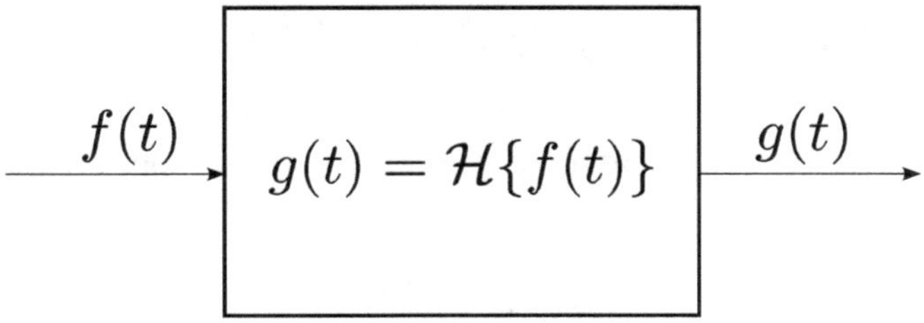

Figure 2.1: A system $\mathcal{H}\{.\}$ with the input signal $f(t)$ and the output signal $g(t)$.

puter. Furthermore, data storage in computers has limited precision, which means that the dependent variable must be discrete. Both are a direct consequence of the finite memory and processing speed of computers. This is the reason why discrete system theory is very important in practice.

Signals can be further categorized into deterministic and stochastic signals. For a deterministic signal, the whole waveform is known and can be written down as a function. In contrast, stochastic signals depend randomly on the independent variable, e. g., if the signal is corrupted by noise. Therefore, for practical applications, the stochastic properties of signals are very important. Nevertheless, deterministic signals are important to analyze the behavior of systems. A short introduction into stochastic signals and randomness will be given in Sec. 2.4.3.

This chapter is presents basic knowledge on how to represent, analyze, and process signals. The correct processing of signals requires some math and theory. A more in-depth introduction into the concepts presented here can be found in [3]. The application to medical data is treated in [2].

2.1.2 Systems

Signals are processed in processes or devices, which are abstracted as **systems**. This includes not only technical devices, but natural processes like attenuation and reverberation of speech in transmission through air as well. Systems have signals as input and as output. Inside the system, the properties of the signal are changed or signals are related to each other. We describe the processing of a signal using a system with the operator $\mathcal{H}\{\cdot\}$ that is applied to the function f. A graphical representation of a system is shown in Fig. 2.1.

An important subtype is the **linear shift-invariant system**. Linear shift-invariant systems are characterized by the two important properties of linearity and shift-invariance (cf. Geek Box 2.1 and 2.2).

Another property important for the practical realization of linear shift-invariant systems is causality. A causal system does not react to the input

Geek Box 2.1: Linear Systems

The linearity property of a system means that linear combinations of inputs can be represented as the same linear combination of the processed inputs

$$\mathcal{H}\{af(t)\} = a\mathcal{H}\{f(t)\} \tag{2.1}$$
$$\mathcal{H}\{f(t) + g(t)\} = \mathcal{H}\{f(t)\} + \mathcal{H}\{g(t)\}, \tag{2.2}$$

with constant a and arbitrary signals f and g. The linearity property greatly simplifies the mathematical and practical treatment, as the behavior of the system can be studied on basic signals. The behavior on more complex signals can be inferred directly if they can be represented as a superposition of the basic signals.

Geek Box 2.2: Shift-Invariant Systems

Shift-invariance denotes the characteristic of a system that its response is independent of shifts of the independent variable of the signal. Mathematically, this is described as

$$g_1(t) = \mathcal{H}\{f(t)\} \tag{2.3}$$
$$g_2(t) = \mathcal{H}\{f(t-\tau)\} \tag{2.4}$$
$$g_1(t-\tau) = g_2(t), \tag{2.5}$$

for the shift τ. This means that shifting the signal by τ followed by processing with the system is identical to processing the signal with the system followed by a shift with τ.

before the input actually arrives in the system. This is especially important for signals with time as the independent parameter. However, non-causal systems do not pose a problem for the independent parameter space, e. g., image filters that use information from the left and right of a pixel. Geek Box 2.3 presents examples for the combination of different system properties.

Linear shift-invariant systems are important in practice and have convenient properties and a rich theory. For linear shift-invariant systems, the abstract operator $\mathcal{H}\{\cdot\}$ can be described completely using the impulse response $h(t)$ (cf. Sec. 2.2.2) or transfer function $H(\xi)$ (cf. Sec. 2.3.2). The impulse response is combined with the signal by the operation of convolution. This is sufficient to describe all linear shift-invariant systems.

Geek Box 2.3: System Examples

Here are some examples of different systems analyzed w. r. t. linearity, shift-invariance, and causality. $f(t)$ represents the input and $g(t)$ the output signal.

- $g(t) = 10f(t)$: linear, shift-invariant, causal
- $g(t) = \sin(f(t))$: non-linear, shift-invariant, causal
- $g(t) = 3f(t+2)$: linear, shift-invariant, non-causal
- $g(t) = f(t) - 2f(t-1)$: linear, shift-invariant, causal
- $g(t) = f(t) \cdot e^{(-0.5t)}$: linear, not shift-invariant, causal

2.2 Convolution and Correlation

This section describes the combination of signals in linear-shift-invariant systems, i. e., convolution or correlation. Before discussing signal processing in detail, we will first start by revisiting important mathematical concepts that will be needed in the following chapters.

2.2.1 Complex Numbers

Complex numbers are an extension to real numbers. They are defined as $z = a + bi$. a is called the real part of z and b the imaginary part. Both act as coordinates in a 2-D space. i is the imaginary unit that spans the second dimension of this space. The special meaning of i is that $i^2 = -1$. This makes complex numbers important for many areas in mathematics, but also in many applied fields like physics and electrical engineering. To extract the coordinates of the complex number, we use the following definitions

$$a = \mathrm{Re}\,(z) \tag{2.6}$$
$$b = \mathrm{Im}\,(z)\,. \tag{2.7}$$

We can directly write $z = \mathrm{Re}\,(z) + \mathrm{Im}\,(z)\,i$. Another important definition is the complex conjugate $\bar{z}$, which is the same number as z except with the opposite sign for the imaginary part $\bar{z} = a - bi$.

Real numbers are the subset of the complex numbers for which $b = 0$, i. e., no imaginary part. Geometrically, this means that real numbers are defined on a one-dimensional axis, whereas the complex numbers are defined on a 2-D plane. The geometric interpretation of complex numbers is also helpful to see the equivalence of the Cartesian coordinate notation $z = a + bi$ and the polar coordinate notation $z = A\,(\cos\phi + i\sin\phi)$ of complex numbers. The

Geek Box 2.4: Complex Numbers and Geometric Interpretation

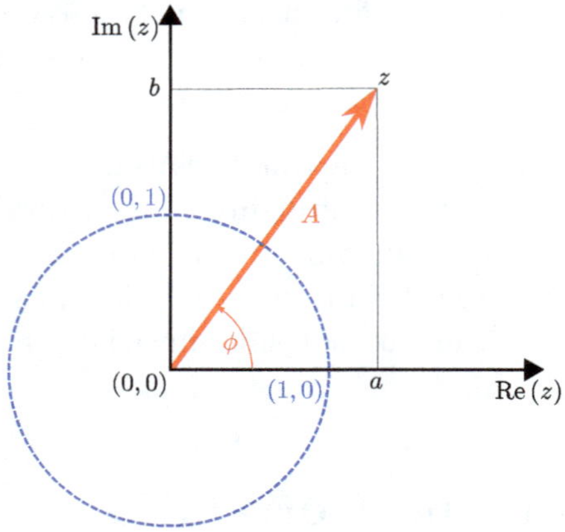

If a point on the 2-D plane is seen as a position vector, A is the length of the vector and ϕ the angle relative to the real axis. The two notations can be converted to each other using the following formulas:

$$A = \sqrt{a^2 + b^2}$$

$$\phi = \begin{cases} \arctan \frac{b}{a}, & \text{if } a > 0 \\ \arctan \frac{b}{a} + \pi, & \text{if } a < 0 \text{ and } b \geq 0 \\ \arctan \frac{b}{a} - \pi, & \text{if } a < 0 \text{ and } b < 0 \\ \frac{\pi}{2}, & \text{if } a = 0 \text{ and } b > 0 \\ -\frac{\pi}{2}, & \text{if } a = 0 \text{ and } b < 0 \\ \text{undefined}, & \text{if } a = 0 \text{ and } b = 0 \end{cases}$$

$$a = A \cos \phi$$

$$b = A \sin \phi$$

polar coordinates consists of magnitude A and angle ϕ (cf. Geek Box 2.4). For system theory, an important property of complex numbers is Euler's formula

$$\exp(i\phi) = e^{i\phi} = \cos(\phi) + i \sin(\phi). \quad (2.8)$$

Using this relation, a complex sum of sine and cosine can be expressed conveniently using a single exponential function. This leads directly to the exponential notation of complex numbers $z = Ae^{i\phi}$. We will use the complex numbers and different notations in Sec. 2.3.

Description	Equation
Linearity	$g(t) * (a \cdot f(t) + b \cdot h(t)) = a((g * f)(t)) + b((g * h)(t))$
Shift-invariance	$g(t) * f(t - \tau) = (g * f)(t - \tau)$
Commutativity	$g(t) * f(t) = f(t) * g(t)$
Associativity	$g(t) * ((f * h)(t)) = ((f * g)(t)) * h(t)$
Distributivity	$f(t) * (g(t) + h(t)) = (f * g)(t) + (f * h)(t)$

Table 2.1: Some mathematical properties of convolution. a, b are constants.

2.2.2 Convolution

As mentioned above, convolution is the operation that is necessary to describe the processing of any signal with a linear shift-invariant system. Convolution in the continuous case is defined as

$$g(t) = (h * f)(t) = \int_{-\infty}^{\infty} h(\tau) f(t - \tau) \, \mathrm{d}\tau. \tag{2.9}$$

In order for the convolution to be well-defined, some requirements for the functions h and f must be fulfilled. For the infinite integral to exist, h and f must decay fast enough towards infinity. This is the case if one of the functions has compact support, i. e., it is 0 everywhere except for a limited region. As an example, the convolution of a square input function $f(t)$ with an Gaussian function $h(t)$ is investigated in Geek Box 2.5. Further mathematical properties of convolution are listed in Table 2.1.

A common basic signal is the Dirac function which is also called delta function or impulse function. It is a infinitely short, infinitely high impulse.

$$\delta(t) = \begin{cases} \infty, & \text{if } t = 0 \\ 0, & \text{otherwise} \end{cases} \tag{2.10}$$

It is impossible to describe the Dirac function using classical functions. It requires the use of generalized functions or distributions, which is out of the scope of this introduction. The Dirac function is usually represented graphically as an arrow of length 1, see Fig. 2.2.

Sequences of Dirac pulses are useful to select only certain points of a function like a sifter (cf. Figure 2.3). The sifting property of the Dirac function is given by integrating the product of a function and a time-delayed Dirac function

Geek Box 2.5: Convolution Example

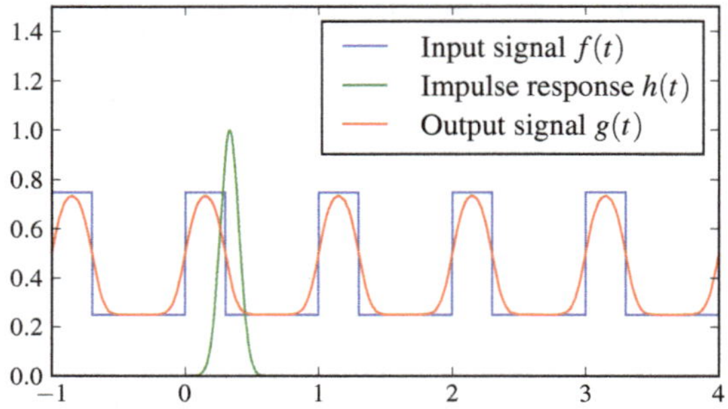

For the definition of the square function, the Heaviside step function is useful to shorten the notation

$$H(t) = \begin{cases} 0, & \text{if } t < 0 \\ 1, & \text{otherwise} \end{cases}.$$

Then, the square function and the Gaussian are defined as

$$f(t) = k_1 + k_2 \sum_{n=-\infty}^{\infty} H(t - nT) - H(t - nT - k_3)$$
$$h(t) = \frac{1}{\sqrt{2\pi\sigma}} e^{-\frac{1}{2}\left(\frac{t}{\sigma}\right)^2},$$

with the offset k_1, the amplitude k_2, the duty-cycle k_3, and the period T of the square function and the standard deviation σ of the Gaussian. The convolution with a Gaussian results in a smoothing of the edges of the square function.

$$\int_{-\infty}^{\infty} f(t)\delta(t - T)\,\mathrm{d}t = f(T).$$

With the sifting property, the element at $t = T$ can be selected from the function, which is equivalent to sampling the function at that time point.

The sift property is useful for convolution of an arbitrary function and the Dirac function.

$$f(t) * \delta(t - T) = \int_{-\infty}^{\infty} f(\tau)\delta(t - T - \tau)\,\mathrm{d}\tau = f(t - T) \tag{2.11}$$

Consequently, the Dirac function is the identity element of convolution.

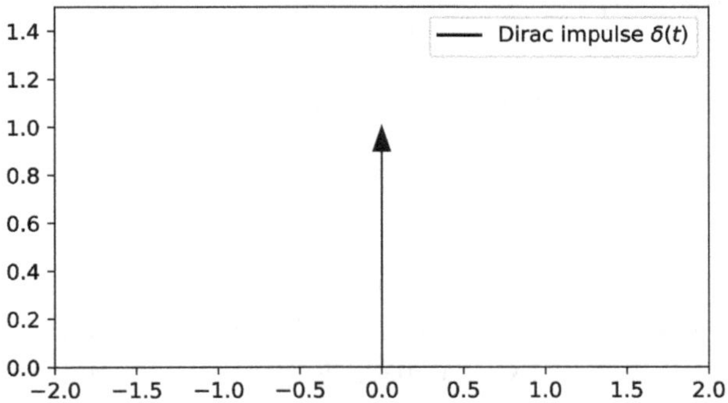

Figure 2.2: Graphical representation of the Dirac function $\delta(t)$. The arrow symbolizes infinity.

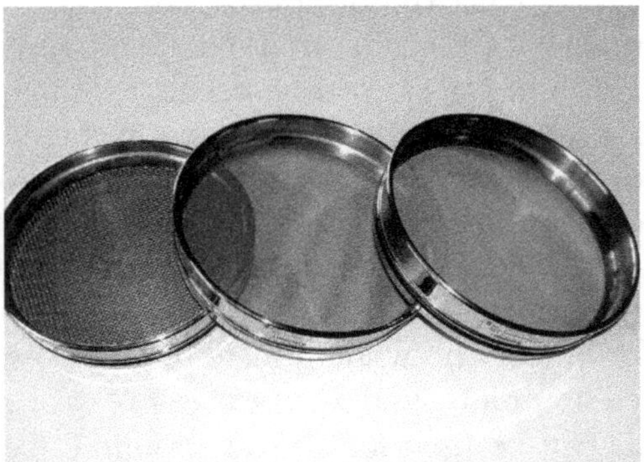

Figure 2.3: Laboratory sifters are used to remove undesired parts from discrete signals. Sequences of Dirac pulses can be applied in a similar way. Image courtesy of BMK Wikimedia.

The response of a system to a Dirac function on the input is called the impulse response of the system $h(t) = \mathcal{H}\{\delta(t)\}$. Using the superposition principle, every other signal can be represented as a linear combination of infinitely many Dirac functions. Therefore, the output of a system to any input signal is computed by convolution of the input signal $f(t)$ with the impulse response $h(t)$.

$$g(t) = f(t) * h(t) \tag{2.12}$$

For medical applications, an important example of a linear shift-invariant system is an imaging system. The output of an imaging system is often modeled as a linear shift-invariant system. The impulse response of an imaging system is called point spread function. It describes how a single point, i. e., a Dirac impulse, is spread on the sensor plane by the specific imaging system. The point spread function is a description of the behavior of the system.

2.2.3 Correlation

Another basic operation to combine a signal and a system is correlation

$$g(t) = (h \star f)(t) = \int_{-\infty}^{\infty} h^*(\tau) f(t+\tau)\,\mathrm{d}\tau, \tag{2.13}$$

where h^* is the complex conjugate of h. The main difference to convolution is that the input signal f is not mirrored before combination with h, i. e., $f(t+\tau)$ instead of $f(t-\tau)$. Correlation is a way to measure the similarity of two signals.

An application of correlation is the matched filter. The matched filter is specifically designed to have a high response for a specific deterministic signal or waveform $f(t)$. It is **matched** to that signal. The matched filter is directly computed by correlation with the desired signal. Alternatively, convolution with an impulse response of the mirrored, complex conjugate of the desired deterministic signal $h(t) = f^*(-t)$ can be used.

Technical uses for correlation can be found in signal transmission and signal detection. For a medical example, the heartbeats of a person can be detected in an Electrocardiogram (ECG) using correlation with a template QRS complex (QRS complex denotes the combination of three of the graphical deflections seen on an ECG). In image processing, a certain deterministic signal is searched for across the whole image. In this case, the deterministic signal is often called template and the process of searching is called template matching. This can be used for the detection of specific structures and tracking of structures over time. Geek Box 2.6 puts the correlation in signal processing in relation to the statistical correlation coefficient.

2.3 Fourier Transform

Up to this point, all operations and mathematical definitions were performed in continuous domain. Also, we have not discussed the relation between discrete and continuous representations which are important to understand the concept of sampling. In the following, we will introduce the Fourier transform and related concepts which will allow us to deal with exactly such problems.

2.3.1 Types of Fourier Transforms

A cosine wave f of time t with amplitude A, frequency ξ, and phase shift φ can be described by the following three equivalent parametrizations.

Geek Box 2.6: Relation to the Statistical Correlation Coefficient

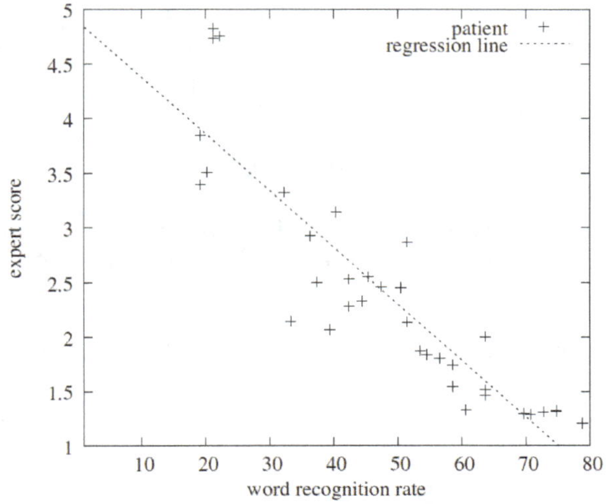

In statistics, the so-called Pearson correlation coefficient r [5] is a measure of agreement between two sets of observations $\boldsymbol{x}$ and $\boldsymbol{y}$. Coefficient r is defined in the interval $[-1, 1]$ and if $|r| = 1$, a perfect linear relationship between the two variables is present. It is computed in the following way:

$$r(\boldsymbol{x}, \boldsymbol{y}) = \frac{\sum_n (x_n - \bar{x})(y_n - \bar{y})}{\sigma_x \sigma_y}$$

Here, we use $\bar{x}$, $\bar{y}$, σ_x, and σ_y to denote the respective mean values and standard deviations. If we assume the standard deviations to be equal to 1 and the means equal to 0, we arrive at the following equation:

$$r(\boldsymbol{x}, \boldsymbol{y}) = \sum_n x_n \cdot y_n$$

This is identical to the discrete version of correlation for real inputs for $t = 0$. Also note that this can be considered simply as an inner product $\boldsymbol{x}^\top \boldsymbol{y}$.

The image at the top of the page shows a scatter plot between two variables *word recognition rate* and *expert rater*. Each point (x_n, y_n) denotes one patient for whom both of the two variables were measured. The closer the two are to the dotted line, the better their agreement. Here, their dependency is negative as if one variable is high, the other is low and vice versa. $r \approx -0.9$ in this example. Please refer to [4] for more details.

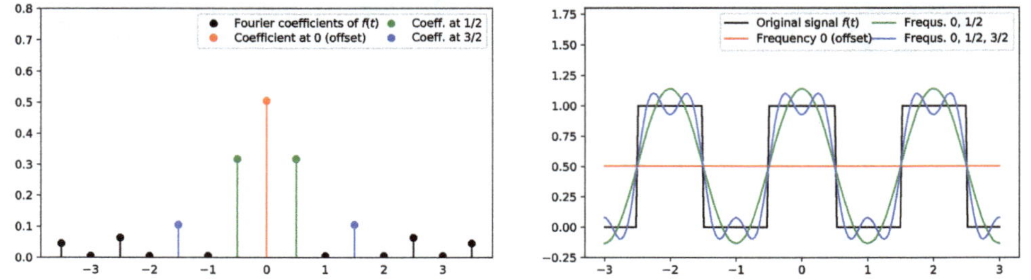

(a) Fourier coefficients, weights of trigonometric functions approximating the signal $f(t)$

(b) Periodic signal and approximations using different numbers of Fourier coefficients

Figure 2.4: Approximation of a periodic signal using a weighted sum of trigonometric functions

$$
\begin{aligned}
f(t) &= A \cdot \cos(2\pi\xi t + \varphi) && A, \varphi \in \mathbb{R} \\
&= a \cdot \cos(2\pi\xi t) + b \cdot \sin(2\pi\xi t) && a, b \in \mathbb{R} \\
&= c \cdot \mathrm{e}^{2\pi i\xi t} + \bar{c} \cdot \mathrm{e}^{-2\pi i\xi t} && c \in \mathbb{C}
\end{aligned}
$$

In Geek Box 2.7, we show how the parameters a, b, and c are related to A and φ.

A **Fourier series** (cf. Geek Box 2.8) is used to represent a continuous signal using only discrete frequencies. As such a Fourier series is able to approximate any signal as a superposition of sine and cosine waves. Fig. 2.4(b) shows a rectangular signal of time. The absolute values of its Fourier coefficients are depicted in Fig. 2.4(a). As can be seen in Fig. 2.4(a), the Fourier coefficients decrease as the frequency increases. It is therefore possible to approximate the signal by setting the coefficients to 0 for all high frequencies. Fig. 2.4(b) includes the approximations for three different choices of sets of frequencies.

The Fourier series, which works on periodic signals, can be extended to aperiodic signals by increasing the period length to infinity. The resulting transform is called **continuous Fourier transform** (or simply Fourier transform, cf. Geek Box 2.9). Fig. 2.5(b) shows the Fourier transform of a rectangular function, which is identical to the Fourier coefficients at the respective frequencies up to scaling (see Fig. 2.5(a)).

The counter part to the Fourier series for cases in which time domain is discrete and the frequency domain is continuous is called the **discrete time Fourier transform** (cf. Geek Box 2.10). It forms a step towards the **discrete Fourier transform** (cf. Geek Box 2.11) which allows us to perform all previous operations also in a digital signal processing system. In discrete space, we can interpret the Fourier transform simply as a matrix multiplication with a complex matrix $\boldsymbol{F}$

Name	Function	Fourier transform
Rectangular	$\mathrm{rect}(at) = \begin{cases} 0 & \text{if } \lvert at\rvert > \frac{1}{2} \\ \frac{1}{2} & \text{if } \lvert at\rvert = \frac{1}{2} \\ 1 & \text{if } \lvert at\rvert < \frac{1}{2} \end{cases}$	$\mathcal{F}\left[\mathrm{rect}(t)\right](\xi) = \frac{1}{\lvert a\rvert}\,\mathrm{sinc}(\frac{\xi}{a})$
Triangular	$\mathrm{tri}(t) = \begin{cases} 1 - \lvert t\rvert & \text{if } \lvert t\rvert < 1 \\ 0 & \text{if } \lvert t\rvert \leq 1 \end{cases}$	$\mathcal{F}\left[\mathrm{tri}(t)\right](\xi) = \mathrm{sinc}^2(\xi)$
Gaussian	$\mathrm{gauss}(t) = \mathrm{e}^{-at^2}$	$\mathcal{F}\left[\mathrm{gauss}(t)\right](\xi) = \sqrt{\frac{\pi}{a}}\mathrm{e}^{-\pi^2\xi^2/a}$

Table 2.2: Fourier transforms of popular functions. Here we use the definition $\mathrm{sinc}(x) = \frac{\sin(\pi x)}{\pi x}$. Note that a convolution of two rectangular functions yields a triangular function as $\mathcal{F}\left[\mathrm{rect}(t) * \mathrm{rect}(t)\right] = \mathrm{sinc}^2(\xi)$.

$$\boldsymbol{k} = \boldsymbol{F}\boldsymbol{n} \tag{2.14}$$

where the signal $\boldsymbol{n}$ and the discrete spectrum $\boldsymbol{k}$ are vectors of complex values. The inverse operation is then readily found as

$$\boldsymbol{n} = \boldsymbol{F}^H\boldsymbol{k} \tag{2.15}$$

where $\boldsymbol{F}^H$ is the Hermitian, i. e., transposed and element-wise conjugated, of $\boldsymbol{F}$. Geek Box 2.12 shows some more details on how to find these relations. Fig. 2.5 shows all types of Fourier transforms introduced in this section in comparison. Tab. 2.2 shows the Fourier transforms of popular functions.

In computer programs, discrete Fourier transforms are implemented very efficiently using fast Fourier transform (FFT). This approach reduces the number of computations from the order of N^2 to the order of $N \log N$, if N is the length of the signal. In the next section, we will see why convolution and correlation also benefit from this efficiency.

2.3.2 Convolution Theorem & Properties

The convolution of two functions f and g is defined as in Sec. 2.2.2, and $\cdot$ denotes point-wise multiplication. The convolution theorem states that a convolution of two signals in space is identical to a point-wise multiplication of their spectra (see Equation 2.24). The opposite also holds true (see Equation 2.25).

$$\mathcal{F}\{f * g\} = F \cdot G \tag{2.24}$$

$$\mathcal{F}\{f \cdot g\} = F * G \tag{2.25}$$

Geek Box 2.7: Equivalent Cosine Representations

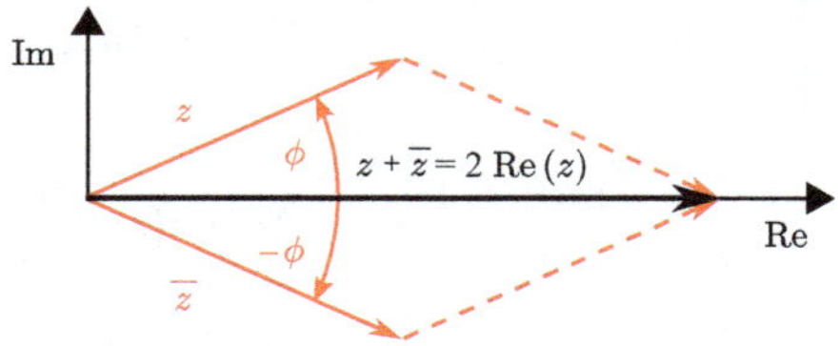

Oscillations of the same frequency can be represented in several equivalent ways. In the following, we make use of the complex numbers introduced in Sec. 2.2.1 and the correspondence between a sum of complex exponentials and the real part $z+\overline{z} = 2\,\mathrm{Re}(z)$ to convert the different representations into the same expression.

Amplitude and phase shift, where we define $c = \frac{1}{2}A\mathrm{e}^{i\varphi}$:

$$\begin{aligned} f(t) &= A \cdot \cos(2\pi\xi t + \varphi) = \mathrm{Re}\left(A \cdot \mathrm{e}^{2\pi i\xi t + i\varphi}\right) \\ &= \mathrm{Re}\left(A \cdot \mathrm{e}^{i\varphi} \cdot \mathrm{e}^{2\pi i\xi t}\right) = \underline{\underline{\mathrm{Re}\left(2c \cdot \mathrm{e}^{2\pi i\xi t}\right)}}. \end{aligned}$$

Sum of cosine and sine functions, where we define $c = \frac{1}{2}(a - ib)$:

$$\begin{aligned} f(t) &= a \cdot \cos(2\pi\xi t) + b \cdot \sin(2\pi\xi t) \\ &= a \cdot \cos(2\pi\xi t) + b \cdot \cos(2\pi\xi t - \pi/2) \\ &= \mathrm{Re}\left(a \cdot \mathrm{e}^{2\pi i\xi t}\right) + \mathrm{Re}\left(b \cdot \mathrm{e}^{2\pi i\xi t - \pi/2}\right) \\ &= \mathrm{Re}\left(a \cdot \mathrm{e}^{2\pi i\xi t}\right) + \mathrm{Re}\left(b \cdot \mathrm{e}^{2\pi i\xi t} \cdot \mathrm{e}^{-i\pi/2}\right) \\ &= \mathrm{Re}\left(a \cdot \mathrm{e}^{2\pi i\xi t}\right) + \mathrm{Re}\left(-ib \cdot \mathrm{e}^{2\pi i\xi t}\right) \\ &= \mathrm{Re}\left((a - ib) \cdot \mathrm{e}^{2\pi i\xi t}\right) = \underline{\underline{\mathrm{Re}\left(2c \cdot \mathrm{e}^{2\pi i\xi t}\right)}}. \end{aligned}$$

Sum of complex exponentials:

$$\begin{aligned} f(t) &= c \cdot \mathrm{e}^{2\pi i\xi t} + \bar{c} \cdot \mathrm{e}^{-2\pi i\xi t} \\ &= \mathrm{Re}\left(c \cdot \mathrm{e}^{2\pi i\xi t}\right) + i\,\mathrm{Im}\left(c \cdot \mathrm{e}^{2\pi i\xi t}\right) + \mathrm{Re}\left(c \cdot \mathrm{e}^{2\pi i\xi t}\right) - i\,\mathrm{Im}\left(c \cdot \mathrm{e}^{2\pi i\xi t}\right) \\ &= \underline{\underline{\mathrm{Re}\left(2c \cdot \mathrm{e}^{2\pi i\xi t}\right)}}. \end{aligned}$$

Geek Box 2.8: Fourier Series

The Fourier series (Equation 2.17) represents a periodic signal of period T by an infinite weighted sum of shifted cosine functions of different frequencies. The Fourier coefficients c are calculated using Equation 2.16.

$$c[k] = \frac{1}{T}\int_{d}^{d+T} f(t)\ \mathrm{e}^{-2\pi itk/T}\,\mathrm{d}t \qquad k \in \mathbb{Z} \tag{2.16}$$

$$f(t) = \sum_{k=-\infty}^{\infty} c[k]\ \mathrm{e}^{2\pi itk/T} \qquad t \in \mathbb{R} \tag{2.17}$$

The coefficients $c[k]$ and $c[-k]$ together form a shifted cosine wave with frequency $\xi = \frac{|k|}{T}$ (see Geek Box 2.7). It follows that $c[-k] = \overline{c[k]}$:

$$\begin{aligned} c[k]\ \mathrm{e}^{2\pi itk/T} + c[-k]\ \mathrm{e}^{-2\pi itk/T} &= c[k]\ \mathrm{e}^{2\pi itk/T} + \overline{c[k]}\ \mathrm{e}^{-2\pi itk/T} \\ c[-k]\ \mathrm{e}^{-2\pi itk/T} &= \overline{c[k]}\ \mathrm{e}^{-2\pi itk/T} \\ &\Rightarrow c[-k] = \overline{c[k]} \end{aligned}$$

Geek Box 2.9: Continuous Fourier Transform

Given a time-dependent signal f, its Fourier transform F at frequency ξ is defined by Eq. (2.18). The inverse Fourier transform is defined by Eq. (2.19).

$$F(\xi) = \int_{-\infty}^{\infty} f(t)\ \mathrm{e}^{-2\pi it\xi}\,\mathrm{d}t \qquad \xi \in \mathbb{R} \tag{2.18}$$

$$f(t) = \int_{-\infty}^{\infty} F(\xi)\ \mathrm{e}^{2\pi it\xi}\,\mathrm{d}\xi \qquad t \in \mathbb{R} \tag{2.19}$$

In general, $f(t)$ can be a complex signal. We will, however, only consider the case where $f(t)$ is real-valued. The continuous Fourier transform is symbolized by the operator $\mathcal{F}$.

Geek Box 2.10: Discrete-time Fourier Transform

The spectrum (i. e., continuous Fourier transform) of a band-limited signal that is sampled equidistantly and sufficiently dense with distance T can be calculated using the discrete-time Fourier transform (DTFT) defined by Equation 2.20. The inverse transform is given by Equation 2.21. For details about the required sampling distance see Sec. 2.4.2.

$$F_{\frac{1}{T}}(\xi) = \sum_{n=-\infty}^{\infty} f[n]\, \mathrm{e}^{-2\pi i \xi n T} \qquad \xi \in \mathbb{R} \tag{2.20}$$

$$f[n] = T \int_{d}^{d+\frac{1}{T}} F_{\frac{1}{T}}(\xi)\, \mathrm{e}^{2\pi i \xi n T}\, \mathrm{d}\xi \qquad n \in \mathbb{Z} \tag{2.21}$$

Fig. 2.5(c) shows the DTFT of a band-limited function and the Fourier transform. The DTFT is identical to the Fourier transform up to scaling except that it is periodic with period $1/T$.

Geek Box 2.11: Discrete Fourier Transform

The spectrum of a periodic and band-limited signal can be calculated with the discrete Fourier transform (DFT) as defined by Equation 2.22. The signal can be reconstructed with the inverse DFT as defined by Equation 2.23.

$$F[k] = \sum_{n=0}^{N-1} f[n]\, \mathrm{e}^{-2\pi i n k/N} \qquad k \in \mathbb{Z} \tag{2.22}$$

$$f[n] = \frac{1}{N} \sum_{k=0}^{N-1} F[k]\, \mathrm{e}^{2\pi i n k/N} \qquad n \in \mathbb{Z} \tag{2.23}$$

Fig. 2.5(d) shows the DFT and the Fourier series of a band-limited signal. The DFT is identical to the Fourier series up to scaling except that it is periodic with period $1/N$.

Geek Box 2.12: Discrete Fourier Transform as Matrix

A discrete Fourier transform can be rewritten as a complex matrix product. To demonstrate this, we start with the definition of the discrete Fourier transform:

$$
\begin{aligned}
F[k] &= \sum_{n=0}^{N-1} f[n]\ \mathrm{e}^{-2\pi i n k/N} \\
&= \sum_{n=0}^{N-1} \mathrm{e}^{-2\pi i n k/N}\ f[n]
\end{aligned}
$$

Now, we replace the summation with an inner product of two vectors $\boldsymbol{\xi}_k$ and $\boldsymbol{n}$ (cf. Geek Box 2.6):

$$
F[k] = (\mathrm{e}^0, \mathrm{e}^{-2\pi n k/N}, \ldots, \mathrm{e}^{-2\pi i(N-1)k/N}) \begin{pmatrix} f[0] \\ f[1] \\ f[2] \\ \vdots \\ f[N-1] \end{pmatrix} = \boldsymbol{\xi}_k^\top \boldsymbol{n}
$$

We see that $\boldsymbol{\xi}_k$ is a discretely sampled wave at frequency k. This equation can now be interpreted as the k-th row of a matrix vector product. Thus, we can rewrite the entire discrete Fourier transform of all K frequencies to

$$
\boldsymbol{k} = \begin{pmatrix} F[0] \\ F[1] \\ \vdots \\ F[K-1] \end{pmatrix} = \begin{pmatrix} \boldsymbol{\xi}_0^\top \\ \boldsymbol{\xi}_1^\top \\ \vdots \\ \boldsymbol{\xi}_{K-1}^\top \end{pmatrix} \boldsymbol{n} = \boldsymbol{F}\boldsymbol{n}
$$

As such, each row of the above matrix multiplication computes a correlation between a wave of frequency k for all K frequencies under consideration. Furthermore the relation $\boldsymbol{F}^H = \boldsymbol{F}^{-1}$ holds if $\boldsymbol{F}^H$ is scaled with $\frac{1}{N}$. Hence, $\boldsymbol{F}$ forms an orthonormal basis. If we continue this line of thought, we can also interpret a Fourier transform as a basis rotation. In our case, we do not rotate by a certain angle, but we project our time-dependent signal into a frequency resolved time-independent space.

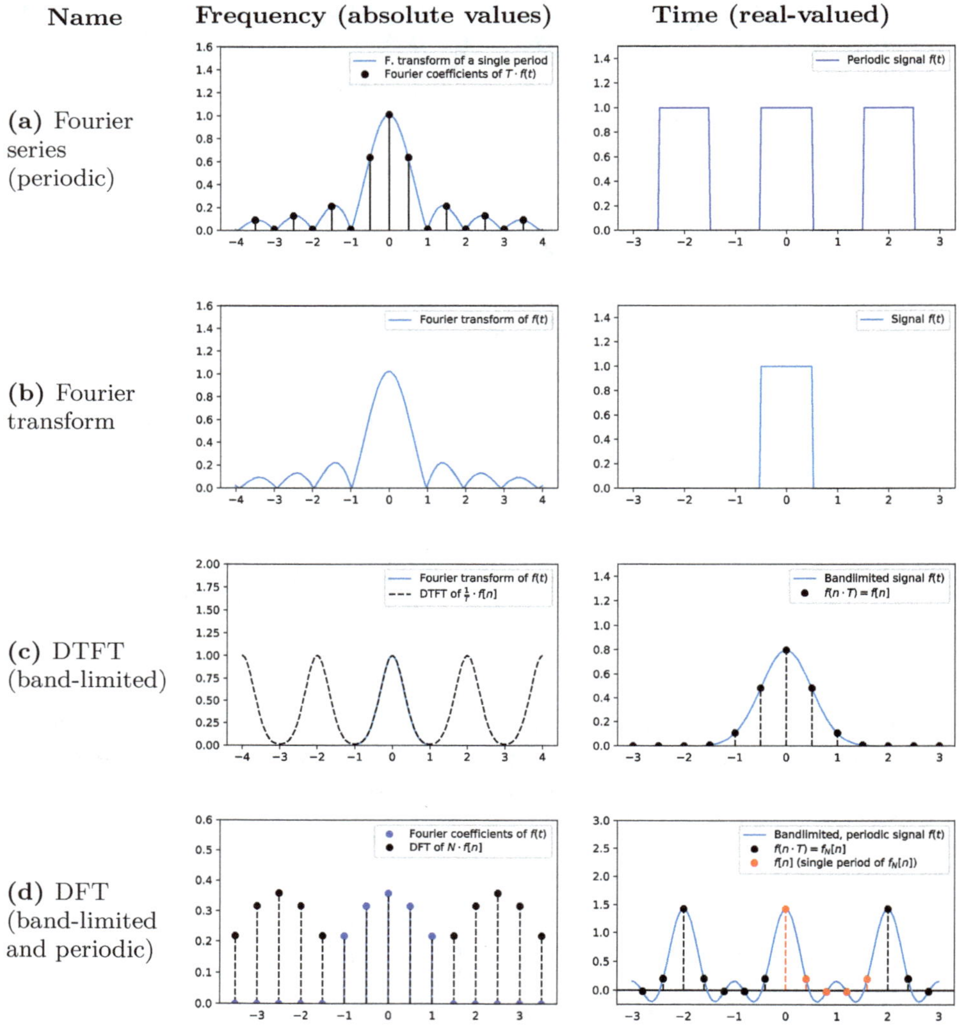

Figure 2.5: Different types of Fourier transforms.

A similar theorem exists for the DFT. Let $\boldsymbol{C}_h$ denote the matrix that performs the convolution with discrete impulse response $\boldsymbol{h}$, and $\boldsymbol{f}$ be a discrete input signal. Then system output $\boldsymbol{g}$ is obtained as

$$\boldsymbol{g} = \boldsymbol{h} * \boldsymbol{f} = \boldsymbol{C}_h \boldsymbol{f} = \boldsymbol{F}^H \boldsymbol{H} \boldsymbol{F} \boldsymbol{f}.$$

where $\boldsymbol{H}$ is a diagonal matrix that contains the Fourier transformed coefficients of $\boldsymbol{h}$. Note that $\boldsymbol{F}$ and $\boldsymbol{F}^H$ can be implemented efficiently by means of FFT. In addition to the convolution theorem, the Fourier transform has other notable properties. Some of those properties are listed in Table 2.3.

Description	Time	Frequency
Linearity	$a \cdot f(t) + b \cdot g(t)$	$a \cdot F(\xi) + b \cdot G(\xi)$
Shift	$f(t-a)$	$e^{-2\pi i a \xi} F(\xi)$
Scaling	$f(at)$	$\frac{1}{\lvert a \rvert} F\left(\frac{\xi}{a}\right)$
Derivative	$\frac{d^n f(t)}{dt^n}$	$(2\pi i \xi)^n F(\xi)$
Convolution theorem (see Sec. 2.3.2)	$(f * g)(t)$	$F(\xi) \cdot G(\xi)$
Dual of the convolution theorem	$f(t) \cdot g(t)$	$(F * G)(\xi)$

Table 2.3: Effects of modifications of a signal in time on the Fourier transform.

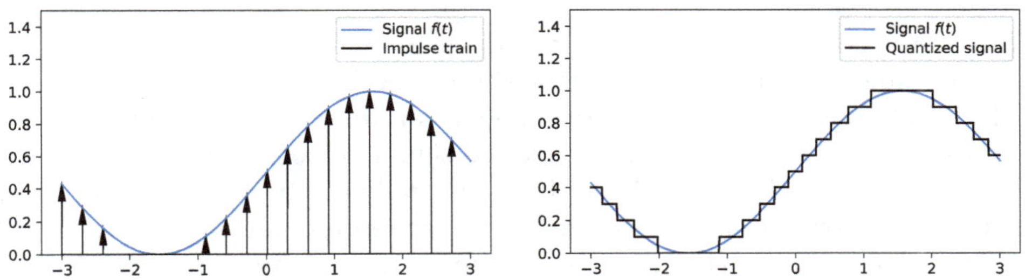

(a) Sampling as convolution with an impulse train. **(b)** Quantization of a continuous signal to discrete values.

Figure 2.6: Discrete system theory

2.4 Discrete System Theory

2.4.1 Motivation

As already indicated in the introduction, discrete signals and systems are very important in practice. All signals can only be stored and processed at fixed discrete time instances in a digital computer. The process of transforming a continuous time signal to a discrete time signal is called **sampling**. In the simplest and most common case, the continuous signal is sampled at regular intervals, which is called uniform sampling. The current value of the continuous signal is stored exactly at the time instance where the discrete time signal is defined. This can be modeled by a convolution with an impulse train, see Fig. 2.6(a). At first glance, it looks like a lot of information is discarded in the process of sampling. However, under certain requirements, the continuous time signal can be reconstructed exactly. Further details are given in Sec. 2.4.2.

As we have already seen with the discrete Fourier transform, most methods introduced in this Chapter can be equally applied to discrete signals. We denote discrete signals using brackets [] instead of parentheses (), as we already did in the Geek Boxes. Integrals must be replaced by infinite sums, for example for the discrete convolution

$$g[n] = (h * f)[n] = \sum_{k=-\infty}^{\infty} h[k]f[n-k]. \tag{2.26}$$

In the discrete case, the Dirac function takes on a simple form.

$$\delta[n] = \begin{cases} 1, & \text{if } n = 0 \\ 0, & \text{otherwise} \end{cases} \tag{2.27}$$

Note that in contrast to the continuous Dirac function, it is possible to exactly represent and implement the discrete Dirac function.

In addition to the discrete independent variable, the dependent variable can also be discrete. This means that the signal value $f(t)$ or $f[n]$ can only take values of certain levels. Apart from naturally discrete signals, all signals must be converted to a fixed discrete value for representation and processing in digital computers. For example, image intensities are often represented in the computer using 8 bit, i. e., 256 different intensities, or 12 bit which corresponds to 4096 different levels. The process of transforming a continuous-valued signal to a discrete-valued signal is called **quantization**. In most cases, a uniform quantization is sufficient, which means that the discrete levels have equal distance from each other. The continuous-valued signal is rounded to the nearest discrete level available, see Fig. 2.6(b). The error arising during this process is called quantization noise. Some more details on noise and noise models are given in Sec. 2.4.3.

2.4.2 Sampling Theorem

The Nyquist-Shannon sampling theorem (or just sampling theorem) states that a band-limited signal, i. e., a signal where all frequencies above ξ_B and below $-\xi_B$ are zero, can be fully reconstructed using samples $1/(2\xi_B)$ apart. If we consider a sine wave of frequency ξ_B, we have to sample it at least with a frequency of $2\,\xi_B$, i. e. twice per wavelength.

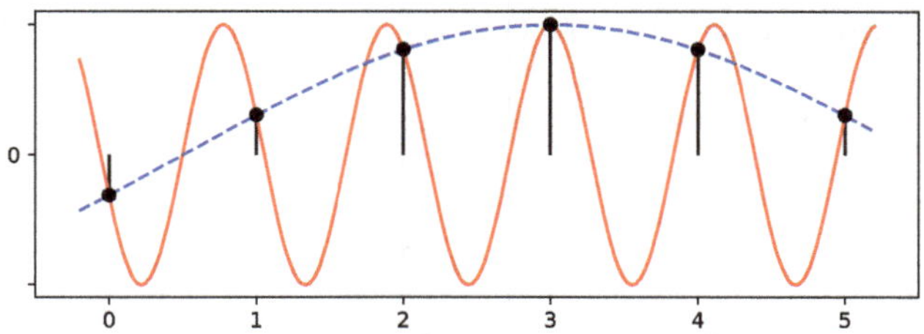

Figure 2.7: Sampling a sine signal with a frequency below $2\,\xi_B$ will cause aliasing. The reconstructed sine wave shown with blue dashes does not match the original frequency shown in red.

Formally, the theorem can be derived using the periodicity of the DTFT (see Fig. 2.5(c)). The DTFT spectrum is a periodic summation of the original spectrum, and the periodic spectra do not overlap as long as the sampling theorem is fulfilled. It is therefore possible to obtain the original spectrum by setting the DTFT spectrum to zero for frequencies larger than B. The signal can then be reconstructed by applying the inverse Fourier transform. We refer to [3] for a more detailed description of this topic.

So far, we have not discussed how the actual sampling frequency $2\,\xi_B$ is determined. Luckily such a band limitation can be found for most applications. For example, even the most sensitive ears cannot perceive frequencies above 22 kHz. As a result, the sampling frequency of the compact disc (CD) was determined at 44.1 kHz. For the eye, typically 300 dots per inch in printing or 300 pixels per inch for displays are considered as sufficient to prevent any visible distortions. In videos and films, a frame rate of 50 Hz is often used to diminish flicker. High fidelity devices may support up to 100 Hz.

If the sampling theorem is not respected, *aliasing* occurs. Frequencies above the Nyquist frequency are wrapped around due to the periodicity and appear as lower frequencies. Then, these high frequencies are indistinguishable from the true low frequencies. Fig. 2.7 demonstrates this effect visually.

2.4.3 Noise

In many cases, acquired measurements or images are corrupted by some unwanted signal components. Common noise sources are quantization and thermal noise. Additional noise sources occur in the field of medical imaging, due to the related image acquisition techniques.

We can often find a simple model of the noise corrupting the image. The model does not represent the physical noise causes, but it approximately describes the errors that occur in the final signal. An additive noise model is commonly denoted as

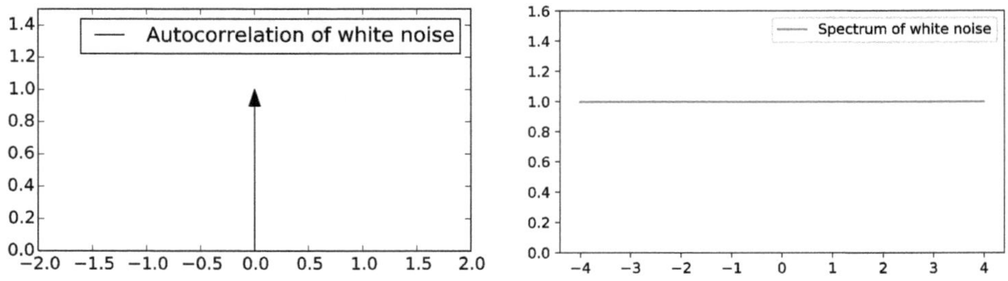

(a) Autocorrelation **(b)** Spectrum

Figure 2.8: Example of a white noise function

$$f(t) = s(t) + n(t) \tag{2.28}$$

where $s(t)$ is the underlying desired signal. We observe the signal $f(t)$, which is corrupted by the noise $n(t)$. For the statistics of the noise, we can use various models e. g., a Gaussian noise distribution $p(n(t)) = \mathcal{N}(n(t)|\mu_n, \Sigma_n)$. Another property of noise is its temporal or spatial correlation. This can be described by correlating the signal with itself, which is called *autocorrelation function*. An extreme case is white noise. White noise is temporally or spatially uncorrelated, meaning the autocorrelation function is a Dirac impulse. The spectrum of white noise is constant, i. e., it contains all frequencies to the same amount as a white light source would contain all visible wavelengths (cf. Fig. 2.8).

2.5 Examples

To conclude this chapter, we want to show the introduced concepts of convolution and Fourier transform on two example systems. A simple system is a smoothing filter, that allows only slow changes of the signal. This is called a low-pass filter. It is an important building block in many applications, for example to remove high-frequency noise from a signal or to remove signal parts with high-frequency before down-sampling to avoid aliasing.

The filter coefficients of a low-pass filter are visualized in Fig. 2.9(a). The low-pass filter has a cutoff frequency of $\frac{\pi}{2} \frac{\text{rad}}{\text{sample}}$ and a length of 81 coefficients. The true properties of the low-pass filter are best perceived in the frequency domain, as displayed in Fig. 2.9(b). Note that the scale of the y-axis is logarithmic. In this context, values of 0 indicate that the signal can pass unaltered. Small values indicate that the signal components are damped. In this example, high frequencies are suppressed by several orders of magnitude. An ideal low-pass filter is a rectangle in the Fourier domain, i. e., all values below the cutoff frequency are passed unaltered and all values above are set

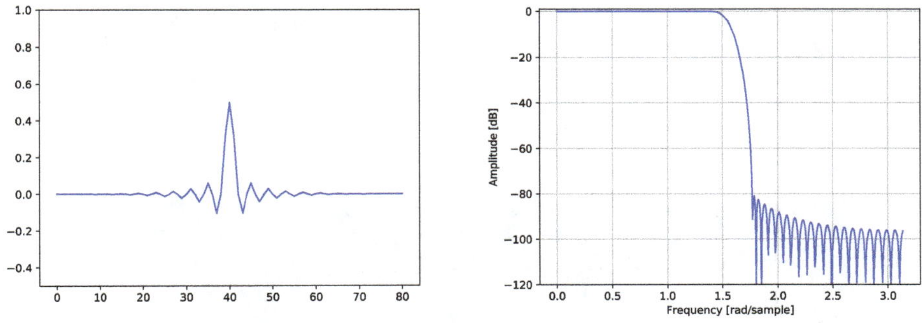

(a) Time domain coefficients

(b) Spectrum

Figure 2.9: Example of a low-pass filter

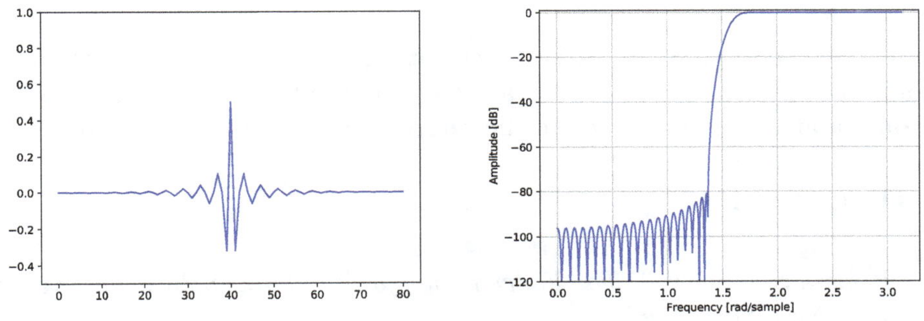

(a) Time-domain coefficients

(b) Spectrum

Figure 2.10: Example of a high-pass filter

to 0. In our discrete filter, we can only approximate this shape. In the time-domain, the coefficients are samples of a sinc function, which is the inverse Fourier transform of a rectangular function in Fourier domain (cf. Tab. 2.2). The opposite of the low-pass filter is the high-pass filter, shown in Fig. 2.10. Here, frequencies below the cutoff frequency are suppressed, whereas frequencies above are unaltered. Note that the time domain versions of high- and low-pass filters are difficult to differentiate.

Finally, we show how a signal with high and low frequency components is transformed after convolution with a high-pass and a low-pass filter. The signal in Fig. 2.11 is a sine with additive white noise. Thus, noise is distributed equally in the whole frequency domain. A large portion of the noise can be removed by suppressing frequency components where no signal is present. Consequently, the cutoff frequency of the filters is slightly above the frequency of the sine function. As a result, the output of the high-pass filter is similar to the noise and the output of the low-pass filter is similar to the sine. In our

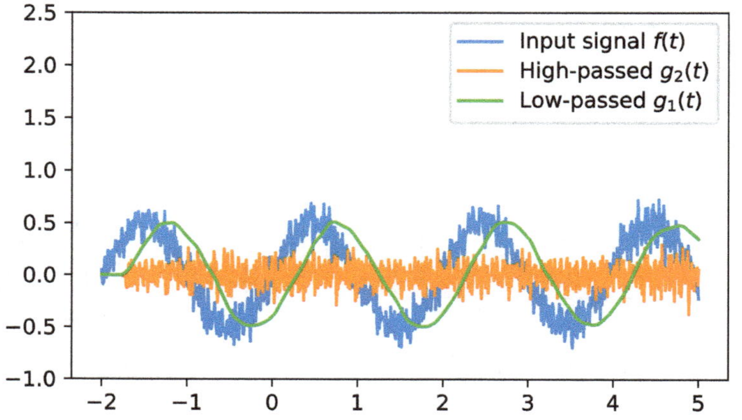

Figure 2.11: Sine signal with additive noise after processing with a low-pass filter and a high-pass filter.

example, we chose a causal filter which introduces a time delay in the filter output. A causal filter can only react to past inputs and needs to collect a certain amount of samples before the filtered result appears at the output.

Further Reading

[1] Ronald N Bracewell. *The Fourier transform and its applications.* McGraw-Hill, New York, 1986.

[2] Olaf Dössel. *Bildgebende Verfahren in der Medizin. Von der Technik zur medizinischen Anwendung.* Vol. 1. 2000.

[3] Bernd Girod, Rudolf Rabenstein, and Alexander Stenger. *Einführung in die Systemtheorie.* Vol. 4. Teubner Stuttgart, 1997.

[4] Andreas Maier. *Speech of children with cleft lip and palate: Automatic assessment.* Logos-Verlag, 2009.

[5] Karl Pearson. "Mathematical contributions to the theory of evolution.—on a form of spurious correlation which may arise when indices are used in the measurement of organs". In: *Proceedings of the royal society of london* 60.359-367 (1897), pp. 489–498.

3

Medical Imaging Devices and Image Processing

Author: David Bernecker

In the previous section, we have described common signal processing methods that may be applied to any kind of signal. In this chapter, we will adopt these concepts to the domain of image processing as it is commonly performed in medical imaging devices.

3.1 Images and Histograms

Before introducing common methods used in image processing, we first have to introduce a representation for images.

3.1.1 Images as Functions

In image processing, an image is usually regarded as a function f that maps image coordinates x, y to intensity values. This simplifies the introduction of derivatives of images which we will later use to detect edges. Furthermore, it is useful for the theoretical description of image filtering. The image coordinates

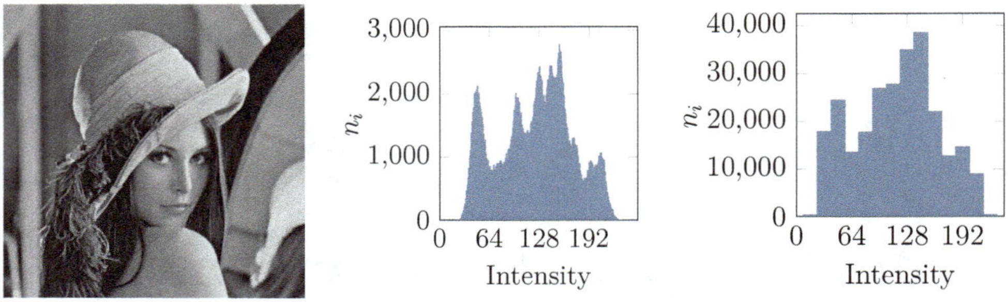

(a) Example grayscale image.

(b) Histogram of the example image with 256 bins.

(c) Histogram of the example image with 16 bins.

Figure 3.1: Histograms

x, y are defined over the discrete image domain $\Omega \subset \mathbb{Z}^2$. For gray-value images, $f(x, y)$ is a scalar function whereas for color images it is a vector consisting of the color channels, e.g., $\boldsymbol{f}(x, y) = (f_r(x, y)\ f_g(x, y)\ f_b(x, y))^\top$ for RGB images.

3.1.2 Histograms of Images

Histograms provide information about the distribution of the intensity values of an image and are frequently used in image segmentation and in image enhancement. A histogram $h(i)$ consists of several *bins* that contain single intensity values or ranges of intensities. For each bin i the number of occurrences n_i of the corresponding intensity values in the image are counted. The histogram may either contain these number of occurrences directly or it can be normalized that the sum over all bins equals one (L_1-normalization). Fig. 3.1 shows an example grayscale image and two histograms with different numbers of bins.

In the context of histograms we can also introduce the cumulative distribution function (CDF) $\mathrm{cdf}(i) = \sum_{j=0}^{i} h(j)$. The CDF sums up the histograms entries and can be calculated for regular as well as normalized histograms.

3.2 Image Enhancement

For visual inspection, it is often beneficial to change the contrast of an image. For example, a computer monitor can only display 8 bit (i.e., 256 different values) for each color channel. For an appropriate display of an image with a larger color depth, the intensity values therefore have to be scaled to this

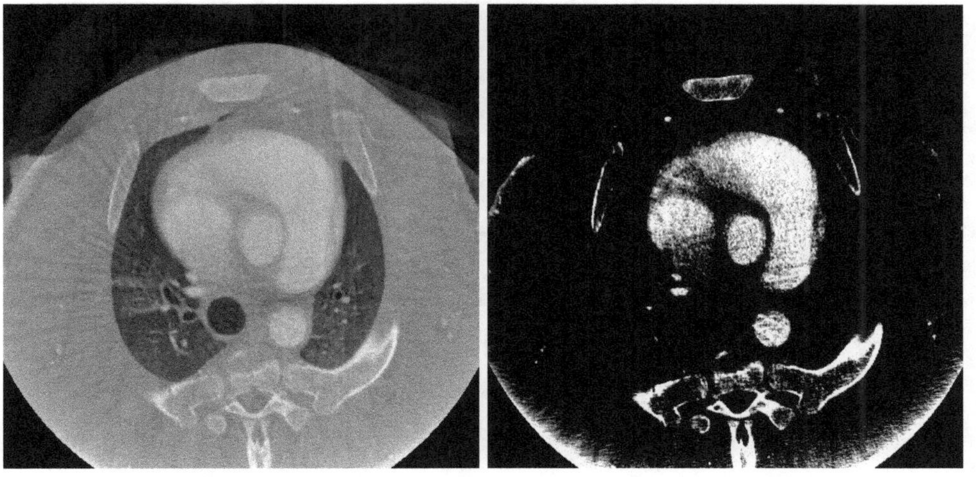

Figure 3.2: Effect of window and level on a C-arm CT slice: The image on the left shows a slice of an animal experiment displaying −1000 to 1000 HU. In this range, the materials air, soft tissue, contrast agent, and bone are displayed. The image on the right shows the same slice in the range from 200 to 500 HU. Now, only contrast agent and bone are visible. Image courtesy of Stanford University.

range in a meaningful way. The easiest way of doing this is by applying a function to the intensity values

$$f'(x, y) = g(f(x, y)). \tag{3.1}$$

3.2.1 Window and Level

In images that have significantly more gray values than 8 bit, semi-automatic adjustment of the display using window and level functions is common. In CT, the gray values have known physical properties and allow interpretation of the material. This effect is diplayed in Fig. 3.2. The image on the left hand side displays the Hounsfield unit (HU) from −1000 to 1000 (cf. Tab. 8.1). This range covers the materials air, soft tissue, contrast agent, and bone. The image on the right shows exactly the same slice. The displayed range is now from 200 to 500 HU which shows only contrast agent in the heart and cortical bone. Note that the image was obtained from a C-arm system which shows significantly lower image quality than conventional CT.

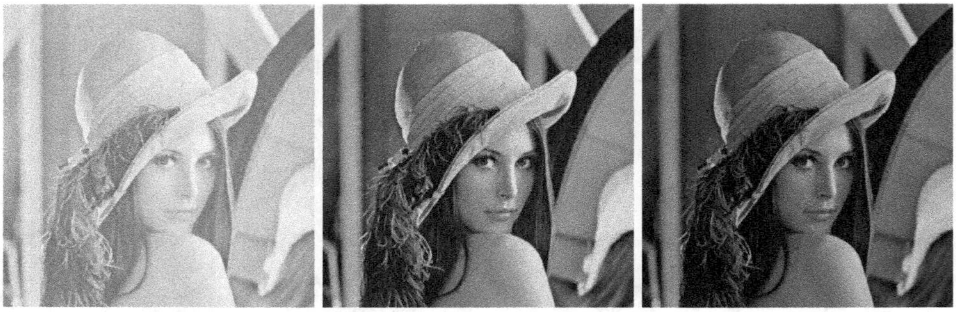

(a) $\gamma = 0.5$ (b) Original image (c) $\gamma = 2$

Figure 3.3: Gamma correction

3.2.2 Gamma Correction

A common choice for g is the use of a power-law, i. e., $g(f) = A \cdot f^\gamma$ (The constant A is used for normalizing the resulting intensities). This type of contrast enhancement is called gamma correction and is adapted to how the human eye perceives images. The result of applying a gamma correction on an image is shown in Fig. 3.3, for both a value of γ smaller and larger than 1.0. As this transformation is the same for all pixel locations, it is called a *global* transformation. Other types of functions auch as log may also be used for g.

3.2.3 Histogram Equalization

A different approach to enhance the display of an image is *histogram equalization.* Often the intensity values found in an image are restricted to a small range of the possible values (i. e., one narrow peak in the histogram). Histogram equalization transforms the image such that all intensity values are equally distributed in the enhanced image. An equal distribution of intensity values is equal to a linear CDF $cdf_{\text{linear}}(i) = a \cdot i$ with the slope a depending on the number of pixels in the image. Fig. 3.4 shows an example for histogram equalization.

3.3 Edge Detection

Edge detection is a common problem in image processing. What we perceive as edges in an image are strong changes between neighboring intensities. Since

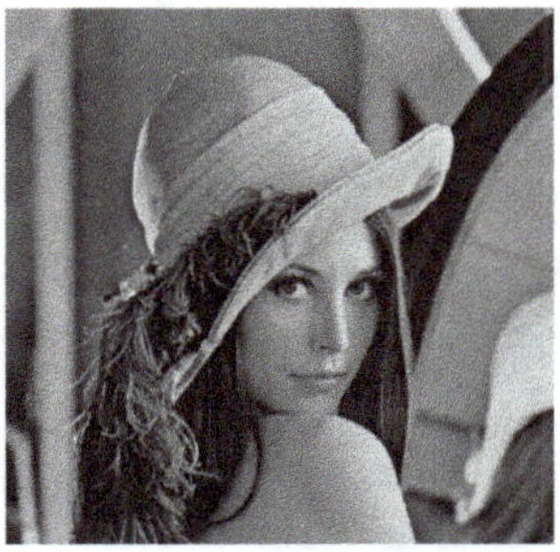

(a) Input image.

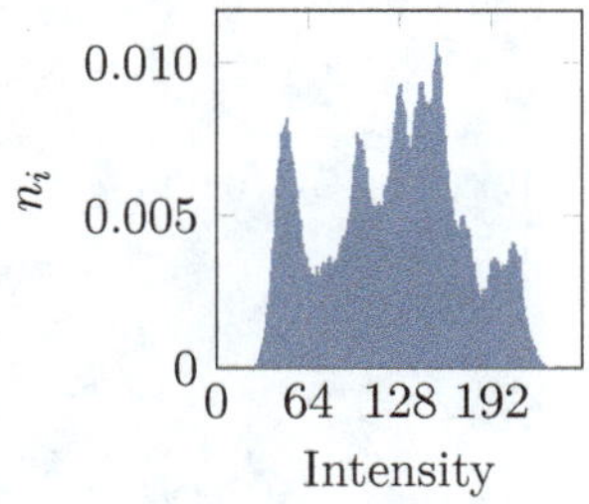

(b) Normalized histogram of the input image. Note the large empty areas for high and low intensity values.

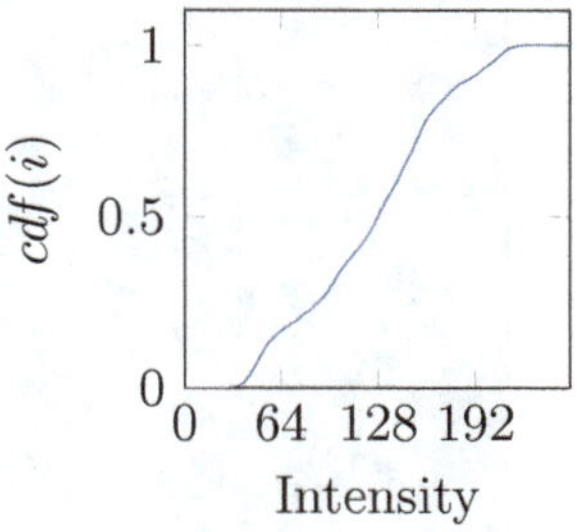

(c) CDF of the histogram of the input image.

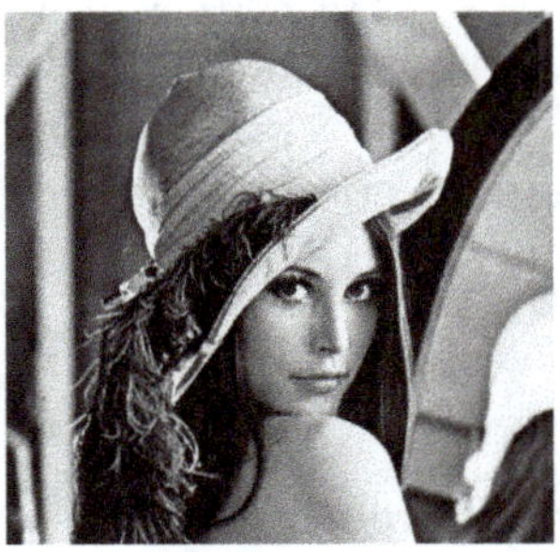

(d) The resulting image after applying a histogram equalization.

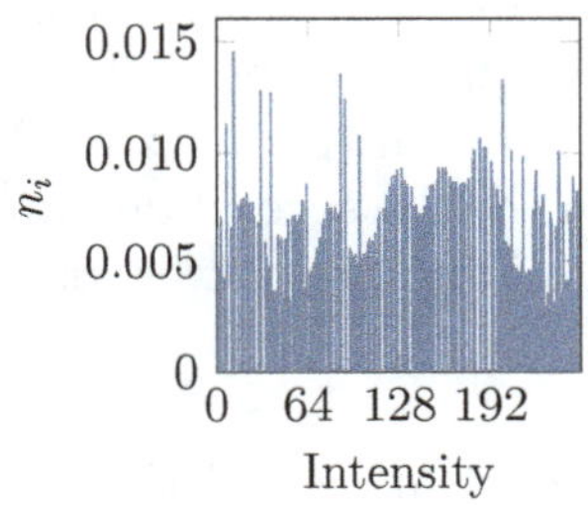

(e) The histogram of the image after histogram equalization. Note how the intensity values now occupy a larger range of values.

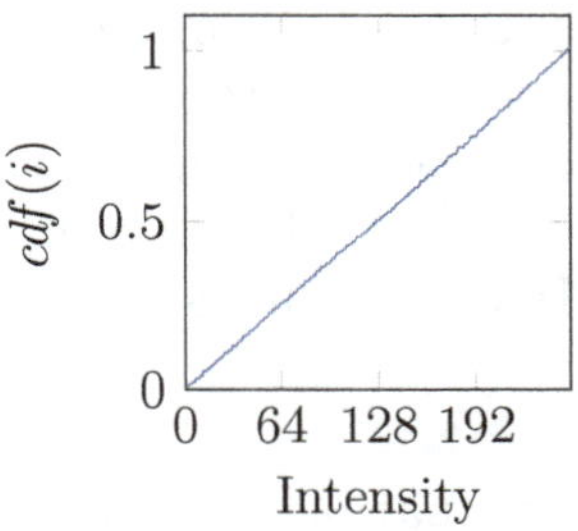

(f) CDF of the equalized histogram, which is now linear.

Figure 3.4: Histogram equalization.

images can be interpreted as functions, we can find these changes by taking the *derivative* of an image. For continuous functions $f(x)$, the derivative is defined by the difference quotient

$$f'(x) = \lim_{h \to 0} \frac{f(x+h) - f(x)}{h}. \tag{3.2}$$

An image, however, is defined as a function over discrete coordinates, where the above formula is not defined. In this case, a derivative can be calculated by using *finite differences*, an approximation that is similar to the difference quotient. The simplest derivatives we can calculate is the *forward difference*:

$$\Delta_x f(x) = f(x+1) - f(x). \tag{3.3}$$

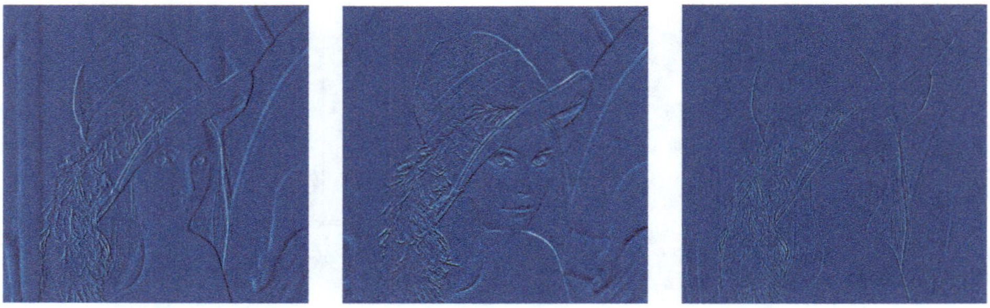

(a) First derivative in x-direction (b) First derivative in y-direction (c) Second derivative in x-direction

Figure 3.5: Derivatives of an image. The image intensities are normalized for better visualization. A neutral gray indicates a derivative of zero. Darker and brighter intensities correspond to negative and positive values of the derivative, respectively. (a) and (b) show the first derivative in x and y-direction respectively. Note how in (b) horizontal lines are more pronounced (e. g., the tip of the hat). In (c) the second derivative in x-direction is shown. Here, thin lines (e. g., of the hair) are better visible.

Comparing the continuous derivative and the forward difference, we can see that only the meaning of h has changed. While for the derivative of a continuous function, h goes to 0, it is replaced by the constant spacing (usually $h = 1$) in the discrete approximation.

In contrast to the continuous case, many different approximations can be used for the discrete derivative. Along the same line as for the forward difference, we can define the *backward-* and *central differences*

$$\nabla_x f(x) = f(x) - f(x-1) \tag{3.4}$$

$$\delta_x f(x) = f(x+1) - f(x-1) \tag{3.5}$$

The difference between these approximations is their applicability at the borders of the image, and in the accuracy of their approximation. The central difference, for example, is a more accurate approximation. While these three approximations are often used in practice, more complicated ones can be constructed. By using more values of the function, i. e., $f(x + 2h)$, $f(x + 3h)$, etc., these approximations become more accurate.

Analogous to the first order derivative, we can also calculate the second order derivative using finite differences

$$\delta_x^2 f(x) = f(x+h) - 2f(x) + f(x-h) \tag{3.6}$$

Fig. 3.5 shows the derivatives of an example image.

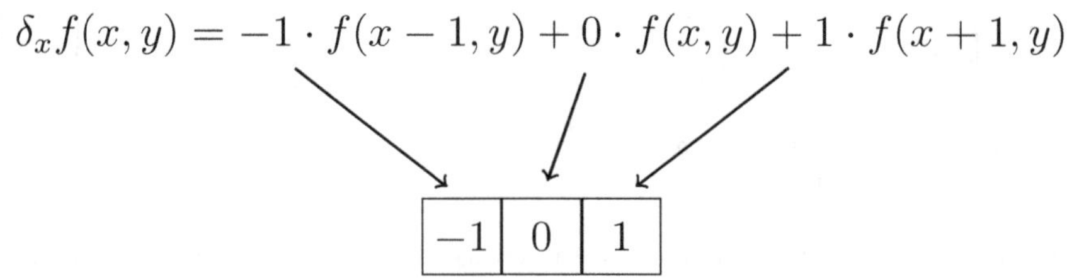

Figure 3.6: Construction of the central difference filter from Eq. (3.5).

3.4 Image Filtering

Filters play an important role in image processing. In this section, we introduce filters by using edge detection as a first example. Next, we stress the importance of the properties of linearity and shift invariance of filters.

In the previous section, we introduced the derivatives of images to identify edges in an image. However, we did not specify how the derivatives can be calculated efficiently for an image. In practice this is done by representing the derivatives as discrete filter kernels (see below).

3.4.1 Filtering – Basics

Filters can be applied to images in order to process them, e. g., for noise reduction. The transformation of the image is determined by the *filter kernel* $h(i,j)$, a rectangular patch of size $w_k \times h_k$ (the point $(0,0)$ is assumed to be at the center of the kernel). At each location in the image, the kernel is applied, and the resulting value is the new value at the center position of the kernel. Fig. 3.6 shows the filter kernel corresponding to the central difference along the direction of the x-axis, and how it is constructed from Eq. (3.5). Some other possible filter kernels for calculating derivatives are shown in Fig. 3.7.

In mathematical terms, a filter $\mathcal{H}$ is treated as an operator that is applied to the input image

$$\mathcal{H}(f(x,y)) = r(x,y)\,, \tag{3.7}$$

where r is the resulting filtered image.

When filters are linear and shift-invariant (cf. Geek Box 3.1), they can be efficiently calculated by convolution. The filtering of an image $f(x,y)$ with the filter kernel $k(i,j)$ can then be expressed as

$$\mathcal{H}\{f(x,y)\} = f * h = \sum_{i=-\frac{w_k}{2}}^{\frac{w_k}{2}} \sum_{j=-\frac{h_k}{2}}^{\frac{h_k}{2}} f(x-i, y-j)h(i,j)\,. \tag{3.8}$$

(a) Central difference **(b)** Forward difference **(c)** Backward difference **(d)** Second order

Figure 3.7: The derivative filters corresponding to the finite differences introduced in Sec. 3.3. The red circles mark the support of the filter.

Geek Box 3.1: Linearity and Shift-invariance of 2-D Filters

Analogous to the 1-D operators introduced in Sec. 2.1.2, filters can possess some important properties such as shift-invariance and linearity. For 2-D images, a filter $\mathcal{H}$ is linear, when a scaling of the input of the filter corresponds to a scaling of the output, and when filtering an image that is the sum of two images f_1, f_2 is the same as when filtering the two images separately and then adding the results

$$\begin{aligned}\mathcal{H}\{\alpha \cdot f(x,y)\} &= \alpha \cdot \mathcal{H}\{f(x,y)\}\\ \mathcal{H}\{f_1(x,y) + f_2(x,y)\} &= \mathcal{H}\{f_1(x,y)\} + \mathcal{H}\{f_2(x,y)\}\,.\end{aligned}$$

Filters are shift-invariant, when the filter does not change when we shift it over an image, i. e., the filter is independent of the position in the image it is applied to

$$\mathcal{H}\{(f(x - x_0, y - y_0)\} = r(x - x_0, y - y_0)$$

For small images and kernels, this expression is usually calculated for each pixel of the filtered image individually. For large images, however, we can use the property of the Fourier transformation that a convolution in the spatial domain is a multiplication in the frequency domain (cf. Geek Box 3.2).

3.4.2 Linear Shift-invariant Filters in Image Processing

We now take a look at some linear shift-invariant filters that are often used in image processing.

Average / Mean / Box Filter

This is the most basic filter. Each element of the kernel has the same value. In order to prevent a change in the range of intensities, the kernel should be

Geek Box 3.2: 2-D Fourier Transform

In the previous chapter, the Fourier transform for 1-D signals (cf. Sec. 2.3) was introduced. The transformation can also be defined for 2-D signals, i. e., images. The Fourier transform $F(\mu, \nu)$ and its inverse transform for continuous functions $f(x, y)$ is defined by

$$F(\mu, \nu) = \iint_{-\infty}^{\infty} f(x, y) e^{-2\pi i(\mu x + \nu y)} \, \mathrm{d}x \, \mathrm{d}y$$
$$f(x, y) = \iint_{-\infty}^{\infty} F(\mu, \nu) e^{2\pi i(\mu x + \nu y)} \, \mathrm{d}\mu \, \mathrm{d}\nu \, .$$

As before in the 1-D case, this transform can also be discretized, which is needed for transforming images. For an image f of size $w_f \times h_f$, the discrete Fourier transform and the inverse Fourier transform are given by

$$F(\mu, \nu) = \sum_{x=0}^{w_f - 1} \sum_{y=0}^{h_f - 1} f(x, y) e^{-2\pi i(\mu x / w_f + \nu y / h_f)}$$
$$f(x, y) = \frac{1}{w_f h_f} \sum_{\mu=0}^{w_f - 1} \sum_{\nu=0}^{h_f - 1} F(\mu, \nu) e^{2\pi i(\mu x / w_f + \nu y / h_f)}$$

The convolution theorem that was introduced for the 1-D Fourier transform also exists for the 2-D case

$$\mathcal{F}\{f * g\} = F \cdot G$$
$$\mathcal{F}\{F * G\} = f \cdot G$$
$$\mathrm{DFT}\{f * g\} = F \cdot G$$

and allows us to filter an image with a filter kernel by multiplying their Fourier transforms and then applying the inverse Fourier transform to the result.

normalized, which leads to the filter kernel shown in Fig. 3.8. The averaging (or mean filter or box filter) blurs an image and can be used to reduce noise in an image. There are, however, better filter choices for this task, as the averaging filter leads to "ringing" artifacts near edges.

$\frac{1}{9}$	$\frac{1}{9}$	$\frac{1}{9}$
$\frac{1}{9}$	$\frac{1}{9}$	$\frac{1}{9}$
$\frac{1}{9}$	$\frac{1}{9}$	$\frac{1}{9}$

(a) Averaging filter of size 3×3

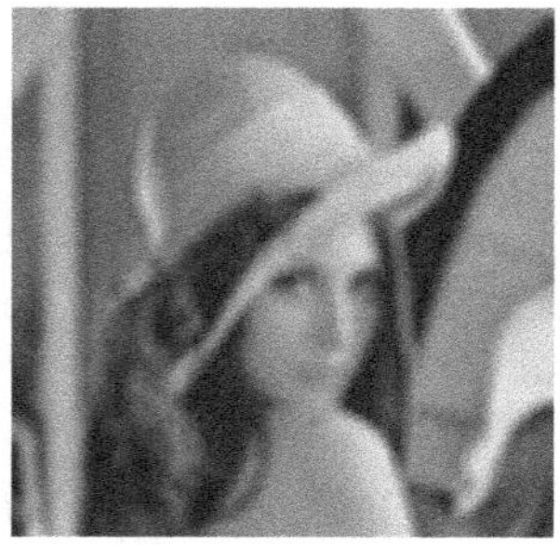

(b) Blurred version of lena

Figure 3.8: Lena after mean filtering

$\frac{1}{16}$	$\frac{1}{8}$	$\frac{1}{16}$
$\frac{1}{8}$	$\frac{1}{4}$	$\frac{1}{8}$
$\frac{1}{16}$	$\frac{1}{8}$	$\frac{1}{16}$

(a) Gaussian filter kernel of size 3×3

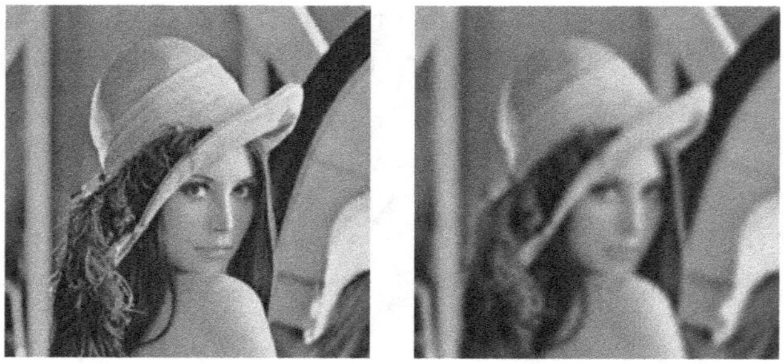

(b) Gaussian filter of size 15x15 and $\sigma = 1$ applied.

(c) Gaussian filter of size 15x15 and $\sigma = 5$ applied.

Figure 3.9: Lena after Gaussian filtering

Gaussian filter

A better choice for blurring an image than the averaging filter is the Gaussian filter. This filter puts a higher weight to values near its center. The values of the kernel can be calculated by the isotropic, zero-mean 2-D Gaussian function

$$h(i,j) = N \cdot e^{-\frac{i^2+j^2}{2\sigma^2}} \tag{3.9}$$

where N is used to normalize the kernel. The parameter σ determines how strong the image is blurred. A small value puts the emphasis on the central pixels when applying the filter, whereas for a large value the weights of neighboring pixels are larger. A typical Gaussian filter and the effect of different values of σ are shown in Fig. 3.9.

−1	0	1
−1	0	1
−1	0	1

(a) Prewitt kernel

−1	0	1
−2	0	2
−1	0	1

(b) Sobel kernel

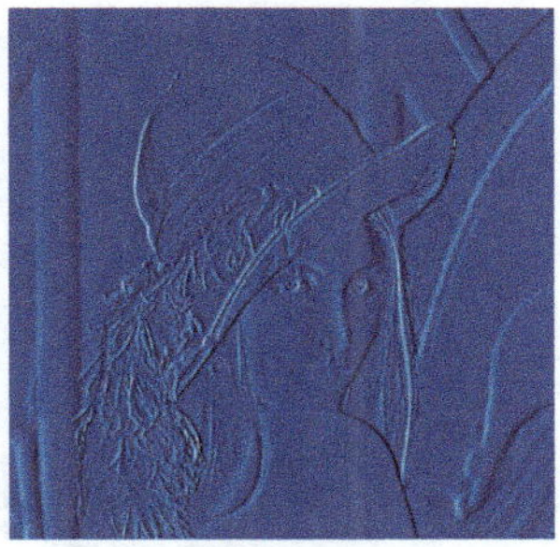

(c) Sobel Lena

Figure 3.10: Prewitt and Sobel

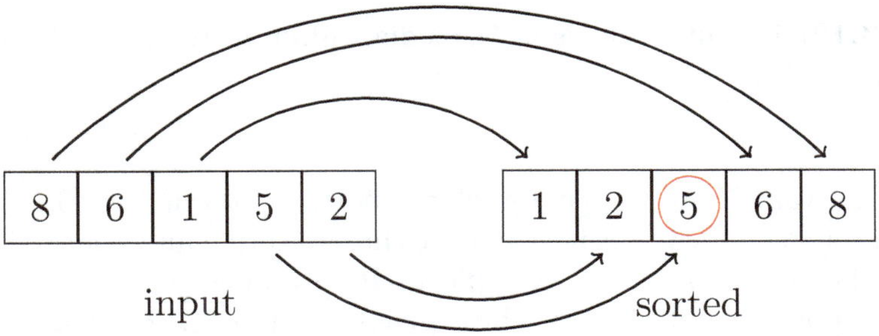

Figure 3.11: Calculating the median (red circle) of an array. The array is first sorted. The median then is the middle value of the array.

Prewitt and Sobel filter

The Prewitt and Sobel filters are combinations of a blurring and a derivative filter. In practice, image noise leads to many falsely detected edges, when one of the derivative filters in Fig. 3.7 is used. It therefore either makes sense to slightly blur the image before the edges are found (not too much, otherwise the edges vanish), or to use the Prewitt and Sobel filters.

The Prewitt filter corresponds to blurring the image with the averaging filter before calculating the derivative. The Sobel filter can be thought of as a combination of a Gaussian filter and the central derivative. Example filter kernels are shown in Fig. 3.10(a) and Fig. 3.10(b), respectively.

3.4.3 Nonlinear Filters – the Median Filter

There exist of course other filters that are not linear and shift-invariant. The most often used one is the median filter. The median of a set of numbers

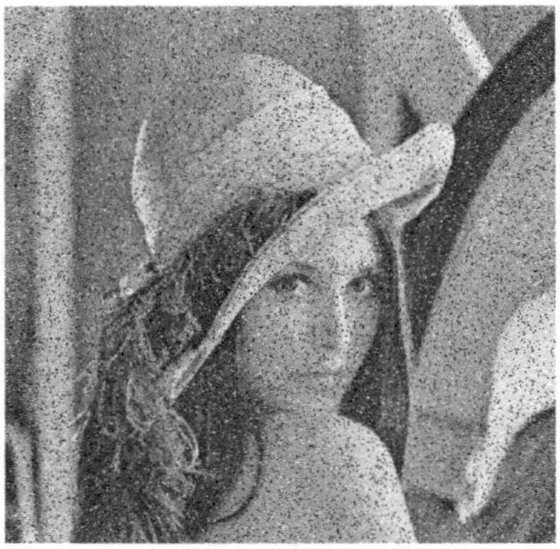

(a) Image corrupted by salt-and-pepper noise.

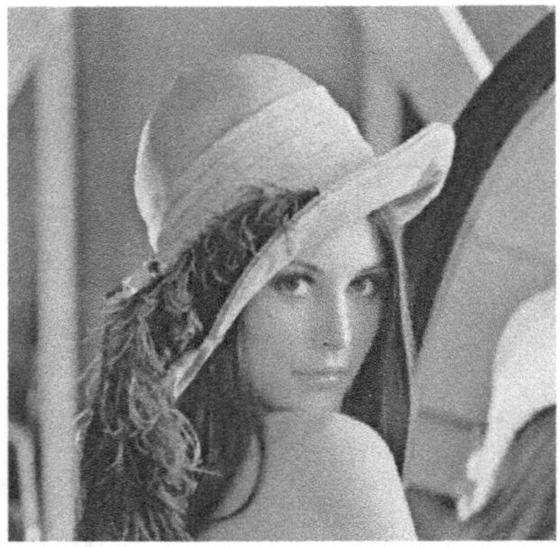

(b) Median filtered image (3×3 kernel).

Figure 3.12: Example for using a median filter to reduce salt-and-pepper noise in an image.

is the value that is at the center of the sorted set (cf. Fig. 3.11) and the median filter sorts the intensity values within its kernel and places the median value at the center. It is for example used to reduce salt-and-pepper noise (sparsely appearing black and white pixels, cf. Fig. 3.12) or in general for noise reduction as it preserves edges better than the averaging or Gaussian filter. However, since the median filter is not linear and shift-invariant, it cannot be applied using convolution and is therefore not as computationally efficient. In fact, for each location in the image, the surrounding pixels have to be sorted individually to calculate the median value.

3.5 Morphological Operators

Morphological operators are operators on sets, so in order to introduce them for images, we have to treat images as sets. So far, we have treated images as discrete functions. They can, however, also be treated as sets that contain tuples $(x, y, f(x, y))$ of coordinates and intensity values as their elements

$$\mathrm{F} = \Big\{ \big(x_0, y_0, f(x_0, y_0)\big),\ \big(x_1, y_1, f(x_1, y_1)\big),\ \ldots,\ \big(x_n, y_n, f(x_n, y_n)\big) \Big\}. \tag{3.10}$$

A morphological operator now consists of a *structuring element* (which is an image/set) and the operation itself. Structuring elements are sets, where the values usually have binary values corresponding to back- and foreground:

$$\mathrm{S} = \Big\{ \big(x_0, y_0\big), \big(x_1, y_1\big), \ldots, \Big\} \tag{3.11}$$

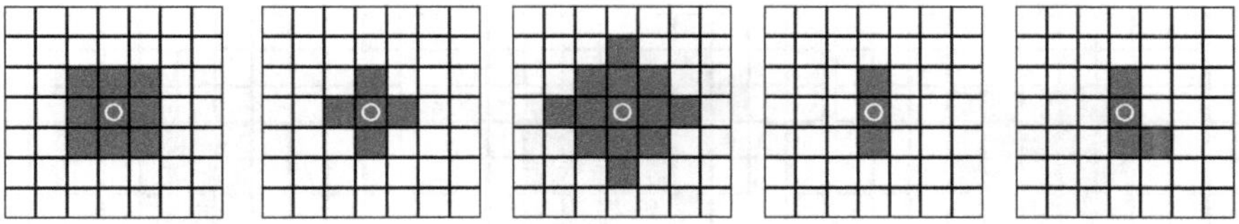

(a) Block (b) Cross (c) Diamond (d) Bar (e) L-shaped

Figure 3.13: Example structuring elements, foreground pixels are dark green, background pixels white. The center is marked by a white circle.

Depending on the goal, different shapes and sizes are used, of which some common ones are shown in Fig. 3.13. As operations themselves, there are four basic ones: erosion, dilation, opening, and closing, where the opening and closing operations actually are compositions of erosion and dilation.

Morphological operators are often applied to binary images, i. e., segmented images, where only foreground and background are distinguished (cf. Sec. 3.6). Thus, images that only contain pixels that are marked with a specific value, i. e.,

$$\mathrm{F}_{\text{bin}} = \Big\{(x,y) \mid f(x,y) = 1\Big\} \tag{3.12}$$

The basic idea behind binary morphological operations is, that the structuring element is shifted over the binary image. The image is then transformed by the operation, depending on how the structuring element fits to the shapes visible in the image, or how it misses them. For all operations, the structuring element S has to be shifted over the image and we will denote the structuring element at image coordinates (x, y) as

$$\mathrm{S}_{(x,y)} = \Big\{(x+i, y+j) \mid (i,j) \in \mathrm{S}\Big\}. \tag{3.13}$$

Binary Erosion

Using the set notation for images and structuring elements, erosion of an image F with the structuring element S can be written as

$$\mathrm{F}_{\text{bin}} \ominus \mathrm{S} = \big\{(x,y) \mid \mathrm{S}_{(x,y)} \subseteq \mathrm{F}_{\text{bin}}\big\}. \tag{3.14}$$

This means that the eroded image contains foreground values only where the whole structuring element falls in the foreground region of the image. This is illustrated in Fig. 3.14 where a rectangular shape is eroded with a cross shaped structuring element.

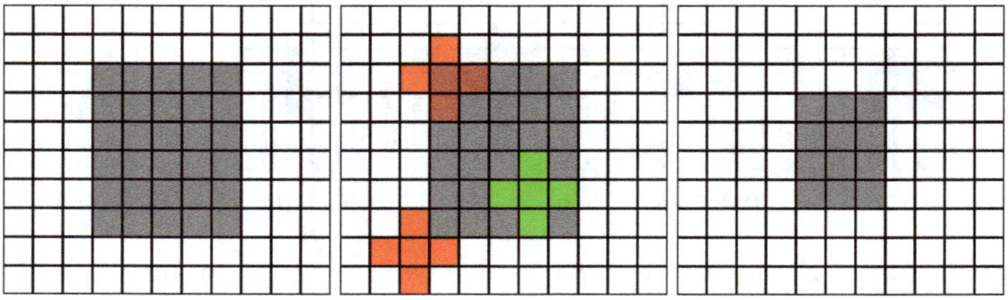

(a) Input image. (b) Structuring element overlaid at several positions. (c) Eroded image.

Figure 3.14: An example for binary erosion with a cross shaped structuring element. (b) shows the structuring element overlaid at several positions. A green structuring element means that the center of the structuring element will be foreground in the eroded image, a red structuring element means that it will be a background pixel. Note that the structuring element is only green when it is completely covered by the block.

Binary Dilation

Using the set notation, binary dilation of an image F with the structuring element S can be written as

$$\mathrm{F}_{\text{bin}} \oplus \mathrm{S} = \left\{(x,y) \mid \mathrm{S}_{(x,y)} \cap \mathrm{F}_{\text{bin}} \neq \emptyset\right\}, \tag{3.15}$$

This means that in the dilated image all pixel locations where the overlap between the structuring element and the foreground pixels in the image is not empty will be a foreground pixel. This is illustrated with an example in Fig. 3.15.

Binary Opening

Opening is a composition of erosion and dilation. The image is first eroded and the result is then dilated with the same structuring element S

$$\mathrm{F}_{\text{bin}} \circ \mathrm{S} = (\mathrm{F}_{\text{bin}} \ominus \mathrm{S}) \oplus \mathrm{S}\,. \tag{3.16}$$

This operation can be used to remove single noise pixels, or small extensions of larger structures (cf. Fig. 3.16).

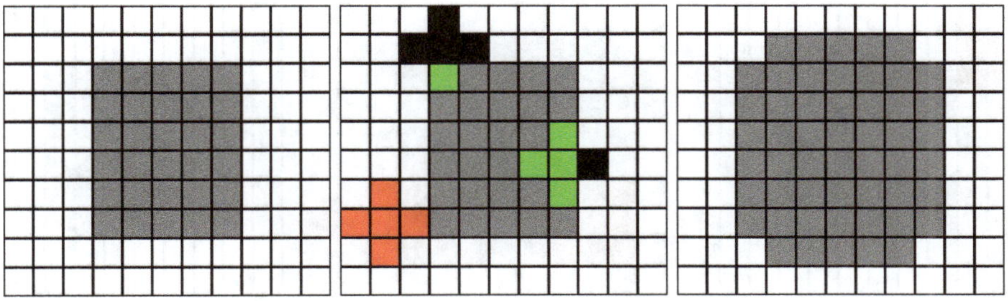

(a) Input image. (b) Structuring element overlaid at several positions. (c) Dilated image.

Figure 3.15: An example for binary dilation with a cross shaped structuring element. (b) shows the structuring element overlaid at several positions. A green structuring element means that the center of the structuring element will be foreground in the eroded image, a red structuring element means that is will be a background pixel. Note that the structuring element is green even when only a part of it overlaps with the block.

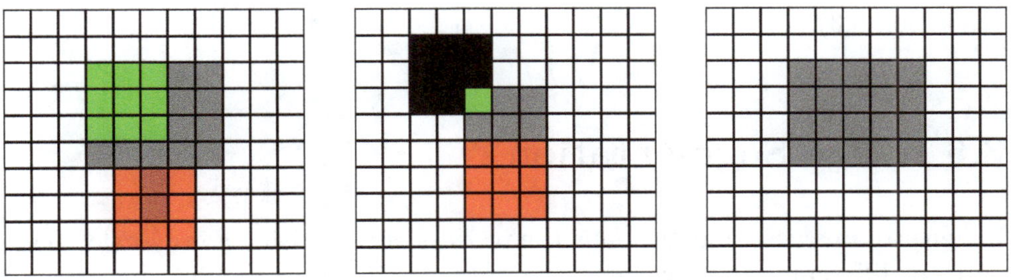

(a) Input image with structuring element overlaid for the erosion. (b) Eroded image with structuring element overlaid for the dilation. (c) Opened image after dilating the eroded image.

Figure 3.16: An example for opening an image with a block shaped structuring element. The image is first eroded and the result is then dilated. Note how the thin extension of the input shape at its bottom is removed by the opening operation.

Binary Closing

Closing, too, is a composition of dilation and erosion. In contrast to opening, the image is, however, first dilated and then eroded with the same structuring element S

$$\mathrm{F_{bin}} \bullet \mathrm{S} = (\mathrm{F_{bin}} \oplus \mathrm{S}) \ominus \mathrm{S}\,. \tag{3.17}$$

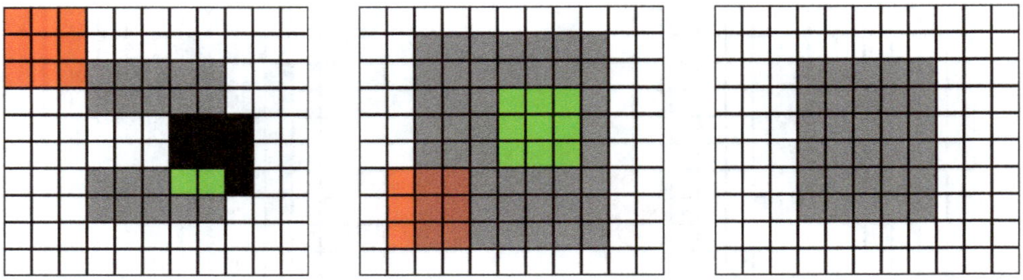

(a) Input image with the structuring element overlaid for the dilation.

(b) Dilated image with structuring element overlaid for the erosion.

(c) Closed image after eroding the dilated image.

Figure 3.17: An example for closing an image with a block shaped structuring element. The image is first dilated and then eroded. Note how the gap between the two blocks is filled by the closing operation.

Closing can be used to fill small gaps in shapes (cf. Fig. 3.17). Note that all of all morphological operators can also be applied on grayscale images (cf. Geek Box 3.3).

3.6 Image Segmentation

In general, image segmentation is the process of converting a grayscale image with L different intensity values (e. g., $L = 256$ for an 8-bit image) into an image with $L_{\text{seg}} \ll L$ gray levels. In the resulting segmented image, the different intensity values partition the image into different regions. This can for example mean a distinction between foreground and background, bones and soft tissue, tumor and healthy tissue or even into several kinds of different tissues. In most applications, however, $L_{\text{seg}} = 2$ and the result is a binary image.

The most basic method for image segmentation is thresholding. For each pixel, its intensity value is compared to a threshold θ, and whether it is larger than the threshold or not, it is assigned to one or the other class.

$$t(x, y) = \begin{cases} 1 & \text{if } f(x, y) \geq \theta \\ 0 & \text{otherwise} \end{cases} \tag{3.20}$$

The only question then is how to choose the threshold value θ. Besides trying different values for θ by hand, the histogram of the image often contains useful information on how to choose the threshold. There are also some algorithms that determine the threshold automatically.

Geek Box 3.3: Grayscale Morphological Operators

Morphological operators can also be defined for grayscale images (and therefore also for color images, where each channel is transformed independently). For opening and closing the same definition as in the binary case can be used. Erosion and dilation, however, have to be redefined since in grayscale images there is no binary decision on what is foreground and what is background.

Grayscale Erosion

Like in the binary case, the structuring element is again shifted over the whole image. The eroded image at location (x, y) is now defined as the minimum in the overlap of the structuring element S at this position and the image F

$$(\mathrm{F} \ominus \mathrm{S})(x, y) = \min_{(i,j)\in \mathrm{S}} f(x+i, y+j)\,. \tag{3.18}$$

Grayscale Dilation

The dilation for grayscale images is defined in a similar way as the maximum in the overlap of structuring element S shifted to the position (x, y) and the image F

$$(\mathrm{F} \oplus \mathrm{S})(x, y) = \max_{(i,j)\in \mathrm{S}} f(x+i, y+j)\,. \tag{3.19}$$

Grayscale Opening / Closing

The grayscale definitions of opening and closing are the same as for the binary case using the grayscale versions of dilation and erosion.

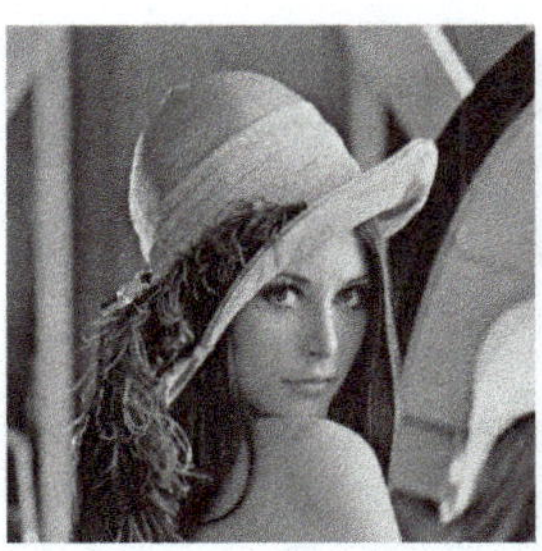
Input Image

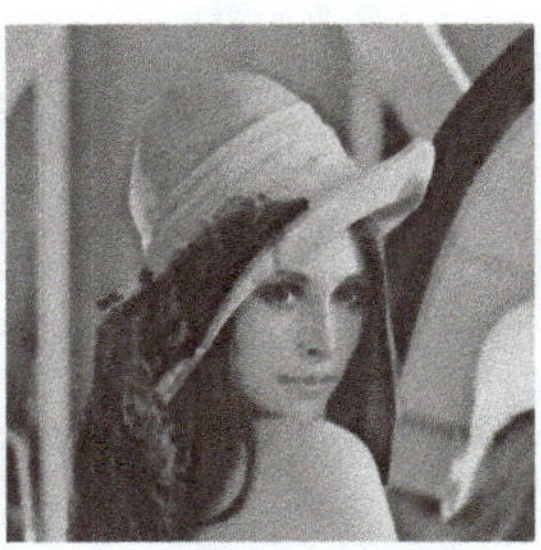
Grayscale Erosion

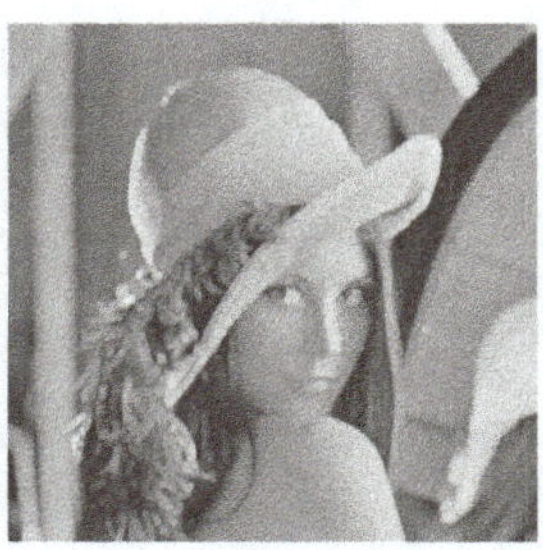
Grayscale Dilation

Bimodal Histograms – Intersection of Gaussians

In many cases the histogram of an image where foreground and background should be separated is bimodal. The assumption here is that the foreground and background both have one characteristic intensity value. Due to shading this leads to two peaks in the histogram (cf. Fig. 3.18). The threshold for separating the two peaks can for example be determined by assuming that the shape of both peaks is Gaussian. In this case, a Gaussian is fit to each peak and the threshold is then determined by locating the intersection of both Gaussians.

Bimodal Histograms – Otsu's Method

Otsu's method is based on the statistical analysis of the image's histogram. The method maximizes the *inter-class variance* σ_b^2 between the foreground and background classes to find the optimal threshold value. To do this, the normalized histogram is used. Let us assume that the image f contains L different intensity values and is of size $w_f \times h_f$. Then the normalized histogram h consists of the values

$$h(i) = \frac{n_i}{w_f \cdot h_f}, \tag{3.21}$$

where n_i is the count of intensity i in the image. For a threshold θ, we can now calculate the probability of a pixel being classified as background (Class 1) or foreground (Class 2)

$$P_1(\theta) = \sum_{i=0}^{\theta} h(i) \tag{3.22}$$

$$P_2(\theta) = 1 - P_1(\theta) = \sum_{i=\theta+i}^{L-1} h(i) \tag{3.23}$$

as a function of the threshold value. We can do the same for the mean values of the intensities belonging to each class

$$\mu_1(\theta) = \frac{1}{P_1(\theta)} \sum_{i=0}^{\theta} (i+1)h(i) \tag{3.24}$$

$$\mu_2(\theta) = \frac{1}{P_2(\theta)} \sum_{i=\theta+1}^{L-1} (i+1)h(i)\,. \tag{3.25}$$

Using these quantities, the inter-class variance can be expressed as

$$\sigma_b^2(\theta) = P_1(\theta)P_2(\theta)\big(\mu_1(\theta) - \mu_2(\theta)\big)^2\,. \tag{3.26}$$

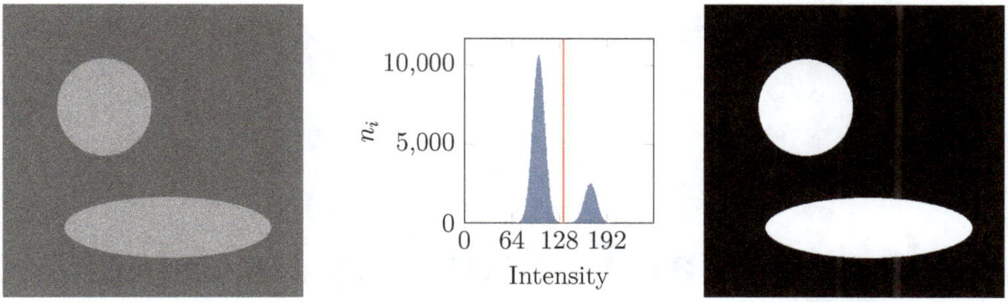

(a) Input image

(b) Histogram of the input image. The threshold value determined with Otsu's method is marked by a red line.

(c) Thresholded image

Figure 3.18: Bimodal histogram thresholding

So maximizing σ_b^2 means that the distance between the mean values of foreground and background is maximized. The optimal threshold θ^* is found by

$$\theta^* = \operatorname*{argmax}_{\theta} \sigma_b^2(\theta), \quad \theta \in [0, L). \tag{3.27}$$

In practice, the number of values θ can take is limited to L different values, and in order to calculate the maximum of σ_b^2, it is sufficient to calculate its values for all possible thresholds. In some cases, the maximum is not unique. When this is the case, the threshold is determined by averaging over the threshold values corresponding to the maximum values of σ_b^2.

Further Reading

[1] Rafael C. Gonzalez and Richard E. Woods. *Digital Image Processing (3rd Edition)*. Upper Saddle River, NJ, USA: Prentice-Hall, Inc., 2006. ISBN: 013168728X.

[2] Richard Szeliski. *Computer Vision: Algorithms and Applications*. 1st. New York, NY, USA: Springer-Verlag New York, Inc., 2010. ISBN: 9781848829343.

4

Endoscopes and Minimally Invasive Surgery

Authors: Sven Haase and Andreas Maier

This chapter points out the key aspects of minimally invasive surgery with particular focus on abdominal surgery using endoscopes. The comparison between minimally invasive and conventional open surgery is illustrated and several procedures are detailed. Moreover, this chapter introduces the term *Image Guidance* and its benefits. Finally, this leads to the motivation why range imaging is of special interest for the next step of modern surgery. As endoscopes are more or less regular cameras that are inserted into the body, we also use this section to introduce the pinhole camera in Geek Box 4.1, elaborate on fundamental mathematical concepts of projection in Geek Box 4.2, and introduce homogeneous coordinates and perspective spaces in Geek Box 4.3. Fig. 4.1 displays an endoscopic image taken in the sigmoid colon which is the part of the large intestine that is closest to the rectum.

4.1 Minimally Invasive Surgery and Open Surgery

One criterion to categorize medical interventions is the degree of invasiveness. Therefore, we distinguish between minimally invasive and open surgery which is illustrated in Fig. 4.2. As the notation suggests, minimally invasive procedures describe medical procedures with little operative trauma. In com-

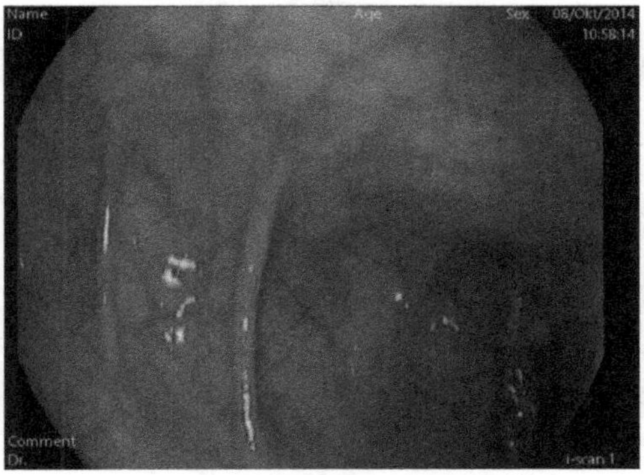

Figure 4.1: View into the colon using an endoscope. Here, the so-called sigmoid colon is under investigation for abdominal pain. The inner walls of the colon appear healthy without any signs of inflammation. Image data courtesy of University Hospital Erlangen, Germany.

parison to conventional open surgery, this leads to a shorter recovery time for the patient and thereby to a reduced hospital stay. In recent years, a variety of minimally invasive alternatives to conventional open surgery have evolved with special focus on pathologies of the heart and the abdomen. In contrast to open surgery, the physician has no direct access to the organs or structures of the human body. On the one hand, this means fewer and smaller scars and less pain for the patient, but on the other hand, without direct access the physician has a limited sense of orientation and usually has to rely on additional imaging techniques. For some medical procedures minimally invasive alternatives are not available as the incision is just too small, e. g., the removal of larger organs or transplantations. For smaller organs such as the kidney or gallbladder, laparoscopic interventions are already performed as a common routine. In terms of operative time, minimally invasive surgery usually takes longer due to the smaller incision and worse orientation. Both open and in most cases minimally invasive surgery require anesthesia during the intervention. Statistical comparison of open and minimally invasive surgery in terms of quality-of-life shows an overall improved result for laparoscopic interventions.

4.2 Minimally Invasive Abdominal Surgery

As one of the most important fields of minimally invasive procedures, the diagnosis and treatment of abdominal pathologies is the main medical application of this chapter. Here, a variety of important special instruments are required:

Geek Box 4.1: Pinhole Camera

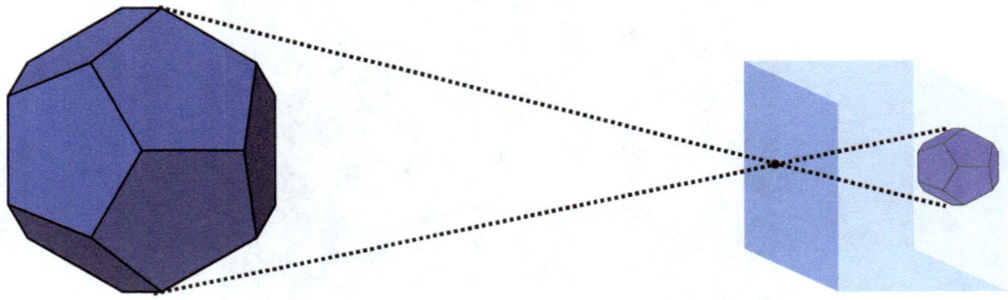

The pinhole camera model is a simple yet powerful model that allows us to describe various effects of the projection process. The model assumes the the outside world is observed using a pinhole. As such the outside world is projected onto a screen on the opposite side of the pinhole. Due to the pinhole, the image of the world is a scaled, upside-down version of the outside world. Doing so, the model allows us to describe perspective, i. e., that the size of the projection is dependent on the distance. In medical imaging and computer vision [2], the pinhole camera model is a widely used assumption. Another convention that is also commonly used is that the screen is virtually placed outside the camera for graphical simplification.

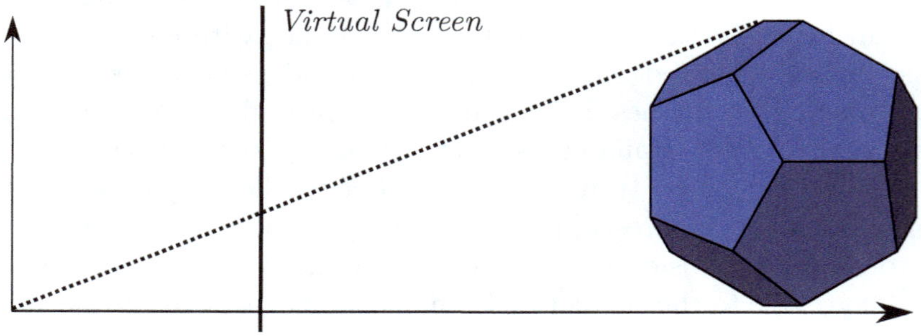

- *Endoscopes*: Depending on the procedure these devices are non-rigid (flexible endoscopes) or rigid (laparoscopes) and serve as a camera inside the human body. Rigid endoscopes have the benefit that the navigation is much more intuitive although the degrees of freedom during the navigation is reduced compared to non-rigid endoscopes.
- *Trocars*: To allow a fast exchange of different instruments a trocar is placed in the human body as a port to the abdominal cavity. For different procedures, different sizes ranging from several milimeters up to a few centimeters are used.

Geek Box 4.2: Mathematical Projection Models

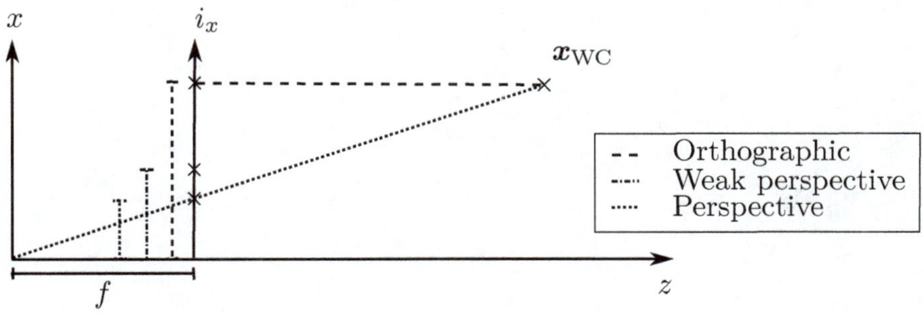

In order to describe camera projections in math, we employ linear algebra and matrix calculus. The figure above compares the projection of a point $\boldsymbol{x}_{\mathrm{WC}} = (x, y, z)^\top$ onto a virtual screen at coordinate $\boldsymbol{i} = (i_x, i_y)^\top$ at focal length f (cf. Geek Box 4.1). For simplicity, we neglect the y components in the figure.
The orthographic projection (dashed line) simply neglects the distance to the screen and finds the projection as

$$\begin{pmatrix} i_x \\ i_y \end{pmatrix} = \begin{pmatrix} 1 & 0 & 0 \\ 0 & 1 & 0 \end{pmatrix} \begin{pmatrix} x \\ y \\ z \end{pmatrix}.$$

Note that this model is not able to describe scaling as it occurs in projective modeling.
In order to alleviate this problem, the weak perspective model (line-dotted line) can be employed. Here we introduce a scalar value k

$$\begin{pmatrix} i_x \\ i_y \end{pmatrix} = \begin{pmatrix} k & 0 & 0 \\ 0 & k & 0 \end{pmatrix} \begin{pmatrix} x \\ y \\ z \end{pmatrix}.$$

that allows us to fix a global, depth independent scaling.
At this point, we observe that we are not able to find a linear model that is able to describe a full perspective projection model (dotted line)

$$\begin{pmatrix} i_x \\ i_y \end{pmatrix} = \begin{pmatrix} \frac{f \cdot x}{z} \\ \frac{f \cdot y}{z} \end{pmatrix} = \begin{pmatrix} ? & ? & ? \\ ? & ? & ? \end{pmatrix} \begin{pmatrix} x \\ y \\ z \end{pmatrix}.$$

for any focal length f.

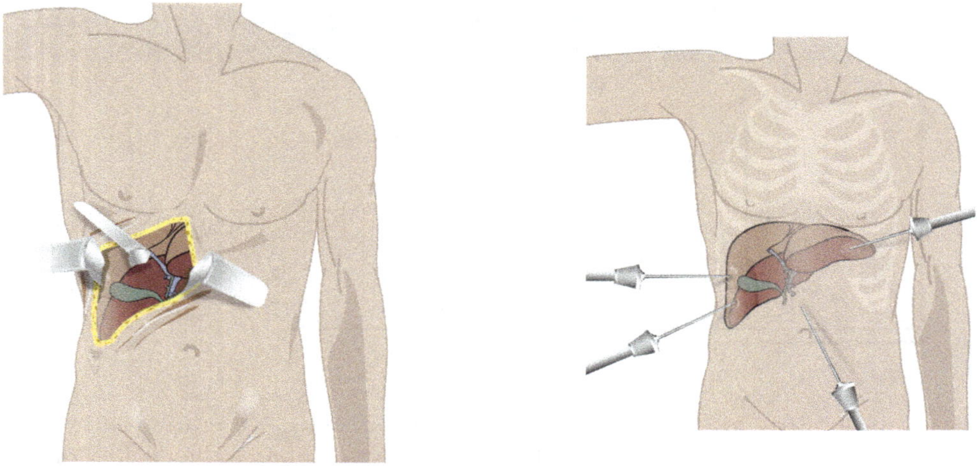

Figure 4.2: Illustrations of a cholecystectomy. The left image shows an open surgery with direct access and the right image shows a minimally invasive approach with endoscopic tools (Courtesy of Prof. Feußner, Technical University Munich, Germany).

- *Surgical instruments*: For the actual procedure, different endoscopic tools are required, e. g., clamps or scissors. Those instruments have a scissor-like grip to control the action at the top of the tool.

The workflow of an endoscopic procedure in general is described by four steps. Usually, the patient has to be anesthetized in a first step. The actual procedure starts with small incisions where the trocars are inserted. Then, the abdomen is insufflated with carbon dioxide gas. This allows the physician to have more room for the procedure. Finally, the endoscope and the tools are inserted through the trocars to start the actual treatment.

4.3 Assistance Systems

Modern surgery companies developed a variety of assistance systems to ease the navigation or to reduce the required manpower for minimally invasive procedures. Usually, several assistants besides the physician are required during the intervention. As the surgeon performs the actual procedure with endoscopic tools, one assistant has to hold the endoscope, one has to hand him the required instruments over, one has to supervise the patient and often a few more are involved for general organization. The remainder of this section introduces some of the available assistance systems in detail.

A very basic and intuitive assistance system is an endoscope holder. These medical devices are available in different complexities, ranging from simple

Geek Box 4.3: Homogeneous Coordinates

In Geek Box 4.2, we have seen that projective transforms cannot be expressed by means of linear transforms in a Cartesian space. However, there exists a class of mathematical spaces in which this is possible. In order to do so, we virtually extend the dimension of our vector $\boldsymbol{x}' = (x', y')^\top$ by an additional component. This way, we create a new *homogeneous* vector

$$\tilde{\boldsymbol{i}} = \begin{pmatrix} \lambda \cdot i_x \\ \lambda \cdot i_y \\ \lambda \end{pmatrix}$$

with $\lambda \neq 0$. Note that $\boldsymbol{i}$ can easily be lifted to homogeneous space by selecting, e. g. $\lambda = 1$. For conversion back to a Cartesian space, one selects simply the last component of a homogenous vector and divides all components by it. Then, the last component can be omitted and the point can be mapped back to the original space. This *projective space* has a number of additional properties, e. g., all points are only equal (denoted by $\hat{=}$), if they map back to the original Cartesian point and points with 0 in the last component cannot easily be mapped back to the original space as they lie at *infinity*. A very good introduction is given in [2].

Using this powerful concept, we can now return to our previous problem and observe

$$\boldsymbol{i} = \begin{pmatrix} i_x \\ i_y \end{pmatrix} = \begin{pmatrix} \frac{f \cdot x}{z} \\ \frac{f \cdot y}{z} \end{pmatrix} \hat{=} \begin{pmatrix} f \cdot x \\ f \cdot y \\ z \end{pmatrix} = \begin{pmatrix} f & 0 & 0 \\ 0 & f & 0 \\ 0 & 0 & 1 \end{pmatrix} \begin{pmatrix} x \\ y \\ z \end{pmatrix}.$$

non-electronic static holders to automatic flexible holders that are navigated with a joystick. In general, these endoscope holders allow a more stable image acquisition as they exclude any jitter induced by a human. However, those systems are often very basic and still have to be navigated by a surgeon, e. g., the *SOLOASSIST*, an electronic assistance arm that is navigated by a joystick and simulates a human arm.

Besides endoscope holders, fully automatic robotic assistance systems are already commercially available. These systems allow the surgeon to be at a separate workstation as illustrated in Fig. 4.3. All commands are directly transmitted to the robot allowing the surgeon to even be at a distant place while performing the procedure. One of the most wide-spread is the *da Vinci* system. It is navigated by grips and pedals that enable various degrees of freedom. For intuitive visualization, this robot acquires stereoscopic images and thereby gives the surgeon a 3-D impression of the scene.

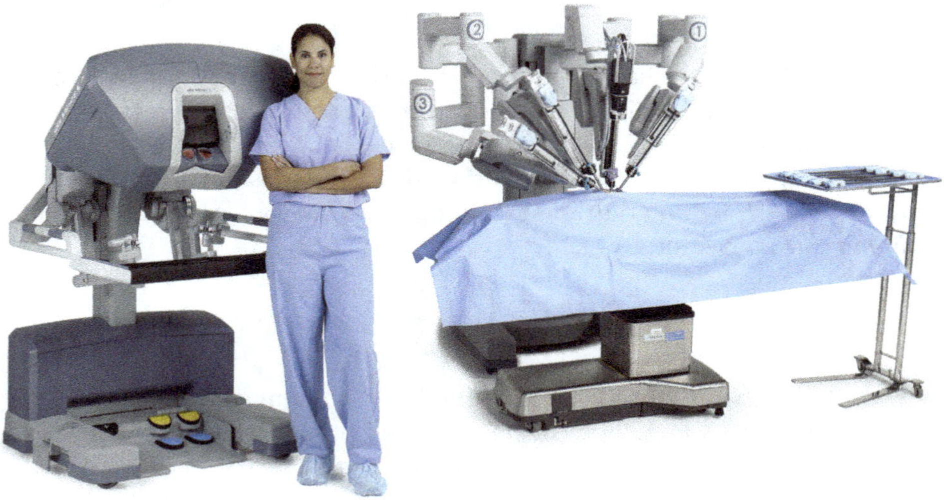

Figure 4.3: The da Vinci assistance system (©2014 Intuitive Surgical, Inc) with the workstation on the left and the distant robotic system on the right.

4.4 Range Imaging in Abdominal Surgery

Although assistance systems for minimally invasive surgery are commercially available, one major problem of endoscopic interventions still remains. The orientation and thereby the navigation within the human body depends on the experience of the surgeon. Due to the lack of intuitive visual comparison to the environment, the narrow field of view induces a loss of depth and size estimation in the abdominal cavity. However, this information is required for diagnosis, e. g., the size of a polyp, and for decision making, e. g., choosing the most reasonable endoscopic instrument. Therefore, a variety of different approaches to compensate for this loss of information were investigated, e. g., adding grids to the endoscope lens or estimating sizes by comparison with known instruments. To achieve more accurate estimations, further approaches considering range images have been investigated. Although these systems can also be utilized to measure sizes or distances, range data acquiring devices also enable completely new projects to assist minimally invasive procedures, e. g., augmenting 3-D range images with preoperative 3-D CT data. Several different techniques have been investigated to acquire endoscopic range images. Besides several *Shape-from-X* approaches, e. g., Shape-from-Shading, the three most popular acquisition techniques are using *stereo vision* setups, *structured light* or time-of-flight (TOF). Today, only stereo endoscopes are commercially available, but the two other techniques are highly investigated by different researchers. This section will focus on the working principle of available range imaging systems.

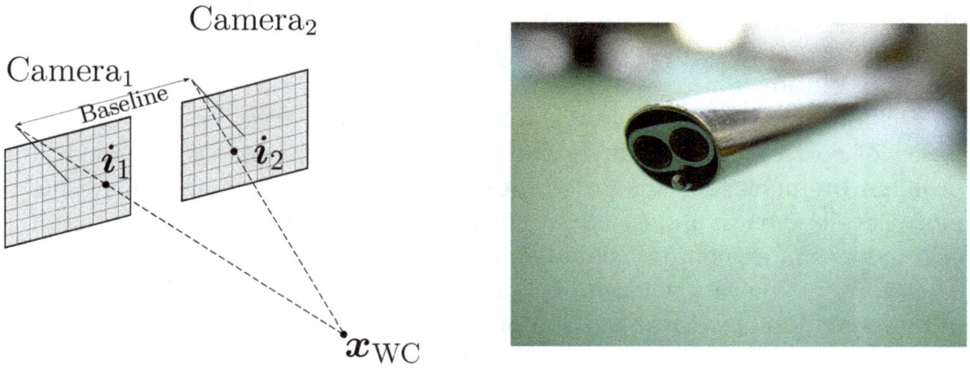

Figure 4.4: The illustration on the left hand side describes a stereo vision setup with two cameras Camera$_1$ and Camera$_2$ that observe a 3-D point $\boldsymbol{x}_{\mathrm{WC}}$. The projection of this point onto each image plane results in a pixel index $\boldsymbol{i}_1$ and $\boldsymbol{i}_2$ which can be computed by a simple pinhole camera model. The right hand side image shows the front view of a stereo endoscope with two apertures to acquire images from two different field of views (close-up view courtesy by Prof. Speidel, National Center for Tumor Diseases, Dresden)).

4.4.1 Stereo Vision

Stereo endoscopes are the most investigated range image acquiring setups in minimally invasive surgery. The principle is also implemented in the da Vinci assistance system. Stereo vision describes an intuitive acquisition technique that is similar to the human vision and depth estimation.

The core concept behind stereo endoscopy is to estimate range information by observing a scene from two different perspectives. Given a known baseline, the framework has to detect the 2-D projections of a 3-D point in both image planes. In theory, using basic trigonometry, the range information of these points can then be calculated by triangulation, see Fig. 4.4. In practice, both lines will probably not intersect and minimizing the distance of both lines will estimate the position of the 3-D point.

The requirements for stereo endoscopy are on the one hand a precisely calibrated device and on the other hand diversified texture information of the observed scene. Accuracy is increased with a wider baseline between both sensors. As this baseline is limited by the diameter of the endoscope, the improved accuracy has to be gained by calculating the corresponding points in both images with higher precision. Corresponding points are calculated by detecting features in both images, e. g., by applying the scale-invariant feature transform (SIFT) or by computing speeded-up robust features (SURF). Matching those feature points results in point pairs that correspond to the same 3-D point in the observed scene. Therefore, the output of a stereo endoscope highly depends on the quality of the two images and on the speed and robustness of the feature detection and matching. The estimated range images of a stereo setup, also called disparity maps, have a scene dependent image resolution.

The bottleneck of this range image acquisition technique is the calculation of corresponding feature points. Hardware manufacturers tackle this problem by increasing image resolution in the sensor domain. This leads to more details even in almost homogeneous regions in the acquired images, but also induces more computational effort to calculate features on both images. Therefore, estimating accurate 3-D range data in real-time is a major issue in stereo endoscopy. Stereo endoscopes are currently the only commercially available and CE certified 3-D endoscopes.

4.4.2 Structured Light

Structured light endoscopy is a novel technique based on stereo vision concepts, but with artificially created feature points instead of those given by textural information. In minimally invasive surgery structured light systems are not yet commercially available.

The working principle of structured light sensors is very similar to stereo vision systems. In comparison to those, structured light systems do not require two cameras observing the scene. The second camera is replaced by a projector that generates a known pattern onto the observed scenario, see Fig. 4.5. The known baseline and corresponding points in the acquired image and the known projection pattern are used to reconstruct 3-D points by triangulation. As the projector generates the pattern that is used to calculate the feature points, structured light is also called an active triangulation technique.

Similar to stereo vision, the baseline between the sensor and the projector and an accurate calibration is required for high quality measurements. As long as the pattern is clearly visible, this technique is independent of texture information of the observed scene. In comparison to stereo vision systems, the feature detection framework can be highly adapted to the projection pattern, as the structure of the feature points is known. The projection pattern should be easy to detect and hard to disturb by the texture of the scene. In conventional structured light setups, stripes or sinusoidal patterns are popular.

As the core concept for structured light is similar to stereo vision, so is its bottleneck of detecting and identifying the feature points of the projected pattern. Furthermore, the smaller the structures of the projected pattern are, the more 3-D points can be reconstructed, but the harder it is to identify those structures in the acquired images.

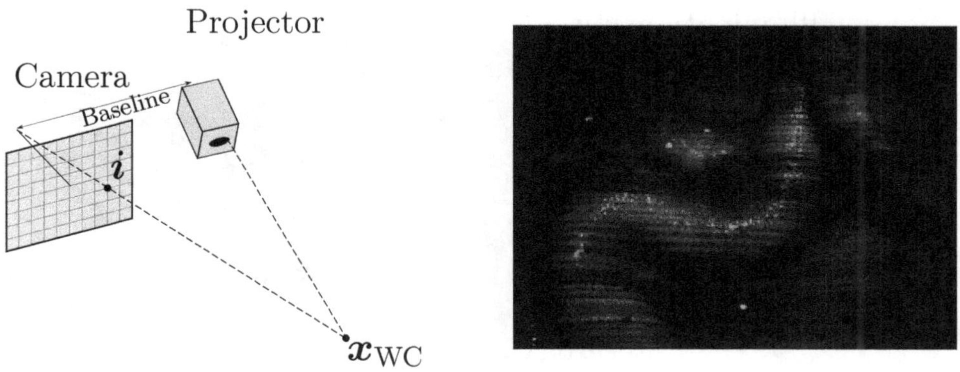

Figure 4.5: The illustration on the left hand side describes a structured light setup with one camera and one projector that generates a known pattern onto the scene. The projection of this point onto the image plane results in a pixel index $\boldsymbol{i}$. Together with the projection pattern the 3-D world $\boldsymbol{x}_{\mathrm{WC}}$ can be reconstructed using triangulation. The right hand side image shows a projection on animal organs.

4.4.3 Time-of-Flight (TOF)

TOF technology [4] tackles the topic of 3-D reconstruction from a completely different field of view. Instead of using acquired color images to find any distinctive structures, reflection characteristics are exploited to physically measure the distances of the observed scene. The first work to introduce this concept is found in [6].

The concept behind TOF technology is to measure a frequency modulated light ray that is sent out by an illumination unit and received by a TOF sensor, see Fig. 4.6. The received sinusoidal signal is sampled at four timestamps to estimate the phase shift Φ between the emitted and the received signal. The radial distance d is then computed by:

$$d = \frac{c}{2f_{\mathrm{mod}}} \cdot \frac{\Phi}{2\pi}, \tag{4.1}$$

where c denotes the speed of light and f_{mod} the modulation frequency.

As the illumination unit can be realized by an light-emitting diode (LED) and the sensor is a simple CMOS or CCD chip, production costs of TOF sensors are rather low. However, due to their novelty compared to stereo vision, current TOF devices exhibit low data quality and low image resolution. Besides the range image, most TOF devices provide additional data, e. g., photometric data, often denoted as the amplitude image and a binary validity mask. Due to its measurement technique, TOF setups do not require

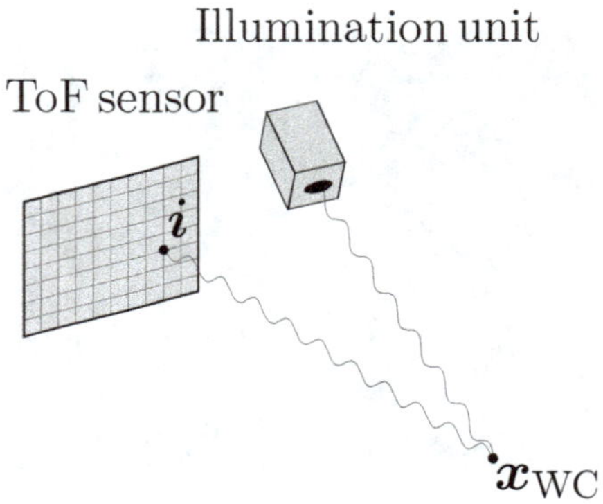

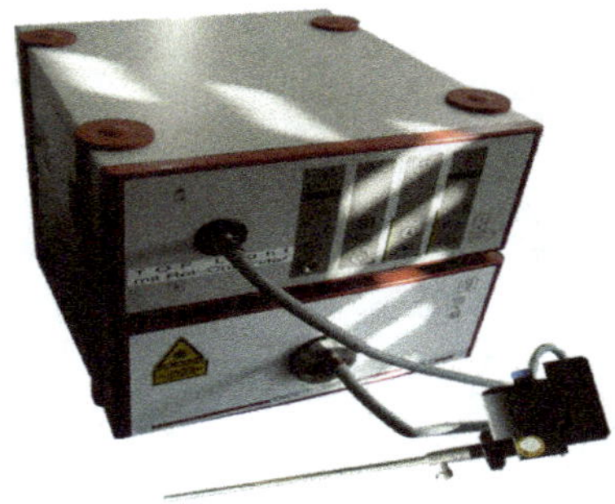

Figure 4.6: The left hand side illustration describes a TOF setup with a single camera and an illumination unit that sends out the modulated light. The reflected signal is then received by the TOF sensor at pixel index $\boldsymbol{i}$. After calculating the phase shift, the radial distance is computed. The right hand side image shows a prototype. The setup includes two separated light sources for the color and the TOF acquisition.

a baseline between the illumination unit and the measuring sensor, which is beneficial for the use in minimally invasive surgery.

Besides the low resolution, systematic errors reduce the data quality extremely. The error sources range from color dependent range measurements over temperature issues of the devices to flying pixels at object boundaries. In minimally invasive procedures, two major issues occur. First, multiple reflection within the abdominal cavity corrupts TOF measurements. Second, inhomogeneous illumination caused by the endoscopic optic hinders accurate range measurements. Still the technology is real-time capable and thereby also suited for live broadcasting [9].

Further Reading

[1] Sven Haase et al. "ToF/RGB Sensor Fusion for 3-D Endoscopy". In: *Current Medical Imaging Reviews* 9.2 (2013), pp. 113–119.

[2] Richard Hartley and Andrew Zisserman. *Multiple view geometry in computer vision*. Cambridge university press, 2003.

[3] K. Kremer. *Minimally Invasive Abdominal Surgery*. Minimally Invasive Abdominal Surgery. Georg Thieme Verlag, 2001. ISBN: 9783131081919.

[4] R. Lange and P. Seitz. "Solid-state time-of-flight range camera". In: *Quantum Electronics, IEEE Journal of* 37.3 (Mar. 2001), pp. 390–397. ISSN: 0018-9197.

[5] L. Maier-Hein et al. “Optical techniques for 3D surface reconstruction in computer-assisted laparoscopic surgery”. In: *Medical Image Analysis* 17.8 (2013), pp. 974–996. ISSN: 1361-8415.
[6] Jochen Penne et al. “Time-of-Flight 3-D Endoscopy”. In: *MICCAI 2009, Part I, LNCS 5761*. Ed. by G.-Z. Yang et al. Vol. 5761. London, 2009, pp. 467–474.
[7] Sebastian Röhl et al. “Dense GPU-enhanced surface reconstruction from stereo endoscopic images for intraoperative registration”. In: *Medical Physics* 39.3 (2012), pp. 1632–1645.
[8] Christoph Schmalz et al. “An endoscopic 3D scanner based on structured light”. In: *Medical Image Analysis* 16.5 (2012), pp. 1063–1072. ISSN: 1361-8415.
[9] Michael Stürmer et al. “3-D tele-medical speech therapy using Time-of-Flight technology”. In: *4th European Congress for Medical and Biomedical Engineering*. Ed. by Marc Nyssen et al. Antwerpen, 2008.
[10] Li-Ming Su et al. “Augmented Reality During Robot-assisted Laparoscopic Partial Nephrectomy: Toward Real-Time 3D-CT to Stereoscopic Video Registration”. In: *Urology* 73.4 (2009), pp. 896–900. ISSN: 0090-4295.
[11] Gyung Tak Sung and Inderbir S Gill. “Robotic laparoscopic surgery: a comparison of the da Vinci and Zeus systems”. In: *Urology* 58.6 (2001), pp. 893–898. ISSN: 0090-4295.
[12] Johannes Totz et al. “Dense Surface Reconstruction for Enhanced Navigation in MIS”. In: *Medical Image Computing and Computer-Assisted Intervention, MICCAI 2011*. Ed. by Gabor Fichtinger, Anne Martel, and Terry Peters. Vol. 6891. Lecture Notes in Computer Science. 2011, pp. 89–96. ISBN: 978-3-642-23622-8.
[13] Nimish Vakil et al. “Endoscopic measurement of lesion size: Improved accuracy with image processing”. In: *Gastrointestinal Endoscopy* 40.2 (1994), pp. 178–183. ISSN: 0016-5107.

5

Microscopes and Microscopy

Authors: Firas Mualla, Marc Aubreville and Andreas Maier

We perceive the physical world around us using our eyes, but only down to a certain limit. Objects with a diameter smaller than 75 μm cannot be recognized by the naked eye, and due to this reason, they remained undiscovered for the most of human history. Entities which belong to this category include cells (diameter of 10 μm), bacteria (1 μm), viruses (100 nm), molecules (2 nm), and atoms (0.3 nm)[1]. In fact, the importance of these micro/nano entities in almost every aspect of our life cannot be sufficiently appreciated. Microscopes are the tools which enable us to extend our vision to the micro-world and, despite the prefix micro- in the name, to the nano-world, too. This chapter takes the reader through the basic principles of the most widely-used light microscopy techniques, their advantages, and their inherent limitations. Further microscope types such as scanning tunneling microscopes or atomic force microscopes are beyond the focus of this text. In contrast to the previous chapter, a pinhole projection model is no longer sufficient to explain

[1] The diameter measurements given here are for a blood cell, a typical bacterium, an influenza virus, a DNA molecule, and a uranium atom.

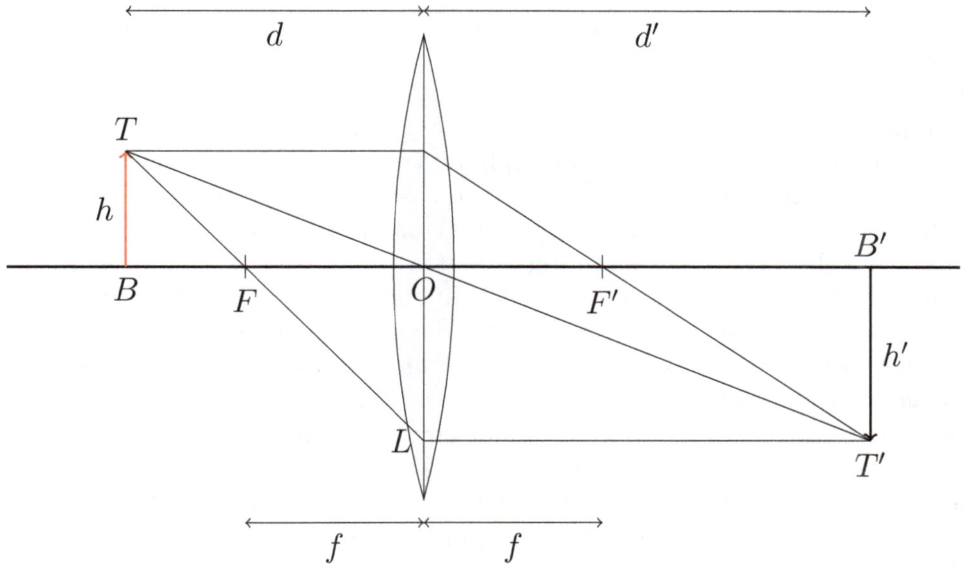

Figure 5.1: Image formation in a converging lens for an object whose distance to the lens is larger than the focal length.

microscopy. Therefore, we introduce the thin lens model as it provides explanations for at least two functionalities: light-gathering and magnification.

5.1 Image Formation in a Thin Lens

Consider an object with height h standing at a distance d in front of a converging lens with a focal length $f < d$. Naturally, the lens creates an image of this object. The question then arises as how we can determine the height of the image h' and its distance d' to the lens. From a *geometrical optics* perspective, the image formation process can be described using three simple rules (cf. Figure 5.1):

1. An incident light ray which passes through the optical center O does not suffer any refraction.
2. An incident light ray parallel to the optical axis is refracted passing through the image focal point F'.
3. An incident light ray which passes through the object focal point F is refracted parallel to the optical axis.

As shown in Figure 5.1, the three rays intersect at a point positioned at distance d' from the lens. Obviously, two rays are sufficient to geometrically construct this intersection point. The image acquired at d' is defined as an *in-*

focus image. On the other hand, an image acquired at a longer or a shorter distance than d', is called *defocused* image. In this context, an image of a point source (such as T in Figure 5.1) is infinitely small at focus (abstracted as a point T' in Figure 5.1), but it is larger than a point for defocused images.

Figure 5.2 shows the result of applying the rules of image formation, i. e., the three rules mentioned above, on the case when the object is within the focal length ($d < f$). As can be seen in the figure, the rays do not converge. However, the ray extensions intersect at a point T', called *virtual* image, from which the rays *appear* to diverge. In contrast, the images formed when $d > f$ are called *real* as they are real convergence points of light rays. Virtual images formed by a converging lens are *upright* while the real images are *upside-down*. Another important difference is that virtual images cannot be projected on a screen, a camera chip, or any other surface. Nevertheless, they can be perceived by the human eye because the eye behaves as a converging lens which recollects the diverged light rays on the retina.

Figure 5.3 shows the result of applying the rules of image formation in a diverging lens when $d < f$. It should be noted, however, that: Contrary to the case of converging lenses, when applying these rules on diverging lenses, the image focus F' is at the side of incident light rays and the object focus F is at the other side of the lens. Similar to the case described in Figure 5.2, the image is upright and virtual. However, in contrast to Figure 5.2, it is demagnified. We obtain this result with a diverging lens when $d > f$ as well.

So far, we could *geometrically* construct the image of an object in a diverging or a converging lens. At this point, we may ask whether there are closed-form equations which relate the object height h to the image height h', or the object-lens distance d to the image-lens distance d'.

Let us consider a converging lens with $d > f$ (cf. Figure 5.1). From the similar triangles TOB and $T'OB'$, one can directly write:

$$\frac{h'}{h} = \frac{d'}{d} \tag{5.1}$$

The same applies for triangles TFB and FOL:

$$\frac{h'}{h} = \frac{f}{d-f} \tag{5.2}$$

Combining Eq. (5.1) and Eq. (5.2) yields:

$$\begin{aligned} \frac{f}{d-f} &= \frac{d'}{d} \\ fd &= d'd - d'f \\ fd + d'f &= d'd \end{aligned}$$

Dividing by fdd' yields the *thin lens equation*:

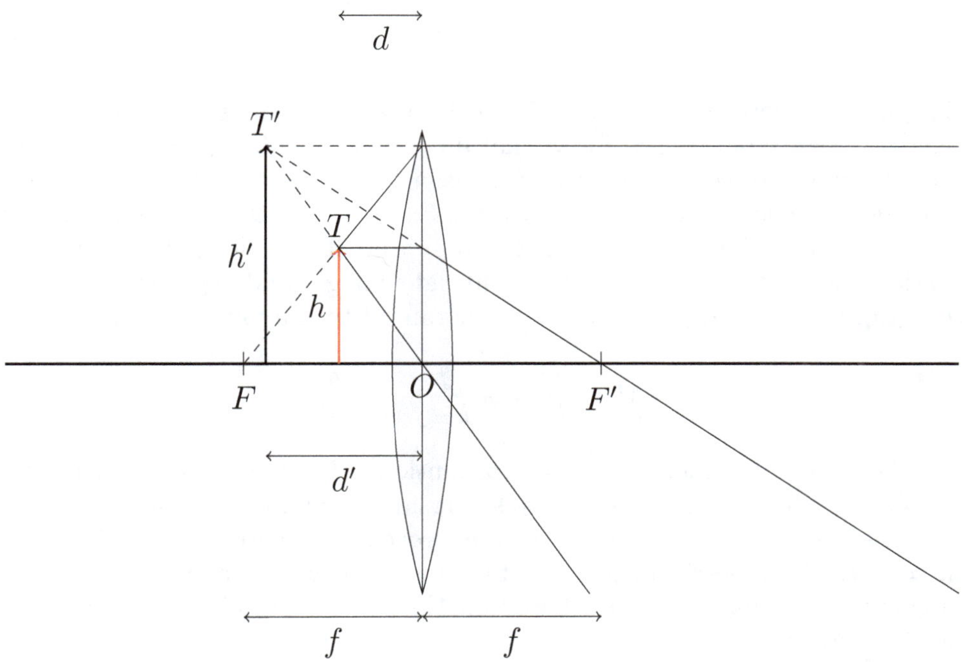

Figure 5.2: Image formation in a converging lens for an object whose distance to the lens is smaller than the focal length.

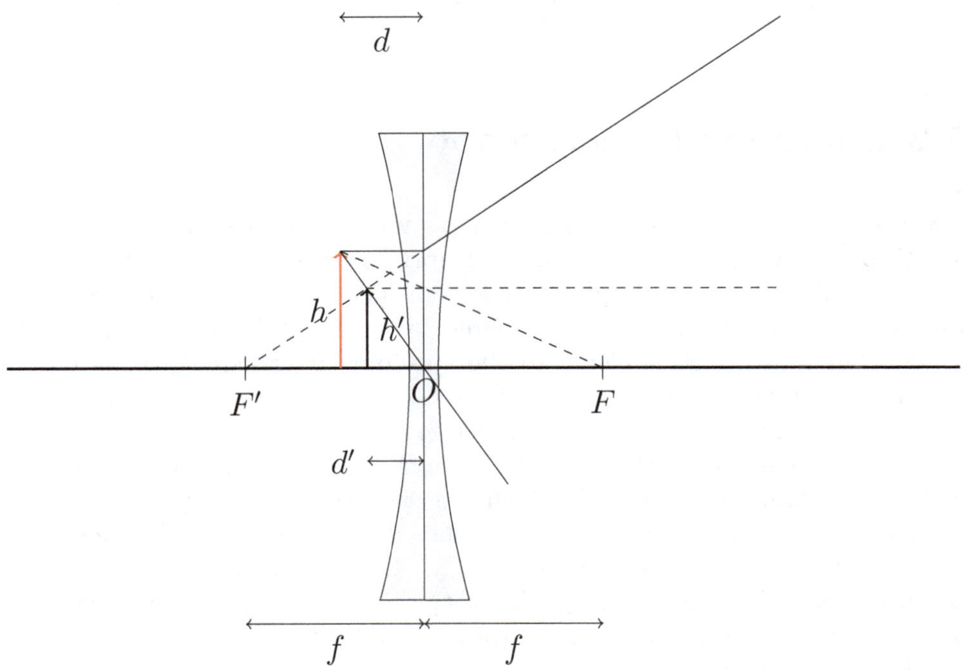

Figure 5.3: Image formation in a diverging lens.

$$\frac{1}{d} + \frac{1}{d'} = \frac{1}{f} \tag{5.3}$$

Eq. (5.3) was derived in this text for real images in a converging lens. Nevertheless, it can be also used for virtual images and/or diverging lenses under the following sign conventions: 1) d' is negative when the image is at the object side of the lens (similar to the case in Figure 5.2), otherwise it is positive. 2) f is negative for diverging lenses. Moreover, if we add a third sign convention stating that h' is positive for upright images and negative otherwise, then Eq. (5.1) and Eq. (5.2) can be generalized to the following form:

$$M = \frac{h'}{h} = -\frac{f}{d-f} = -\frac{d'}{d} \tag{5.4}$$

Based on the above-mentioned sign conventions, the magnification M is positive for upright images and negative for upside-down images. This generalization, i. e., Eq. (5.3) and Eq. (5.4), can be proved to be correct by applying the three rules of geometric image formation and employing triangle similarity for each specific setup. Moreover, based on Eq. (5.4), the following conclusions can be drawn:

- The image of an object in a converging lens is magnified ($|M| > 1$) when $d < 2f$, has the same size of the object when $d = 2f$, and demagnified ($|M| < 1$) when $d > 2f$.
- The image of an object in a diverging lens ($f < 0$) is demagnified.

5.2 Compound Microscope

If you look through a magnifying glass at an object located within the focal length of the lens, you see a magnified upright virtual image of the object. Conceptually, this is a simple microscope. The *compound microscope* (cf. Figure 5.4) extends this basic principle by using at least two converging lenses. The lens which is closer to the specimen is called *objective* lens. It creates a real magnified inverted image G_o of the specimen. This requires that the specimen distance to the objective d_o is in the range $f_o < d_o < 2f_o$, where f_o is the focal length of the objective. The second lens is called *eyepiece* as it is the component through which a user of the microscope observes the sample. The distance of G_o to the eyepiece d_e is, by construction, less than the focal length of the eyepiece ($d_e < f_e$). Consequently, the eyepiece lens creates a magnified virtual image G_e of G_o. Since the image of the first lens is an object for the second one, the total magnification is the product of the two lens magnifications.

In modern microscopes, the objective lens is characterized by its magnification and numerical aperture. The magnification was defined above in

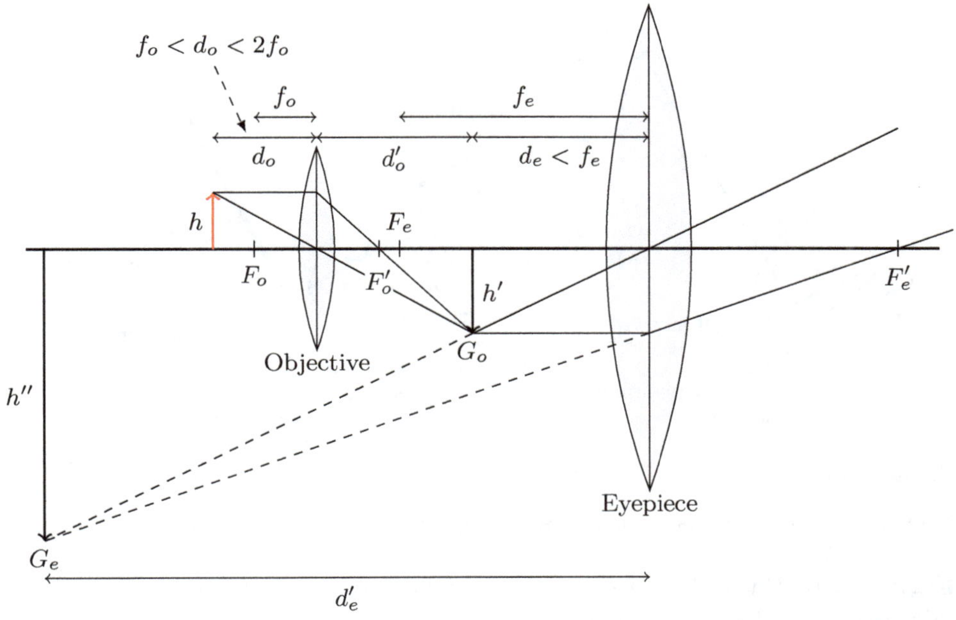

Figure 5.4: Image formation in a compound microscope. Symbols F_o, F'_o, F_e, and F'_e represent the objective object focal point, objective image focal point, eyepiece object focal point, and eyepiece image focal point, respectively. A human observer at the right-hand side of the figure will see the image G_e.

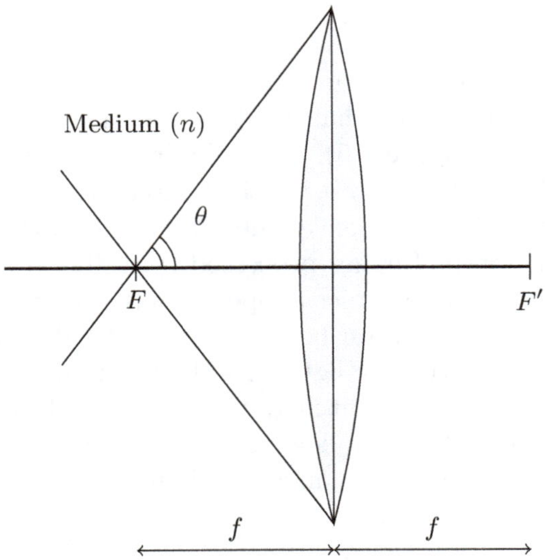

Figure 5.5: The numerical aperture is determined by θ the half angle of the maximum light cone and n the refractive index of the medium between lens and specimen.

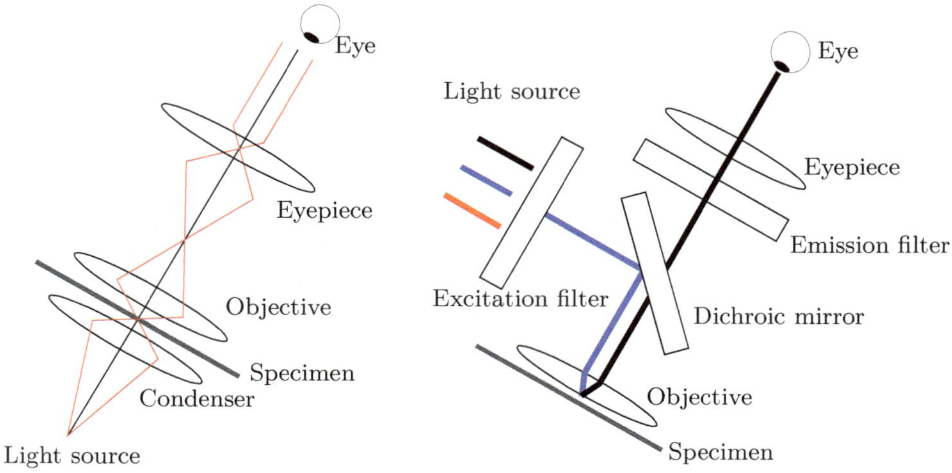

(a) Scheme of a bright field microscope. **(b)** Scheme of a fluorescence microscope.

Figure 5.6: Basic diagrams of a bright field microscope and a fluorescence microscope. Both were drawn after [1].

Eq. (5.4). The numerical aperture quantifies the capability of a lens to gather light. It is defined as follows:

$$\mathrm{NA} = n \ \sin\theta, \tag{5.5}$$

where n is the refractive index of the medium between objective lens and specimen ($n_{\mathrm{air}} \approx 1$) and θ is the half angle of the maximum light cone which the lens can collect (cf. Figure 5.5). Since the image formed by the objective lens is real, it can be captured by a physical detector. For instance, it can be recorded by a CCD chip, and hence, the magnified view can be saved as a digital image which can be further processed by a digital computer.

The principle of compound microscope models the magnification mechanism. Additionally, depending on how the sample is illuminated and which kind of information is carried by light rays, light microscopes can be further classified into subcategories: bright field, fluorescence, phase contrast, quantitative phase, and others. In the following sections, more details will be given about each of the aforementioned microscopic modalities.

5.3 Bright Field Microscopy

Typically, the density and thickness of a specimen are space-variant. Consequently, specimen points absorb light differently, i. e., the energy of light after passing through the specimen is, likewise, space-variant. Figure 5.6(a)

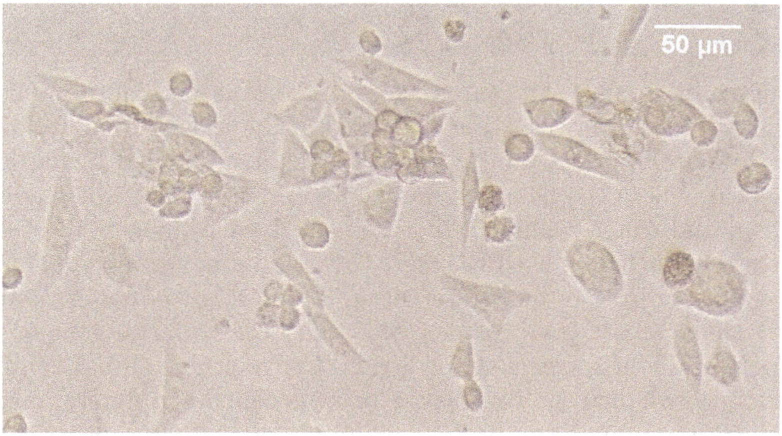

Figure 5.7: A microscopic image of a cell culture: The image was acquired using a Nikon Eclipse TE2000U microscope with a bright field objective of magnification 10× and NA = 0.3.

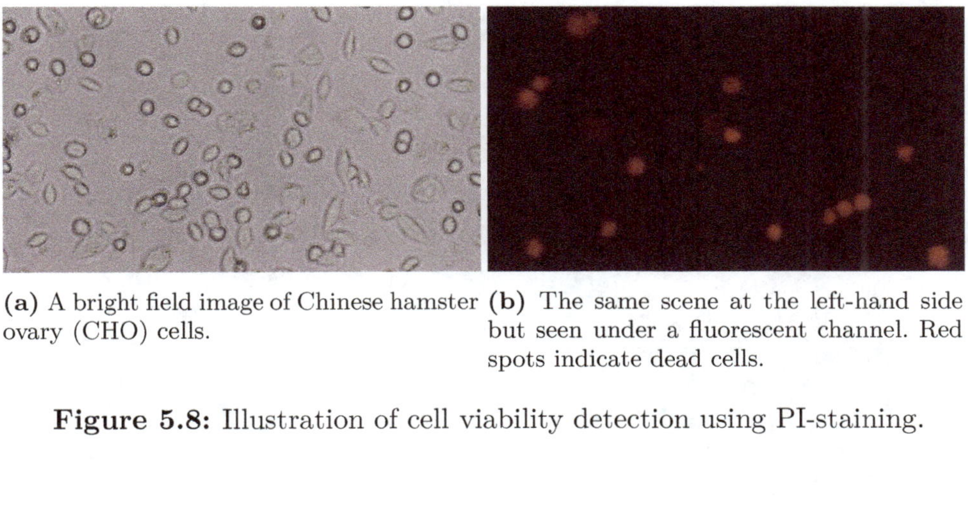

(a) A bright field image of Chinese hamster ovary (CHO) cells.

(b) The same scene at the left-hand side but seen under a fluorescent channel. Red spots indicate dead cells.

Figure 5.8: Illustration of cell viability detection using PI-staining.

schematically shows how this fact can be utilized in a microscopic setup. The *condenser* shown in the figure plays the role of concentrating light coming from a light source at the specimen. The specimen information is encoded in the intensity of light wave which reaches the objective. Background or the part of the scene which does not contain dense objects tends to be bright in the resulting image. This observer impression gave the technique its name. Bright field setup is the number-one choice whenever minimization of expenditure or implementation difficulties are main concerns. An example of a bright field image of cells is shown in Figure 5.7.

In clinical routine cells in suspension are only investigated infrequently. Instead, the most common investigation techniques for bright field microscopy are cytology, where cells and their inner structure are investigated, and histology, where the embedding of cells into the surrounding tissue architecture

Geek Box 5.1: Stains for Histology and Cytology

To highlight cellular structures, sections from tissue biopsies and also cytology slides are often dyed or stained. The most common form of stain in histology is a mixture of two substances called hematoxylin and eosin, where the hematoxylin color stains cell nuclei blue and cytoplasm and other cellular structures are dyed in magenta by eosin. Dyes are furthermore used to assess the amount of certain substances, e. g. copper or iron, or biologic structures adhering to certain biomarkers. Besides a main color, often a secondary (or even third) color with strongly different spectral shape is used to dye other cellular compartments and enhance the contrast, a process called counterstaining.
In order to prepare a sample, it usually undergoes the process of fixation with formaldehyde and embedding in paraffin wax. The fixation stops a great part of the biologic processes and ensures a proper quality of the slide and a slow degradation process. Embedding in a block of wax is a precondition to cutting thin slices of constant thickness, which are then placed on a microscope slide and covered with a coverslip.

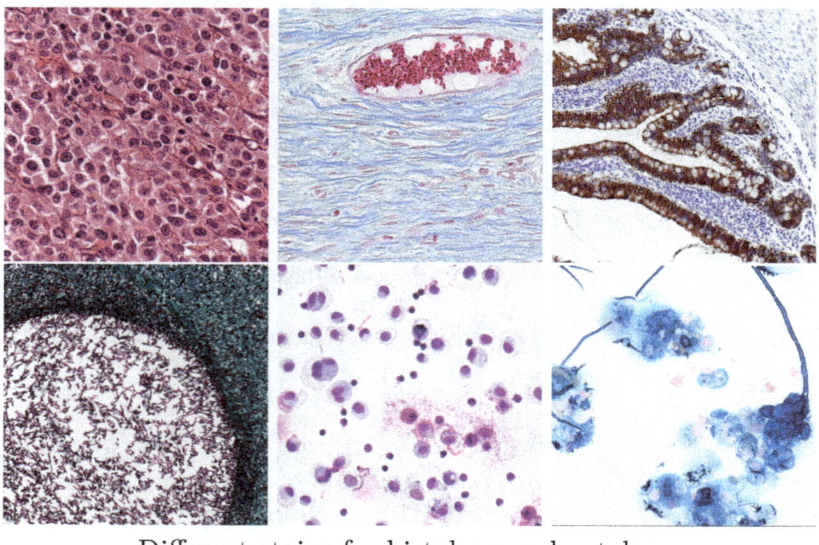

Different stains for histology and cytology.
Top row: Hematoxylin-eosin, Azan, Multi-cytokeratin (AE1, AE3).
Bottom row: Grocott, May-Grünwald-Giemsa, Turnbull Blue.
Images courtesy of FU Berlin, Germany.

is described. For both techniques, staining of the sample plays an important role (see Geek Box on page 77).

5.4 Fluorescence Microscopy

While a bright field microscope utilizes light absorption of a sample, a fluorescence microscope makes use of another natural phenomenon called, unsurprisingly, fluorescence. Some special materials, when illuminated with light having a specific wavelength, emit light with another wavelength. As shown in Figure 5.6(b), an excitation filter is required to select a part of the electromagnetic spectrum for exciting the fluorescent materials in specimen. Another filter is then utilized to separate the emitted light from that used in the excitation process.

Fluorescence microscopes deliver images of high contrast when compared to bright field images. In addition, due to the fact that fluorescence can be incited by specific biological or physical processes, scientists were able to find many applications of fluorescence microscopy in materials science and cellular biology. To give just one example, a widely-used technique for cell viability detection (cf. Figure 5.8) is based on imaging of a fluorescent dye called propidium iodide (PI). Viable cells are usually selectively permeable, i. e., they do not allow molecules to freely cross the cellular membrane. When a cell dies, this exclusion property is lost allowing PI to leak through the cellular membrane toward cell interior. PI binds then to RNA and DNA inside the penetrated cell which drastically enhances the fluorescence. Therefore, dead cells can be easily distinguished from the non-stained viable cells.

There are at least two shortcomings of fluorescence imaging: Firstly, staining may cause some undesired effects on the sample under study. For instance, it was shown that the dyes used in cell viability detection affect cell stiffness. Secondly, what we see under fluorescence microscopy is the activity of fluorescent dyes which, in general, does not reveal structural information. Moreover, these fluorescent dyes do not always cover the entire imaged object. These two factors lead to incomplete shape information. For confocal laser endomicroscopy, also fluorescent dyes are employed, yet in a different setup which is discussed in Geek Box 5.2.

5.5 Phase Contrast Microscopy

As mentioned earlier, in bright field microscopy, light absorption is responsible for image formation. Objects which absorb light are called *amplitude objects* since they affect light amplitude. Transparent objects, on the other hand, hardly alter the amplitude of light. They, however, delay light wave introducing a phase shift, and thus, they are given the name *phase objects*. We demonstrate this effect visually in Figure 5.10 and introduce the underlying math in Geek Box 5.3.

Geek Box 5.2: Confocal Laser Endomicroscopy

Recently, a novel method of fluorescence microscopy imaging has gained attention in research: In Confocal Laser Endomicroscopy (CLE), a fiber bundle carrying laser light in the cyan color spectrum is inserted into cavities of the human body, usually through the accessory channel of a normal endoscope. With high magnification ratios, it is being used for structural tissue analysis *in vivo*, i. e. in the living patient. Due to the confocal construction, a single focal plane in a defined depth can be visualized as a sharp image since the image is not tainted by scattering light. Prior to the examination, a fluorescent contrast agent is given to the patient intravenously, enriching in the intercellular space and thus making outlining cellular structures possible.

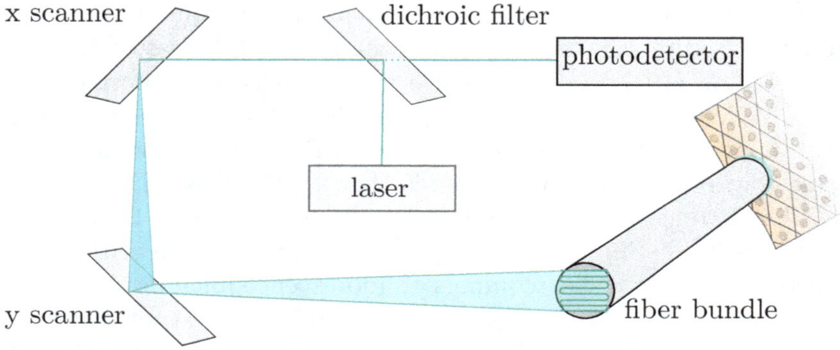

Confocal Laser Endomicroscopy (adapted from [15])

CLE generates video sequences at rates of up to 12 Hz [15] and is clinically used for diagnosis within the gastro-intestinal tract [13]. But its application is not limited there: In the field of neurosurgery, it was shown that a discrimination of brain tumors can be performed on CLE images [9], and it was also successfully used for diagnosis of tumors in the mouth and the upper airways [21, 10].

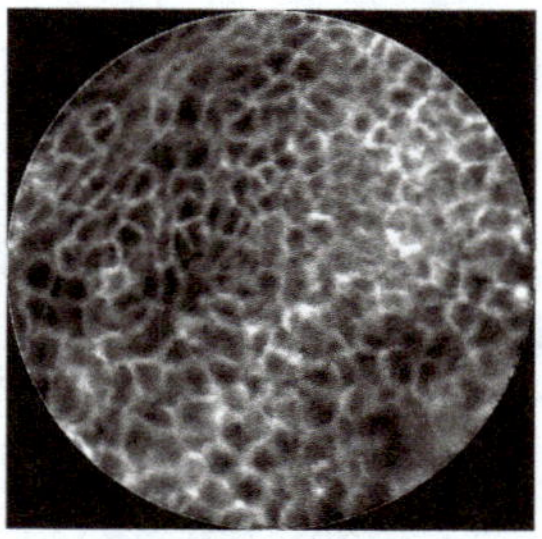

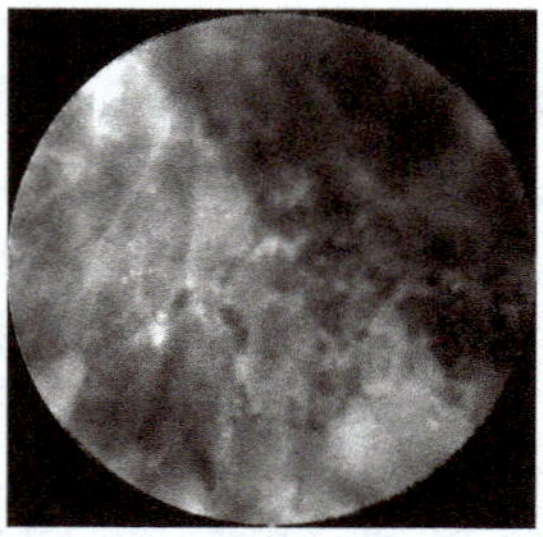

CLE Image of healthy epithelial tissue of the vocal folds (left) and with squamous cell carcinoma (right). Images courtesy of University Hospital Erlangen, Germany.

(a) A bright field image dominated by amplitude objects: CHO cells in suspension.

(b) A bright field image dominated by phase objects: adherent ultra-thin CHO cells.

(c) A phase contrast image of the same scene shown in 5.9(b). In comparison to 5.9(b), cells are clearly visible, albeit surrounded by halo artifacts.

Figure 5.9: Examples of amplitude objects and phase objects in biology.

Typical light detectors such as CCD chips or retina in our eyes can recognize amplitude variations but they are insensitive to phase distortion. In the 1930s, the Dutch physicist Frits Zernike came up with a brilliant trick for converting the invisible phase shift to a visible amplitude change using an optical filter. His contribution is the basis for a long-established technique in laboratories today known as *phase contrast*. Figure 5.9(a) shows a bright field image of a sample dominated by amplitude objects. In this particular example, they are cells in suspension. Figure 5.9(b) also shows a bright field image, but of a sample dominated by phase objects. The sample contains ultra-thin adherent cells. In Figure 5.9(c), the same specimen of Figure 5.9(b) is shown, but under a phase contrast microscope. A considerable improvement in contrast and information content can be clearly seen in the phase contrast image.

5.6 Quantitative Phase Microscopy

In the previous section, phase was employed to obtain more contrast of transparent specimens. At this point, we may ask the following question: what does the numerical phase value tell us about the physical properties of a specimen? As discussed in Geek Box 5.4, we only observe the difference of the phases of two waves and are unable to observe an absolute value.

Phase contrast (cf. Section 5.5) is convenient for *qualitative* unstained imaging of transparent specimens. However, it is not suitable for obtaining *quantitative* phase values for two reasons: Firstly, phase information is perturbed by artifacts, called *phase halos*, in image regions which surround phase objects (cf. Figure 5.9(c)). Secondly, Zernike's approach which links an observed intensity value to the corresponding phase value is valid only for very small phase shifts.

Geek Box 5.3: Wave Equation

Informally speaking, at a point in space $\mathbf{r} = (x, y, z)$, we can imagine the light activity as a particle dancing in time according to $e^{i\omega t}$, where t is time and $\omega = 2\pi\xi$ is the angular frequency which determines light color. In general, this dance is amplitude-scaled and phase-shifted differently at each point in space. Consequently, the wave/particle function $\psi(\mathbf{r}, t)$ can be modeled as follows:

$$\psi(\mathbf{r}, t) = A(\mathbf{r})e^{i(\omega t+\phi(\mathbf{r}))} = A(\mathbf{r})e^{i\phi(\mathbf{r})}e^{i\omega t} = U(\mathbf{r})e^{i\omega t}. \tag{5.6}$$

The term $U(\mathbf{r})$ encodes both amplitude change $A(\mathbf{r})$ and phase shift $\phi(\mathbf{r})$ as a complex number, and is thus called *complex amplitude* of the wave. Eq. (5.6) is not sufficient to describe a wave unless ψ fulfills the celebrated *wave equation*:

$$\frac{\partial^2 \psi}{\partial t^2} = c^2 \nabla^2 \psi, \tag{5.7}$$

where c is the speed of light in the propagation medium, and $\nabla^2 = \frac{\partial^2}{\partial x^2} + \frac{\partial^2}{\partial y^2} + \frac{\partial^2}{\partial z^2}$ is the spatial Laplacian. Assuming that can be factorized as $\psi(\mathbf{r}, t) = \psi_{\mathbf{r}}(\mathbf{r})\psi_t(t)$ (which is the case in Eq. (5.6)), one can derive the *time-independent wave equation*, also known as *Helmholtz's equation*:

$$\nabla^2 U(\mathbf{r}) + k^2 U(\mathbf{r}) = 0, \tag{5.8}$$

where k is defined as $k = \frac{\omega}{c}$ and called *wavenumber*. An important class of solutions for Helmholtz's equation is given by the following complex amplitude:

$$U_\ell(\mathbf{r}) = A_\ell e^{i\ \mathbf{k}^\top \mathbf{r}}. \tag{5.9}$$

In this solution, the amplitude is constant everywhere with a real value A_ℓ whereas the phase is linearly dependent on position $\phi_\ell = \mathbf{k}^\top \mathbf{r} = xk_x + yk_y + zk_z$. In order for Eq. (5.9) to satisfy Helmholtz's equation, $\mathbf{k}$ must fulfill $\sqrt{k_x^2 + k_y^2 + k_z^2} = k$. This fact can be verified by setting $U(\mathbf{r}) = U_\ell(\mathbf{r})$ in Eq. (5.8). Moreover, the locus of points in space for which $U_\ell(\mathbf{r})$ = constant, is a plane with normal vector $\mathbf{k}$. Therefore, waves described by Eq. (5.9) are called *plane waves*.

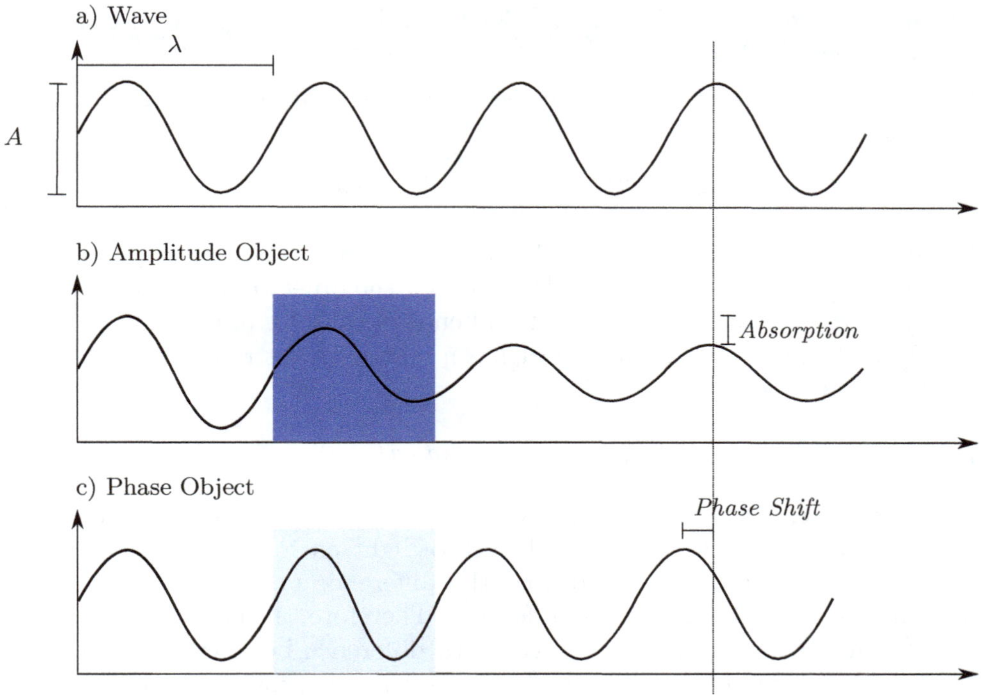

Figure 5.10: If we consider light as a wave with amplitude A and wavelength λ, we observe that amplitude objects reduce the wave amplitude by *absorption*. Phase objects cause a *phase shift* due to differences in the refractive index inside and outside the object.

Quantitative phase microscopy is an umbrella term for a set of techniques by which it is possible to obtain reliable quantitative phase information. Geek Box 5.5 discusses one of the methods to determine quantitative phase in detail: the transport of intensity equation (TIE). Due to the quantitative nature of TIE results, it can be utilized to compute specimen physical descriptors which are difficult to obtain using phase contrast. For instance, it can in principle be used for estimating cell thickness and volume in biological cell cultures. In general, the TIE seems to be attractive when compared to phase contrast for at least two reasons: 1) It is possible to obtain high-contrast phase images using a bright field microscope which is cheap and easy to implement compared to a phase contrast microscope. 2) TIE yields quantitative rather than qualitative phase information. However, every new technique comes with its own problems, and TIE is by no means an exception to this rule. In fact, estimating the axial derivative is very sensitive to the selection of defocus distance Δz. In addition, a TIE solution is prone to be perturbed by a low-frequency bias field which needs to be corrected.

Geek Box 5.4: Phase Shift

In fact, the phase shift introduced by a phase object can be given as follows:

$$\phi_{\mathrm{diff}}(x,y) = k \int_{z_1(x,y)}^{z_2(x,y)} \Delta n\,(x,y,z)\,\mathrm{d}z, \tag{5.10}$$

where k is the wavenumber of the incident light, $\Delta n\,(x,y,z)$ is the difference in the refractive index between the object and surrounding medium, z_1 and z_2 are the start and end coordinates of the light path through the object. If the object has a homogeneous refractive index, Eq. (5.10) reduces to:

$$\phi_{\mathrm{diff}}^{\mathrm{hom}}(x,y) = k \cdot \Delta n \cdot q\,(x,y)\,, \tag{5.11}$$

where $q\,(x,y)$ is the object thickness at (x,y). The product of refractive index with the geometric length of light path is usually termed optical path length. In addition, the difference of two optical path lengths is called optical path difference. Therefore, the numerical value of phase is interpreted as optical path difference between the object and the surrounding medium. The constant k is typically ignored.

5.7 Limitation of Light Microscopy

In Figure 5.1, a *point source* creates a *point image* at focus. This is, however, a result of geometrical optics which does not take the wave nature of light into account. From a wave-optics perspective, light exhibits the properties of waves, and hence, it undergoes diffraction upon encountering a barrier or a slit. In microscopy, this slit is the finite-sized aperture of the objective. Due to the diffraction process, the image of a point source is a pattern known, after Sir George Airy, as *Airy pattern*. As shown in Figure 5.12(a), it is composed of a central spot, known as *Airy disk* (in 2-D), surrounded by multiple diffraction rings. The radius of an Airy pattern, when the image is in its best focus, is:

$$d_{\mathrm{Airy}} = 0.61 \frac{\lambda}{\mathrm{NA}}, \tag{5.14}$$

where $\lambda = \frac{2\pi}{k}$ is the wavelength of incident light. It is noteworthy to mention that d_{Airy} in Eq. (5.14) is given in object-space units. Therefore, in image plane, the radius of the Airy disk is $M \cdot d_{\mathrm{Airy}}$, where M is the magnification.

The *resolving power* of a microscopic system is defined as the minimum distance between two point sources in the object space for which they are still discernible as two points in the image plane. Intuitively, the two points are distinguishable as long as the sum of the two corresponding Airy patterns con-

Geek Box 5.5: Transport of Intensity Equation (TIE)

Teague derived the TIE in 1983 starting from Helmholtz's equation (cf. Eq. (5.8)) under the approximation of a slowly varying field along the z-axis:

$$-k\frac{\partial I(x,y)}{\partial z} = I(x,y)\cdot\nabla_{\perp}^{2}\phi(x,y) + \nabla_{\perp}I(x,y)\cdot\nabla_{\perp}\phi(x,y)\,, \quad (5.12)$$

where $I(x,y)$ is the at-focus intensity image (related to the complex amplitude in Eq. (5.8) by $I = |U|^2$), and $\nabla_{\perp}$ is the gradient operator in the lateral directions, i. e., in the xy plane. The symbol ϕ denotes the phase difference (cf. Eq. (5.10)), but ϕ was used instead of ϕ_{diff} as the phase appears only in differential terms in the TIE. In other words, the phase in TIE is defined up to an additive constant which makes no difference between ϕ and ϕ_{diff}. This equation can be further simplified if we assume ideal phase objects, i. e., $I(x,y) = \text{constant} = I_0$, to the following form:

$$-k\frac{\partial I(x,y)}{\partial z} = I_0\nabla_{\perp}^{2}\phi(x,y)\,\cdot \quad (5.13)$$

The axial derivative at the left-hand side of Eq. (5.12) or Eq. (5.13) can be measured: First, acquire a *bright field* image at focus I_0. Defocus the microscope by a distance Δz and acquire another image $I(\Delta z)$:

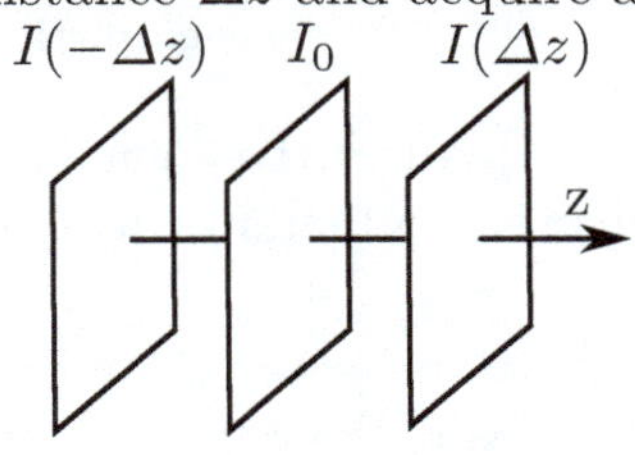

The finite-difference approximation of the derivative is then given by $\frac{I(\Delta z)-I_0}{\Delta z}$. After estimating the axial derivative, the only unknown which is left in the TIE is the phase. Therefore, the TIE can be solved for ϕ yielding a quantitative phase map.

Earlier in this text, it was mentioned that ideal phase objects are invisible in bright field microscopy. In fact, as demonstrated in Figure 5.11, the aforementioned statement is correct only under the condition that the image is acquired at focus. This phenomenon, i. e., the possibility to visualize phase objects in bright field microscopy, can be interpreted in the light of the TIE. The contrast obtained by defocusing is numerically represented by the left-hand side of Eq. (5.13). The right-hand side reveals that this contrast is, in fact, phase information. The employment of defocusing to visualize transparent samples in a bright field setup is sometimes called *defocusing microscopy*.

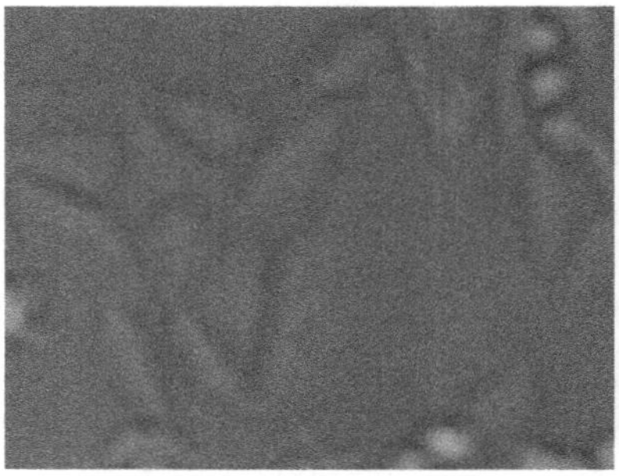

(a) A defocused bright field image of the cell culture: $\Delta z = -15\ \mu$m.

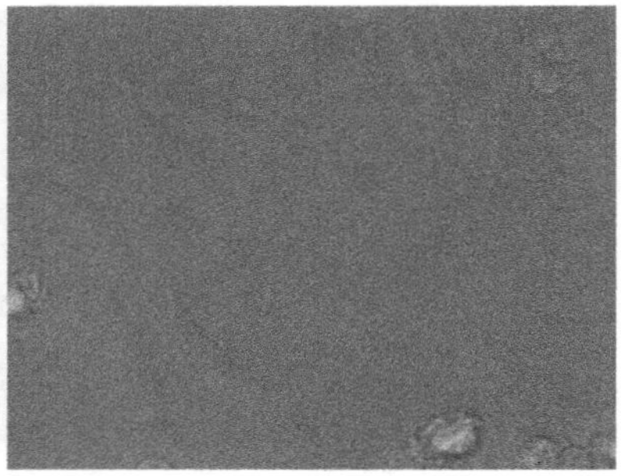

(b) A bright field image of the cell culture at-focus: $\Delta z = 0$.

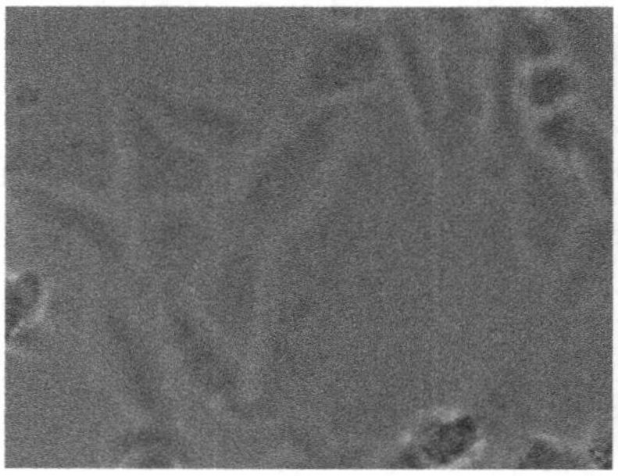

(c) A defocused bright field image of the cell culture: $\Delta z = +15\ \mu$m.

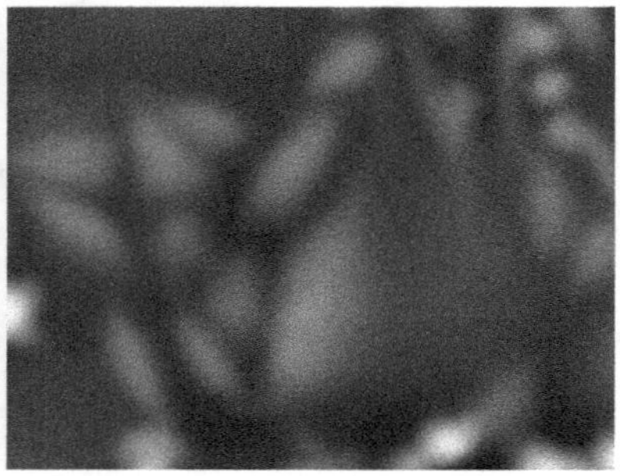

(d) A quantitative phase map obtained by solving the TIE. The bias field was partially corrected using a bias-correction algorithm.

Figure 5.11: Illustration of quantitative phase microscopy using the TIE. The figures show a cell culture of adherent ultra-thin L929 cells.

tains two distinct peaks. However, the condition under which the two peaks are considered *distinct*, can be defined in several ways. This led to different, but similar, definitions of the resolving power. According to Rayleigh, it is given by the radius of Airy disk $d_{\text{min}} = d_{\text{Airy}}$ (cf. Figure 5.12(b)). A slightly different definition, known as *Abbe criterion*, is given as $d_{\text{min}} = 0.5\frac{\lambda}{\text{NA}}$.

In order to enhance microscopic resolution, one needs to employ light of shorter wavelength and/or an objective of higher numerical aperture. Using shorter wavelengths will be considered in the next section. The numerical aperture, as revealed by Eq. (5.5), is theoretically upper-limited by unity when air ($n_{\text{air}} \approx 1$) is the medium between the specimen and the objective. In order to go beyond this limit, microscope manufacturers designed objectives which can function when a medium of higher refractive index such as water ($n_{\text{water}} \approx 1.33$) or oil ($n_{\text{oil}} \approx 1.51$) is embedded between the specimen and the objective. This led to the development of *water immersion objectives* and *oil immersion objectives*.

If we set the wavelength in Eq. (5.14) to the wavelength at the center of the visible spectrum $\lambda_{\text{visible}} \approx 550$ nm and numerical aperture to the theoretical

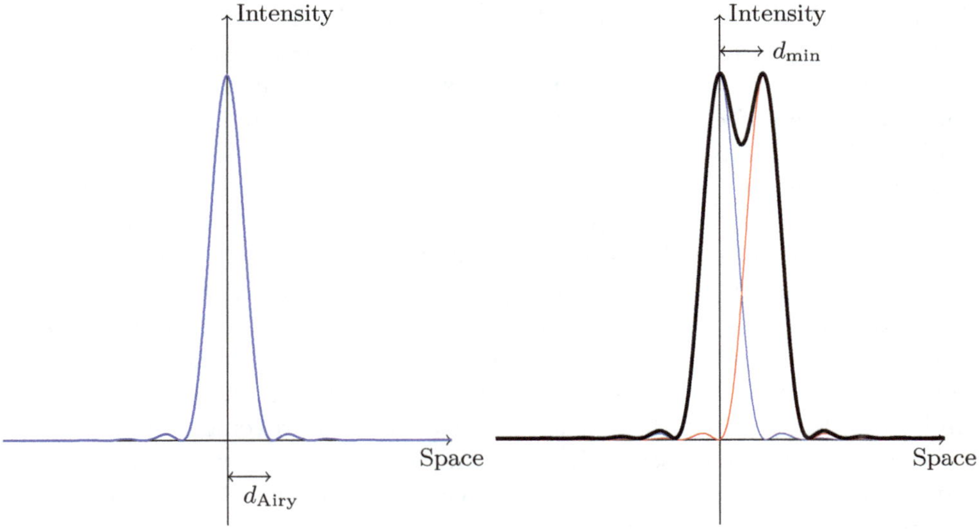

(a) Airy pattern composed of Airy peak with radius d_{Airy} surrounded by diffraction rings.

(b) Rayleigh criterion: Two features with distance less than $d_{\text{min}} = d_{\text{Airy}}$ will be resolved as a single feature.

Figure 5.12: Diffraction barrier: Due to diffraction, the image of a point source is an Airy pattern. The resolving power d_{min} of a microscope is thus limited by the width of this pattern.

upper-bound of oil-immersion numerical apertures $\text{NA}^{\text{best}} = 1.51$, we obtain a Rayleigh resolution of $d_{\text{min}}^{\text{best}} = 222$ nm ≈ 0.2 μm. This value[2] is often cited as the resolution limit of optical microscopy. Two distinct points in object space with a distance less than 0.2 μm will be imaged as a sum of two Airy patterns in which only one distinct peak can be recognized. Increasing the magnification will increase the size of this sum of Airy patterns at the image plane, but the enlarged image remains a single-peak pattern. In other words, beyond a certain limit, increasing the magnification does not resolve new details. This phenomenon is known as *empty magnification.*

5.8 Beyond Light Microscopy

One obvious way of increasing microscopic resolution is using a wavelength which is shorter than the wavelength of visible light. For instance, it is possible to employ ultraviolet (UV) radiation (wavelength in range 300 – 100 nm), soft

[2] Or other close approximations of it depending on the considered upper-limit of numerical aperture and definition of resolving power.

X-ray (10 – 1 nm), hard X-ray (below 1 nm)[3], or electron beams (wavelengths below 5 pm are achievable). Each wavelength range allows us to explore a part of the nano-world, but also imposes a new type of challenges for both microscope manufacturers and users. At the UV wavelengths, glass strongly absorbs light radiation, and thus, in *UV microscopy*, the lenses are made of UV-transparent materials such as quartz. Moreover, at the wavelengths of X-ray radiation, the refractive index of solid substances is very close to the refractive index of air. Since the light-focusing performed by a visible-light lens is inherently a refraction process, these lenses cannot be used to focus X-ray beams. In fact, in *X-ray microscopy*, expensive and impractical devices which are based on diffraction instead of refraction are employed to replace the typical optical lenses. *Electron microscopy* utilizes electromagnetic lenses and cathode rays in order to achieve a drastic improvement in resolution compared to light microscopy. Unlike ultraviolet and X-ray radiation, cathode rays, being electron beams of measurable mass and negative charge, do not belong to the electromagnetic radiation. Therefore, the photon-wave duality, and hence the conception of wavelength, are not directly applicable. One of the major contributions which led to the development of electron microscopy is the theory of Louis de Broglie who stated in his PhD thesis that the particle-wave duality is also valid for matter. According to de Broglie, the wavelength of an electron of mass m_e and speed c_e is given by:

$$\lambda_e = \frac{\rho}{m_e \cdot c_e}, \tag{5.15}$$

where ρ is Planck constant. As an alternative for reflection in optical lenses, in electromagnetic lenses, deflection of electron beams by magnetic fields was exploited to focus the beams. In an electron microscope, similar to a cathode-ray tube, an electron beam is emitted into vacuum by heating the cathode and then accelerated by applying a voltage between the cathode and the anode. The speed of the electrons, and hence the wavelength (cf. Eq. (5.15)), can be controlled by varying the voltage. The first electron microscopes were very similar from a schematic point of view to bright field microscopes. The acquired image is based on the specimen absorption of electrons when transmitted into the sample, and hence, they were given the name *transmission electron microscopes*. A resolution as high as 0.2 nm is achieved by the transmission electron microscopes. A major limitation of this scheme, however, is that only very thin samples can be imaged. *Scanning electron microscopy* was developed to cope with this difficulty. To do so, a primary electron beam is focused by an electromagnetic lens on a very small part of the specimen. This primary beam incites the emission of a secondary electron beam. The intensity of this secondary beam is recorded. Afterwards, the primary beam is moved to another part of the specimen, and the same process is applied.

[3] X-ray and UV radiation, being a part of the electromagnetic spectrum, belong to *invisible* light. The term light microscopy is, however, restricted to visible light in this text.

This is repeated so that the entire specimen is scanned in a raster pattern and the final image is obtained from the recorded values of the secondary beam intensities. Scanning electron microscopy can be used to image thick samples, even though it captures only the surface details. In addition, the secondary beam is accompanied with X-ray emission characteristic to the material which emitted it. Therefore, it is employed to reveal the chemical composition of specimens. Both scanning electron microscopy and transmission electron microscopes work in a vacuum. Consequently, they can be used only for dead specimens. From this perspective, X-ray and traditional light microscopy are preferred over electron microscopy. Although X-ray and electron microscopes provide a considerable improvement of resolution over light microscopes, they are extremely expensive, require large hardware, and mostly involve complicated sample preparation.

5.9 Light Microscopy Beyond the Diffraction Limit

In the past few years, the so-called *superresolution microscopy* became an active research trend. Today, based on this technology, there are microscopes which achieve a resolving power of about 10 nm. While this number is inferior to electron microscopy resolution, the breakthrough lies in the fact that this is achieved using visible light. As stated earlier in this text (cf. Section 5.7), the attainable resolution using visible light is limited to 200 nm. May we then conclude that the theory which led to the diffraction limit in light microscopy is flawed? In fact, superresolution microscopy is based on alternatively turning fluorescent molecules in a specimen on and off. Two adjacent fluorescent molecules with a distance less than 200 nm will not be resolved as two points in a superresolution microscope when both of them are turned on simultaneously. However, this will be the case, i. e., they will be resolved as two points, if only one of them is activated at a specific time, and in addition, there is a mechanism to control this activation process. Superresolution microscopy techniques differ in the way in which this on/off switching is implemented. Major technologies in this field today include: stimulated emission depletion (STED), reversible saturable optical fluorescence transitions (RESOLFT), and stochastic optical reconstruction microscopy (STORM).

Further Readings

[1] B. Alberts et al. *Lehrbuch der Molekularen Zellbiologie.* Wiley-VCH, 2005.

[2] R. Ali et al. "On the Use of Low-Pass Filters for Image Processing with Inverse Laplacian Models". In: *Journal of Mathematical Imaging and Vision* (2010), pp. 1–10.

[3] Marc Aubreville et al. "Automatic Classification of Cancerous Tissue in Laserendomicroscopy Images of the Oral Cavity using Deep Learning". In: *Scientific Reports* 7.1 (2017), s41598–017.

[4] Douglas E Chandler and Robert W Roberson. *Bioimaging: current concepts in light and electron microscopy.* Jones & Bartlett Publishers, 2009.

[5] Guy Cox. *Optical imaging techniques in cell biology.* CRC Press, 2012. ISBN: 978-1-4398-4825-8.

[6] Louis De Broglie. "The wave nature of the electron". In: *Nobel lectures* 12 (1929), pp. 244–256.

[7] Charles A DiMarzio. *Optics for Engineers.* Crc Press, 2011.

[8] Richard Feynman, Robert Leighton, and Matthew Sands. *The Feynman Lectures on Physics.* Second. Vol. 1. Boston: Addison-Wesley, 1963.

[9] Sebastian Foersch et al. "Confocal Laser Endomicroscopy for Diagnosis and Histomorphologic Imaging of Brain Tumors In Vivo". In: *PloS one* 7.7 (July 2012), e41760.

[10] Miguel Goncalves et al. "Value of confocal laser endomicroscopy in the diagnosis of vocal cord lesions". In: *European Review for Medical and Pharmacological Sciences* 21 (2017), pp. 3990–3997.

[11] J.W. Goodman. *Introduction to Fourier Optics.* Second. MaGraw-Hill, 1996.

[12] Stefan W Hell. "Microscopy and its focal switch". In: *Nature methods* 6.1 (2008), pp. 24–32.

[13] A Hoffman et al. "Confocal laser endomicroscopy: technical status and current indications". In: *Endoscopy* 38.12 (Dec. 2006), pp. 1275–1283.

[14] Alan Lacey. *Light Microscopy in Biology: A Practical Approach.* Second. Oxford University Press, 1999.

[15] Elisabeth Laemmel et al. "Fibered confocal fluorescence microscopy (Cell-viZio) facilitates extended imaging in the field of microcirculation. A comparison with intravital microscopy." In: *Journal of vascular research* 41.5 (Sept. 2004), pp. 400–411.

[16] A.E. Mirsky and J. Brachet. *Cell: Biochemistry, Physiology Morphology. Edited by Jean Brachet [and] Alfred E Mirsky.* Academic Press, 1959.

[17] Firas Mualla et al. "Automatic Cell Detection in Bright-Field Microscope Images Using SIFT, Random Forests, and Hierarchical Clustering". In: *IEEE Transactions on Medical Imaging* 32.12 (2013), pp. 2274–2286. DOI: 10.1109/TMI.2013.2280380.

[18] Firas Mualla et al. "Unsupervised Unstained Cell Detection by SIFT Keypoint Clustering and Self-labeling Algorithm". In: *Lecture Notes in Computer Science, Volume 8675, MICCAI 2014 Proceedings, Part III.* Ed. by P. Golland et al. Boston, MA, USA, 2014, pp. 377–384.

[19] Firas Mualla et al. "Using the Low-Pass Monogenic Signal Framework for Cell/Background Classification on Multiple Cell Lines in Bright-Field Microscope Images". In: *International Journal of Computer Assisted Radiology and Surgery* 9.3 (2014), pp. 379–386. DOI: 10.1007/s11548-013-0969-5.

[20] Douglas B. Murphy. *Fundamentals of Light Microscopy and Electronic Imaging*. John Wiley & Sons, Inc., 2002. ISBN: 9780471234296.

[21] Nicolai Oetter et al. "Development and validation of a classification and scoring system for the diagnosis of oral squamous cell carcinomas through confocal laser endomicroscopy". In: *Journal of Translational Medicine* 14.1 (July 2016), pp. 1–11.

[22] Frank L. Pedrotti, Leno M. Pedrotti, and Leno S. Pedrotti. *Introduction to Optics*. 3rd ed. Benjamin Cummings, 2006. ISBN: 0131499335.

[23] Gabriel Popescu. *Quantitative Phase Imaging of Cells and Tissues*. McGraw-Hill, 2011.

[24] Simon Schöll et al. "Influence of the phase effect on gradient-based and statistics-based focus measures in bright field microscopy". In: *Journal of Microscopy* 254.2 (2014), pp. 65–74. DOI: 10.1111/jmi.12118.

[25] Michael Reed Teague. "Deterministic phase retrieval: a Green's function solution". In: *JOSA* 73.11 (1983), pp. 1434–1441.

[26] Laura Waller, Lei Tian, and George Barbastathis. "Transport of intensity phase-amplitude imaging with higher order intensity derivatives". In: *Opt. Express* 18.12 (June 2010), pp. 12552–12561.

[27] Qiang Wu, Fatima A. Merchant, and Kenneth R. Castleman. *Microscope Image Processing*. Burlington: Academic Press, 2008.

6

MRI and its Principles

Authors: Felix Lugauer and Jens Wetzl

Modern MRI systems allow physicians to look inside the body without the use of ionizing radiation (see Fig. 6.1). They provide excellent soft-tissue contrast for morphological imaging as well as a range of possibilities for functional imaging, e. g., for visualizing blood flow, tissue perfusion or diffusion processes. In the following chapter, we will outline the physical fundamentals of magnetic resonance (MR), concepts for imaging, common pulse sequences to produce different contrasts as well as some advanced topics related to speeding up the acquisition and for functional imaging.

6.1 Nuclear Magnetic Resonance (NMR)

6.1.1 Genesis of the Resonance Effect

To explain the MR effect, we first look at the example of a compass needle which is subjected to a magnetic field. The needle progressively aligns itself along the direction of the magnetic field by oscillating around it, as shown in Fig. 6.2. The amplitude of the oscillation decreases over time. But the

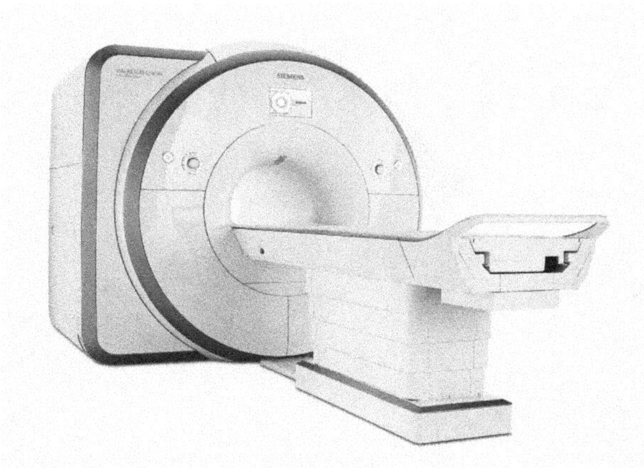

Figure 6.1: A modern MRI scanner can provide both morphological and functional imaging. Image courtesy of Siemens Healthineers AG.

frequency of the oscillation is determined by the strength of the magnetic field and the properties of the needle and remains fixed over time.

Now recall that a radio frequency (RF) wave corresponds to a magnetic field that varies over time. So during its oscillation, our magnetic needle can be seen as an antenna that emits RF waves at the frequency of its oscillation. These emissions stop once the needle has reached a stable position, but by pushing it out of balance, we can cause new RF waves to be emitted. This "push" can also be achieved by means of a magnetic field, one that is applied perpendicularly to the original magnetic field which the needle is aligned with. A Java applet[1] can simulate this process. Broadly speaking, this is the same principle that is applied in MRI to generate images.

The "magnetic needles" in our body commonly used for MRI are hydrogen (^{1}H) nuclei. They have an intrinsic property known as *spin*, visualized as the rotation of a sphere around an axis in Fig. 6.3, which makes them act like small magnets. The endpoints of the axis of rotation can be thought of as the poles of the magnetic needle. In the absence of an external magnetic field, the axes of hydrogen nuclei within the body are randomly distributed, so the sum of all magnetic fields is zero. Subjected to a large magnetic field, denoted by $\boldsymbol{B}_0$, spin axes have the tendency to align in the direction of the magnetic field, similarly to the compass needles. In contrast to a compass, this alignment is only partial, due to random interactions between nuclei (compare Fig. 6.4). Even so, the sum of all spin directions no longer cancels out and will instead point in the direction of the magnetic field. In what follows, we will call this sum of all spin directions the *net (total) magnetization vector* $\boldsymbol{M}$.

Thus, the nuclei inside the body will accumulate to a net magnetization in the presence of a strong magnetic field $\boldsymbol{B}_0$ as the partially aligned spin

[1] `http://drcmr.dk/JavaCompass/`

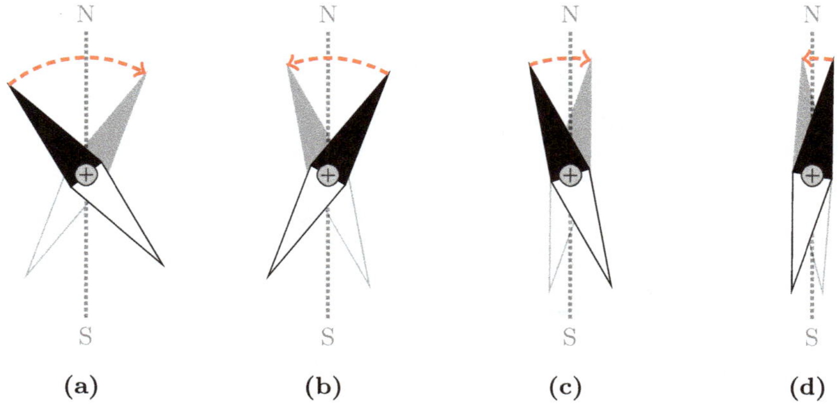

Figure 6.2: Behavior of a compass needle in a magnetic field. The needle oscillates through the "north" position until it reaches a stable position. In real compasses, the magnetic needle is immersed in a fluid to dampen such oscillations.

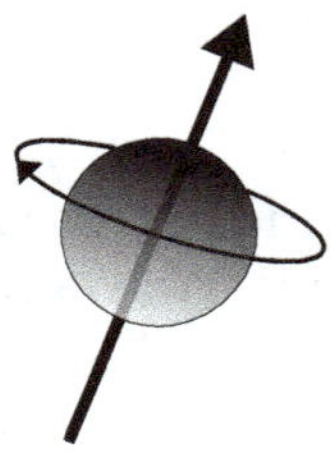

Figure 6.3: Hydrogen nuclei are used for MRI because of their magnetic susceptibility and their vast amount in the human body. An intrinsic property of the hydrogen nuclei is their rotation (spin) which makes them magnetic along the rotational axis.

axes sum up to $\boldsymbol{M}$. Applying, for instance, a field strength of 1 T (tesla) to a million nuclei yields a net magnetization with the magnetic strength of about 3 nuclei, which means that one million partially aligned nuclei make up for only 3 completely aligned nuclei. The induced magnetization $\boldsymbol{M}$ is proportional to the applied field strength of $\boldsymbol{B}_0$ and as there are over 10^{27} hydrogen nuclei in the whole body, the net magnetization accumulates to a measurable magnitude.

In our compass example, we said that the magnetic needle oscillates until it reaches a stable position, and emits RF waves due to this oscillation. The oscillation of the needle is a 2-dimensional motion happening in the plane of the compass. For spin axes, a similar process happens, but the motion is 3-dimensional and is called *precession*. From its initial position, the spin axis rotates around the axis of the strong magnetic field $\boldsymbol{B}_0$. At the same time, the angle between the spin axis and $\boldsymbol{B}_0$ decreases over time, until they are

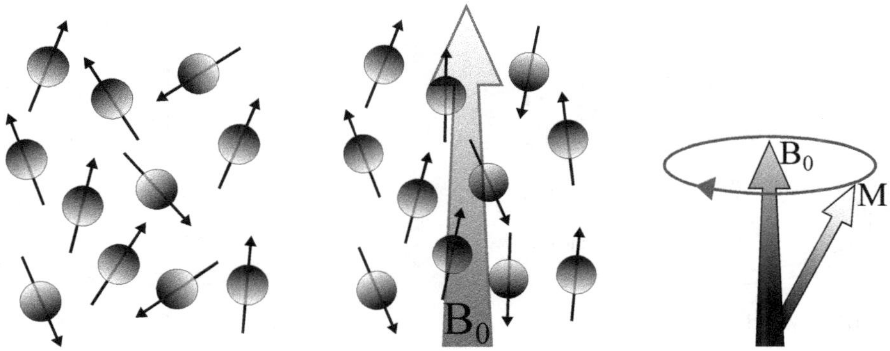

(a) Random spins (b) Partially aligned spins (c) Precession

Figure 6.4: Nuclei axes within the body will point randomly (a) until a strong magnetic field forces their rotation axes to partially align with the applied magnetic field (b). The accumulated magnetization of all spins $\boldsymbol{M}$ precesses around $\boldsymbol{B}_0$ (c).

aligned. The same motion can be observed in reverse with a spinning top, with the spin axis corresponding to the tilt of the spinning top and the axis of $\boldsymbol{B}_0$ corresponding to the direction of gravity[2]. As with the oscillation of the compass needle, the precession causes the emission of RF waves.

We said for the magnetic needle that the frequency of the oscillation is determined by the strength of the magnetic field and the properties of the needle and that it remains fixed over time. The same holds for nuclear spin precession, and the frequency of the precession is

$$f_\ell = \gamma \cdot \|\boldsymbol{B}_0\|, \tag{6.1}$$

also known as the *Larmor frequency*. The *gyromagnetic ratio* γ is the field strength dependent ratio for a specific nucleus, which is 42.576 MHz/T for hydrogen. Using, for instance, a 1.5 T field strength, protons will resonate with a frequency of about 64 MHz. Please note that precession should not be confused with spin, being the rotation of a single nucleus around its own axis.

We will now abstract away from the behavior of individual spins and only consider the net magnetization $\boldsymbol{M}$. Analogously to our compass needle, we will push $\boldsymbol{M}$ out of its stable position, a process which we call *excitation*, to cause the emission of RF waves from the body. The direction of $\boldsymbol{M}$ can be modified through a weaker magnetic field $\boldsymbol{B}_1$ in a direction orthogonal to $\boldsymbol{B}_0$ by applying RF waves from a coil in the resonance frequency of $\boldsymbol{M}$.

In the case of $\boldsymbol{M}$, this is not as straightforward as it was for the compass needle. In the 2-D plane of the compass, there is only one choice for the direc-

[2] MIT Physics Demo: `https://www.youtube.com/watch?reload=9&v=8H98BgRzpOM`

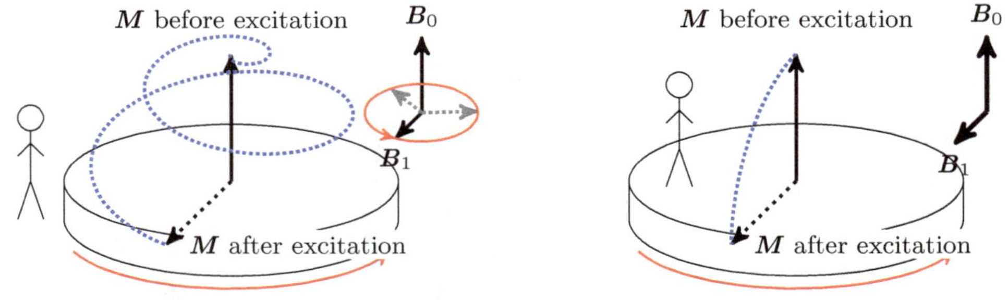

(a) "World" frame of reference **(b)** Rotating frame of reference

Figure 6.5: Excitation of the magnetization vector $\boldsymbol{M}$ viewed from the world (a) and rotating frame of reference (b). The precession is illustrated as a turntable, denoted by the red arrow, on which $\boldsymbol{M}$ is mounted. Viewed from the outside, the combination of the precession and excitation motions looks quite complex and the $\boldsymbol{B}_1$ field rotates in tune to the precession. From the rotating frame of reference, only the simple path of the excitation motion is visible and the $\boldsymbol{B}_1$ field is static. Figure recreated from [9].

tion of the second magnetic field, which is orthogonal to the main magnetic field. $\boldsymbol{M}$ precesses in a 3-D motion around $\boldsymbol{B}_0$, so the second magnetic field $\boldsymbol{B}_1$ must be orthogonal to $\boldsymbol{B}_0$ as well as aligned with the current rotation angle of $\boldsymbol{M}$. But we can simplify things if we change our point of view. Imagine the precession of $\boldsymbol{M}$ by picturing that the vector $\boldsymbol{M}$ is "attached" to a turntable which is rotating around $\boldsymbol{B}_0$. The motion of $\boldsymbol{M}$ as it is being pushed out of balance and precessing at the same time seems complicated, as does the direction of $\boldsymbol{B}_1$ that needs to be applied, see Fig. 6.5(a). Now if we step onto the turntable and look at the motion again, it is much simpler. In this *rotating frame of reference*, the direction of $\boldsymbol{B}_1$ is constant, and we cannot see the precession motion, only the excitation caused by $\boldsymbol{B}_1$, see Fig. 6.5(b).

Once the secondary magnetic field $\boldsymbol{B}_1$ is turned off, the magnetization vector $\boldsymbol{M}$ will slowly return to the equilibrium position by a process called *relaxation*, which is described in the next subsection. During this process, RF waves are emitted from the body and can be received with coils placed near the body surface. This is the signal from which MR images are then generated, as outlined in Sec. 6.2.

6.1.2 Relaxation and Contrasts

This section aims at explaining the concept of relaxation, which is the origin of contrast between different tissues in the resulting images. Relaxation is the process that causes the net magnetization to constantly approach equilibrium,

i. e., resting state again after excitation by an RF pulse. In addition to the dependency on the field strength, the speed of relaxation is tissue dependent as proton interactions are limited for large molecules or dense tissue where water molecule movement is hindered. This means that different tissue, e. g., water and fat, will end relaxation at different time points and, thus, the amount of signal received during relaxation time will differ. This is what gives rise to the contrast between tissue in MR images. To differentiate between different tissues, we will no longer look at the net magnetization vector $\boldsymbol{M}$ of all excited spins but instead overlay our imaging volume with a voxel grid and look at magnetization vectors per voxel.

6.1.2.1 Relaxation

Let's first recap the situation before relaxation starts: The per-voxel magnetization vectors are initially aligned with the main magnetic field $\boldsymbol{B}_0$, which we will now assume to be aligned with the z axis of our coordinate system. As such, each magnetization vector can be split into a *longitudinal* component $\boldsymbol{M}_z$ and a *transversal* component $\boldsymbol{M}_{xy}$ such that $\boldsymbol{M} = \boldsymbol{M}_{xy} + \boldsymbol{M}_z$. So initially, $\|\boldsymbol{M}_{xy}\| = 0$ and $\|\boldsymbol{M}_z\|$ is a positive number dependent on the number of hydrogen nuclei contained within the voxel. During excitation, an RF pulse tips the magnetization vector into the transversal plane, such that $\|\boldsymbol{M}_z\| = 0$ and $\|\boldsymbol{M}_{xy}\|$ is maximal. We call such an RF wave a *90° pulse* because it changes the angle of the magnetization vector by 90°.

Once the 90° pulse ends, relaxation occurs in the form of two independent processes to get back to the equilibrium state. The magnetization vector recovers its longitudinal component, i. e., $\|\boldsymbol{M}_z\|$ tends towards its original magnitude. And, usually much faster, the magnetization vector loses its transversal component, i. e., $\|\boldsymbol{M}_{xy}\|$ tends towards 0. These independent processes happen on different time scales, meaning that the magnitude of the magnetization vector is not constant over time. Fig. 6.6 visualizes the trajectory of a magnetization vector during relaxation. The physical reasons for both relaxation processes are outlined in the following paragraphs.

Recovery of longitudinal magnetization

is achieved by a process called spin-lattice relaxation, whereby the nuclear spins release the energy received from an RF pulse back into the surrounding lattice (tissue), leading towards thermal equilibrium or resting state. The recovery of the longitudinal magnetization follows an exponential function $\|\boldsymbol{M}_z(t)\| = \|\boldsymbol{M}_0\|(1 - \mathrm{e}^{-t/T_1})$, which is characterized by a time constant T_1, which is different for each tissue class. The time constant T_1 is defined as time period for $\boldsymbol{M}_z$ to recover $1 - \frac{1}{\mathrm{e}} \approx 63\,\%$ of its initial magnetization $\boldsymbol{M}_0$. This characteristic number of an exponential function serves to determine the

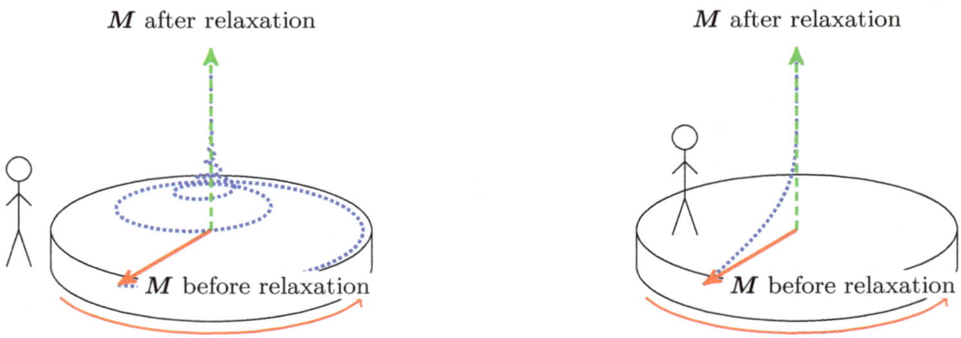

(a) "World" frame of reference

(b) Rotating frame of reference

Figure 6.6: Visualization of the precession and relaxation of white matter with $T_1 = 510\,\text{ms}$ and $T_2 = 67\,\text{ms}$ in the "world" (a) and rotating frame of reference (b). After 90° RF excitation, the magnetization is in the transverse plane (red vector), which is the starting point for the relaxation process. The magnetization then follows the blue trajectory until the resting state (green vector) is reached. Figure recreated and amended from [9].

point in time when the process is considered "finished". The common wisdom is that after $5T_1$, which corresponds to a 99.3 % recovery, the process is as good as done. As an example, white matter has a T_1 of 510 ms while it is 2500 ms for arterial blood. The magnetization recovery for arterial blood is plotted in Fig. 6.7(a).

Decay of transversal magnetization (in theory)

The decay of transversal magnetization is caused by random interactions between nuclei when a perfectly homogenous magnetic field can be assumed. More explicitly, interactions between the magnetic fields of nuclei lead to temporary phase differences. Ultimately, the nuclei move out-of-phase and the overall signal that can be measured along $\boldsymbol{B}_1$ decreases affecting the transversal magnetization $\boldsymbol{M}_{xy}$. Again, the magnetization is an exponential function but this time the exponential time constant T_2 determines the *decay* of $\|\boldsymbol{M}_{xy}(t)\| = \|\boldsymbol{M}_0\|\mathrm{e}^{-t/T_2}$. T_2 is defined as the time after excitation when the signal value is decreased to $\frac{1}{\mathrm{e}} \approx 37\,\%$ of its initial value $\boldsymbol{M}_0$. It is dependent on the tissue density or rather the chemical structure, and, thereby, also characteristic for every tissue. The longitudinal magnetization decay of arterial blood is plotted in Fig. 6.7(b).

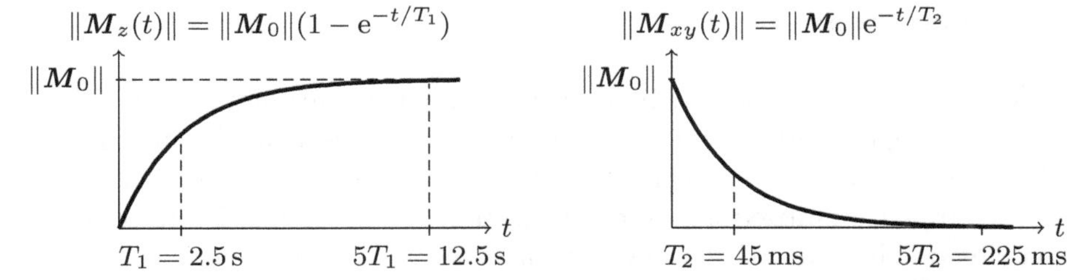

(a) Longitudinal magnetization recovery **(b)** Transverse magnetization decay

Figure 6.7: Plots of the recovery of longitudinal magnetization (a) and the decay of transverse magnetization (b) for arterial blood with $T_1 = 2.5\,s$ and $T_2 = 45\,ms$. As a rule of thumb, the process is considered completed after five times the respective time constant, with over 99 % of the longitudinal magnetization restored after $5T_1$ and less than 1 % of transverse magnetization remaining after $5T_2$.

Decay of transversal magnetization (in practice)

The actual decay happens more quickly, i. e., the received signal in an MRI acquisition decays faster than predicted by T_2. This is due to imperfections in the homogeneity of the main magnetic field $\boldsymbol{B}_0$, which is related to various effects like magnetic susceptibilities and magnet manufacture. T_2^* („T two star") refers to the relaxation which includes the ideal tissue-dependent relaxation due to random interactions between nuclei (T_2) plus the additional loss of signal due to field imperfections. Note that T_2^* is also affected by tissue-dependent magnetic susceptibilities and is always shorter than T_2. However, there exists a measurement method, called *spin echo* that can recover the signal lost through field dependent dephasing of nuclei via refocusing pulses (see Sec. 6.3.1).

Fig. 6.7 compares the exponential course of T_1 recovery and T_2 decay, produced by the signal of arterial blood. Now, we can also fully explain the 3-D visualization of relaxation in Fig. 6.6 which is described by the blue trajectory: the net magnetization vector $\boldsymbol{M}_0$ (green) has been completely tipped into the xy-plane (red vector). As relaxation starts, imagine the length of the red vector to decrease ($\boldsymbol{M}_{xy}$) with an exponential decay defined by T_2, while at the same time the length of the green vector ($\boldsymbol{M}_{xy}$) grows with a speed defined by T_1. Above all, the magnetization vector rotates around the main magnetic field $\boldsymbol{B}_0$ (here, z-direction) with the field strength dependent Larmor frequency.

6.1.2.2 Contrasts

MR images can be controlled by a large number of parameters including the type of sequence and numerous sequence parameters per acquisition. The choice of the contrast or weighting for a particular image is fundamental as it determines the subsequent medical application and hereby its diagnostic significance. There are three major contrasts being distinguished: T_1 weighting, T_2 weighting and proton density (PD) weighting. Weighting is used in the sense that the acquisition parameters were chosen such that image contrast mainly reflects variations due to one of these tissue-inherent properties, for instance, spin-spin relaxation (T_2).

The parameters that control the particular weighting of a spin echo sequence are the *echo time (TE)* and the *repetition time (TR)*. TE is the time delay after an emitted RF pulse until the RF signal is measured. In the meantime, transversal magnetization decay and signal loss will occur due to T_2 relaxation, which means that the TE determines the T_2 weighting of images. For example, a long TE compared to the T_2 of the tissue being captured yields a strong T_2 contrast but only little signal as the signal decay has progressed for a long time.

TR is the period of time between successive RF pulses. Several similar measurements are needed, for instance, to encode multiple lines per image or for advanced imaging protocols. An RF pulse in succession will flip parts of the *available* longitudinal magnetization into the transversal plane. During the following relaxation, the longitudinal magnetization builds up again with a speed determined by T_1. If the time between successive measurement is short (short TR), the available magnetization is used often and cannot recover to equilibrium yielding a relatively small signal per repetition. A long TR, in contrast, will produce a stronger signal as most of the longitudinal magnetization will have recovered by then. However, the contrast in T_1 vanishes entirely if the longitudinal magnetization has fully recovered before the measurement is taken, i. e., TR is significantly longer than T_1 of the tissues. Thus, the T_1 weighting of an image is controlled by TR where a long TR produces a signal-intense limited T_1 weighting and a short TR will amplify the variations between tissue with varying T_1 but with a generally weak signal.

The third type of contrast, proton density weighting, is chosen to minimize both T_1 and T_2 variations. What is then left are variations due to the proton density itself, a tissue specific property which quantifies the number of mobile hydrogen protons per unit volume. As the number of mobile hydrogens bound in water decreases slightly from pure water over fat to solids, a PD-weighted image allows to enhance these variations. A long TR, sufficient for the magnetization to recover to equilibrium state, in combination with a short TE leads to a proton density weighted image. In summary, the following applies for sequences that consist of a simple excite-wait-measure-wait scheme:

	short TE	long TE
short TR	T_1 weighting	—
long TR	PD weighting	T_2 weighting

$\boldsymbol{T_1}$ weighting is determined by a *short* TE to minimize T_2 effects and a *short* TR ($\sim T_1$) at which the longitudinal magnetization has not yet recovered.

$\boldsymbol{T_2}$ weighting can be achieved by a *long* TR to reduce T_1 impact and a *long* TE ($\sim T_2$) to allow the differences in T_2 decay to appear.

PD weighting is given by a *long* TR such that the magnetization can reach equilibrium and measured immediately after the RF pulse (*short* TE).

The missing combination is long TE and short TR, which would result in a contrast mixture of T_1 and T_2 with no clinical use and, additionally, a weak signal amplitude.

6.2 Principles of Magnetic Resonance Imaging

Having introduced the underlying physical phenomenon of MR, we will now look at the *imaging* component of MRI. So far, we cannot localize the source of an emitted radio frequency wave, but only measure the sum of the signals from all spatial locations affected by an excitation.

An important component of an MRI system are the gradient coils, which allow us to impose a linear variation of the otherwise homogeneous magnetic field $\boldsymbol{B}_0$. Three gradient coils oriented in three orthogonal directions, e. g., head-feet, left-right and anterior-posterior, enable such a variation in any spatial direction by a weighted combination of the three.

Two concepts based on the gradient coil system will be explained to allow the spatial localization of emitted RF waves: slice selection and spatial encoding.

6.2.1 Slice Selection

An intuitively understood concept is that of slice-selective excitation. If the gradient coils are used to induce a linear variation of the main magnetic field $\boldsymbol{B}_0$ in head-feet direction, then the Larmor frequency f_ℓ of hydrogen nuclei – where resonance occurs – will be spatially dependent on their offset z along the direction:

$$f_\ell(z) = \gamma \cdot (\|\boldsymbol{B}_0\| + z) \tag{6.2}$$

Depending on the direction of the linear gradient, the Larmor frequency for ^{1}H nuclei in the feet would be lower or higher than that of nuclei in the

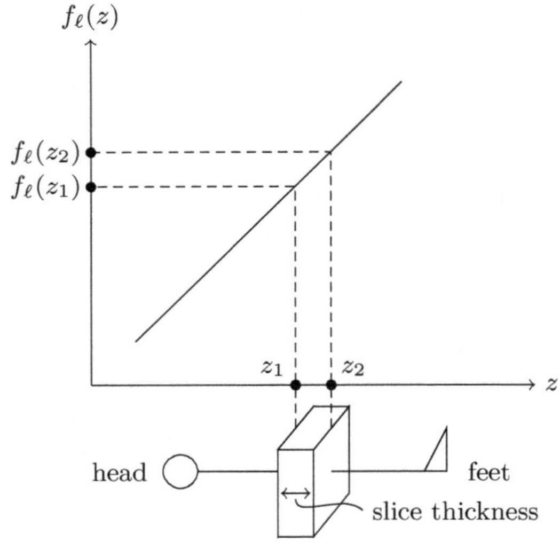

Figure 6.8: A linear variation of the magnetic field in head-feet direction causes the Larmor frequency $f_\ell(z)$ to be spatially dependent on the offset z along the variation direction. An excitation pulse with frequencies in the range of $f_\ell(z_1)$ to $f_\ell(z_2)$ will cause resonance in nuclei that lie within the depicted slice of thickness $|z_1 - z_2|$.

head. Now modifying the frequency of the excitation RF wave allows a slice-selective excitation, only nuclei whose Larmor frequency matches that of the wave will be excited.

If the excitation contains only a single frequency, the corresponding excited slice will be infinitely thin and not enough nuclei will resonate to produce a measurable signal. By emitting a wave containing a range of frequencies, the thickness of a slice can be chosen to provide a good trade-off between spatial resolution and signal-to-noise ratio. A visualization of this concept is shown in Fig. 6.8.

6.2.2 Spatial Encoding

Unfortunately, the slice selection method cannot be extended to encode spatial locations within a slice. Even with multiple gradient fields, we can only select a (possibly oblique) plane, not a single point in 3-D space. Instead, we make use of the phase information of spins in the transversal plane, i. e., the direction they are pointing.

6.2.2.1 One-dimensional Example

We will illustrate this with a 1-D example "image" and later extend the concept to multiple dimensions. Within our example slice, there are more hydrogen nuclei toward the boundaries and less in the middle, represented by the magnitude of the magnetization vectors within each voxel.

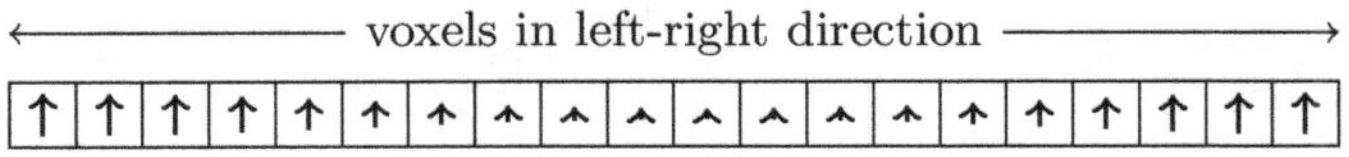

Directly after excitation, all spins within the excited slice point in the same direction. The quantity measurable by our MRI system is the net magnetization, the sum of all spin magnetization vectors within the voxels of the excited slice:

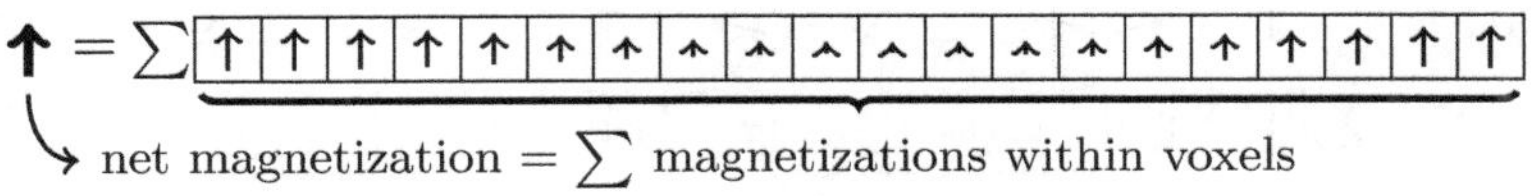

In the absence of any relaxation, all spins would precess at the Larmor frequency implied by the magnetic field strength. Assuming a homogeneous magnetic field, the magnitude of the net magnetization vector would not change:

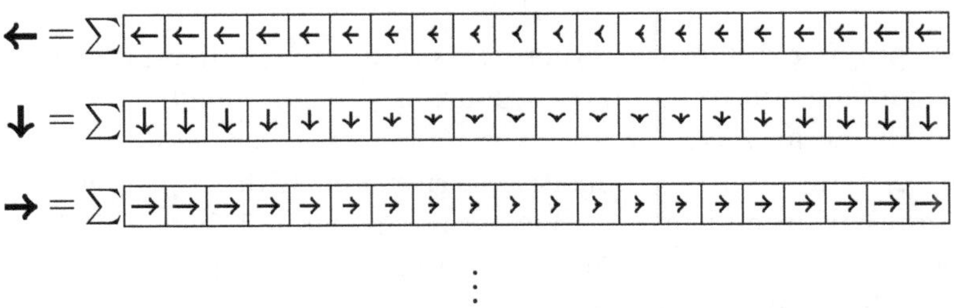

By applying a linear gradient, the precession frequency of spins changes along the direction of the gradient, i. e., spins to the right rotate faster than those on the left. Spins are no longer *in phase*, and the phase shift between adjacent voxels is dependent on the strength of the applied field. This phase shift has an influence on the magnitude of the net magnetization vector and it may even become zero. A graph of the net magnetization magnitude for different gradient field strengths is shown below, with two example "images" showing different phase shifts.

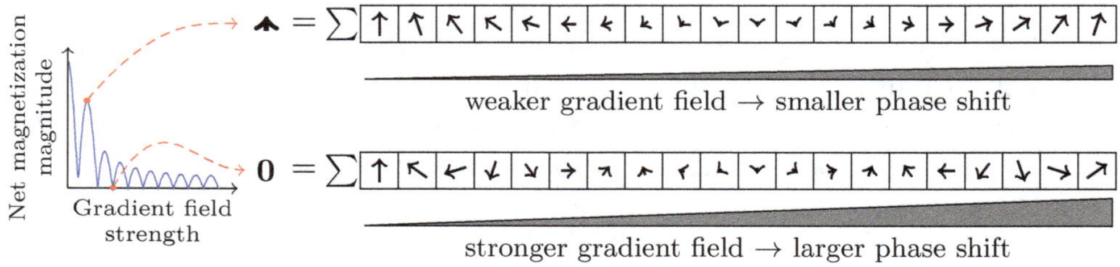

This may seem counterproductive at first sight, but it is the core principle of spatial encoding. If the hydrogen nuclei distribution of the measured tissue matches the "pattern" implied by the phase shift, there will be a measurable net magnetization. The better the match, the higher the magnitude of the net magnetization will be, as shown here:

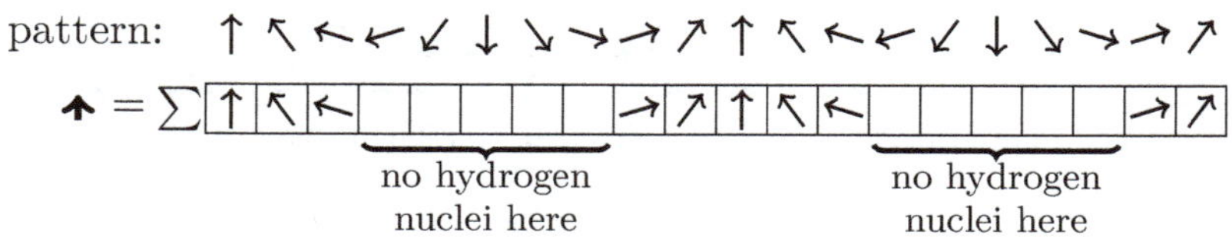

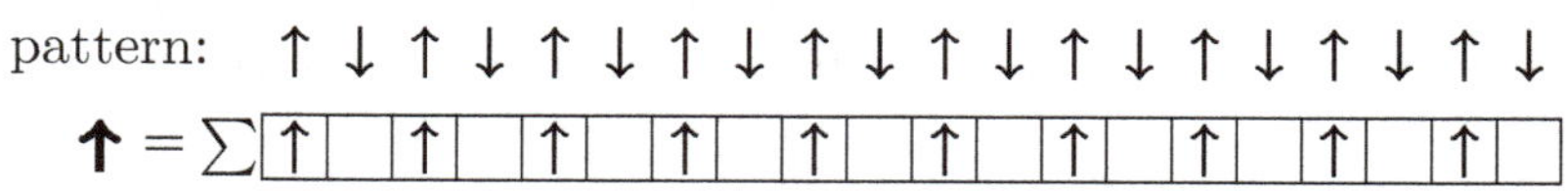

So by applying different gradients, i. e., creating different patterns in the phase orientation of spins, and measuring the net magnetization, i. e., the similarity to the applied pattern, we can get an intermediate representation of the underlying hydrogen density distribution. If done properly, the actual distribution within a slice can then be reconstructed from this intermediate representation. Note that this step happens after slice selection, i. e., the phase encoding is only applied to spins within the slice of interest.

The phase pattern can also be understood in terms of an intensity pattern, by mapping phase angles to gray values. For the two phase patterns shown above, the corresponding intensity patterns are shown here:

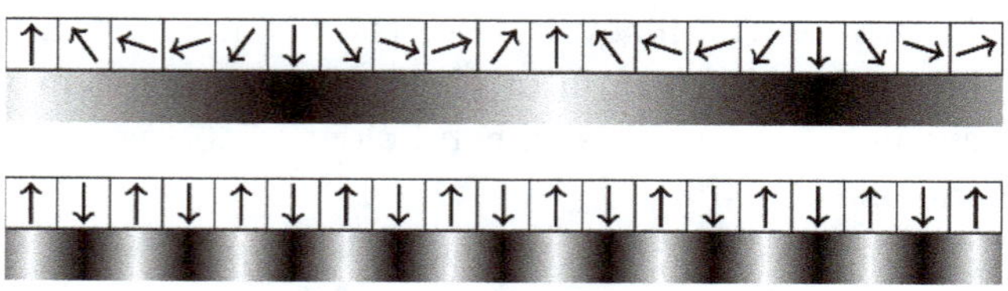

The observations above can also be derived mathematically and demonstrate that we are actually measuring the Fourier transform of the signal (cf. Geek Box 6.1).

Geek Box 6.1: Relation to 1-D Fourier Transform

The phase pattern can be described as a function which maps the offset in right-left direction x to a complex number of magnitude 1 and an angle dependent on x and the phase shift k corresponding to the gradient field strength:

$$p_k(x) = \mathrm{e}^{\mathrm{i}kx} = \cos(kx) + \mathrm{i}\sin(kx) \tag{6.3}$$

The match of the pattern $p_k(x)$ to our image $f(x)$ is performed by a pointwise multiplication and summation, i. e., a correlation. The result is the measured net magnetization $m(k)$ dependent on the phase shift k:

$$m(k) = \int f(x) p_k(x)\, \mathrm{d}x \tag{6.4}$$

$$= \int f(x) \mathrm{e}^{\mathrm{i}kx}\, \mathrm{d}x \tag{6.5}$$

We can now see that the image $f(x)$ we want to compute is the Fourier transform of the measured net magnetization $m(k)$, which is how it can be reconstructed. In other words, phase encoding performs a Fourier decomposition of our image.

6.2.2.2 Generalization to Multiple Dimensions

The concept of phase encoding effortlessly generalizes to more dimensions. For example, to perform spatial localization in two dimensions within an excited slice, e. g., left-right and anterior-posterior, two gradient fields in those directions are applied to create 2-D phase patterns:

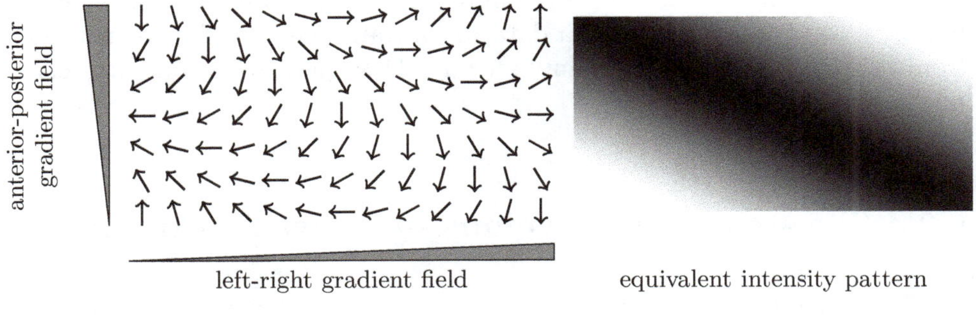

The concept can also be expanded to n-D and comprises again a Fourier transform (cf. Geek Box 6.2)

Geek Box 6.2: Relation to n-D Fourier Transform

In general, the phase shift pattern for an n-D image $f(\boldsymbol{x})$, $\boldsymbol{x} \in \mathbb{R}^n$, dependent on the phase shift in each dimension combined into a vector $\boldsymbol{k}$ is

$$p_{\boldsymbol{k}}(\boldsymbol{x}) = \mathrm{e}^{\mathrm{i}\langle \boldsymbol{x}, \boldsymbol{k} \rangle} = \cos\left(\sum_{j=1}^{n} x_j k_j\right) + \mathrm{i}\sin\left(\sum_{j=1}^{n} x_j k_j\right) \tag{6.6}$$

and the measured net magnetization $m(\boldsymbol{k})$ is the n-dimensional inverse Fourier transform of $f(\boldsymbol{x})$:

$$m(\boldsymbol{k}) = \int f(\boldsymbol{x}) p_{\boldsymbol{k}}(\boldsymbol{x}) \, \mathrm{d}\boldsymbol{x} \tag{6.7}$$

$$= \int f(\boldsymbol{x}) \mathrm{e}^{\mathrm{i}\langle \boldsymbol{x}, \boldsymbol{k} \rangle} \, \mathrm{d}\boldsymbol{x} \tag{6.8}$$

In the literature, a differentiation is often made, naming one of the considered dimensions the *frequency encoding direction* and the remaining $n-1$ dimensions the *phase encoding directions*. The process of spatial encoding is then explained as two separate steps, *frequency encoding* and *phase encoding*. However, the idea behind both is the same – the one outlined above – and the differences are only due to the technical procedure of reading out data with the scanner, which is omitted here.

6.2.3 $\boldsymbol{k}$-space

In the magnetic resonance community, Fourier space is often referred to as $\boldsymbol{k}$-space as a reference to the wavenumber k. The purpose of an MRI examination is to fill the $\boldsymbol{k}$-space with data so that an image can be reconstructed from it. Fig. 6.9 shows an example for a 2-D $\boldsymbol{k}$-space with some associated phase patterns.

6.2.4 Slice-selective vs. Volume-selective 3-D Imaging

Having understood the concepts of slice selection and spatial encoding, two options present themselves for 3-D imaging:

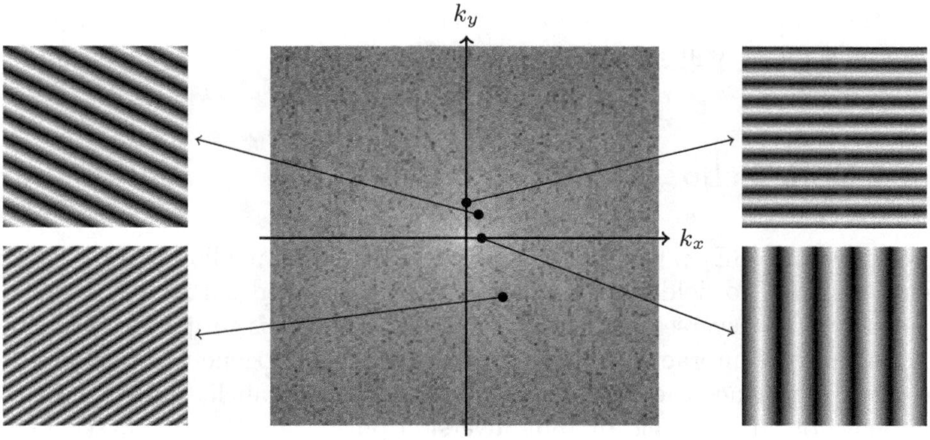

Figure 6.9: Example of a filled 2-D $\boldsymbol{k}$-space, with grey values encoding similarity as dark = low and bright = high, with associated phase patterns for some $\boldsymbol{k}$-space positions.

Slice-selective: Use slice selection to successively acquire, reconstruct, and stack 2-D slices of the desired 3-D volume, using 2-D spatial encoding for localization within each slice.

Volume-selective: Excite the entire volume without slice selection and use 3-D spatial encoding for localization, followed by a 3-D reconstruction.

Both approaches have advantages and disadvantages and the choice for which approach to use is dependent on the intended use of the acquired volume. Slice-selective acquisitions are commonly non-isotropic with high in-plane resolutions $< 1\,\mathrm{mm}$, but with a high slice thickness of several millimeters. Volume-selective acquisitions have an inherent signal-to-noise ratio benefit because more ^{1}H nuclei resonate. They typically feature isotropic resolution which lies inbetween the in-plane resolution and slice thickness of slice-selective acquisitions (for comparable acquisition durations).

6.3 Pulse Sequences

A pulse sequence describes the sequence of RF pulses which are applied in repetition in order to successively acquire the whole $\boldsymbol{k}$-space of an object. This includes order and position of every sample as well as the information how the 3-D gradient coils of the scanner hardware have to be adjusted accordingly. Sequences can look quite complex in a detailed view but they are usually determined by a small number of recurring building blocks such as (partial) flips of longitudinal magnetization via RF excitations, waiting periods and readout gradients.

In the following, we focus on the description of the general concepts of two prominent pulse sequences.

6.3.1 Spin Echo

The spin echo (SE) pulse sequence is widely used as it allows to regain the signal loss due to field imperfections. As we discussed earlier in Sec. 6.1.2, the decay of transverse magnetization after excitation is subject to dephasing due to random interactions and external field inhomogeneities. Apparently, we cannot influence the random interactions between nuclei but we can alter the phase of nuclei using an 180° inversion pulse such that dephased nuclei can end up *in phase* again. For this to work, constant field imperfections are assumed which holds in practice for conventional MRI acquisitions. The principle of the spin echo sequence is shown in Fig. 6.10 and can be summarized to:

1. A 90° RF pulse flips the magnetization into the transversal plane.
2. Dephasing due to random nuclei interactions and field inhomogeneities sets in. Some nuclei will spin slightly faster and others slower due to local field variations. The phases of these nuclei will further diverge over time such that their magnetic moments will cancel each other, resulting in a decay of transversal magnetization.
3. After a waiting period of TE/2, a 180° pulse inverts the magnetization by flipping the dephased vectors along the x (or y) axis. In consequence, the nuclei whose phase trailed behind are now ahead of the main magnetic moment and vice versa.
4. After another waiting period of TE/2, all magnetic moments have refocused and are in phase again as the faster spins have caught up with the lower spinning nuclei by this time. Now, a large signal, so called *spin echo*, which is of negative sign but with the T_2^* effects removed can be measured.
5. Multiple echos can be formed by repeating steps 2–4 as long as some signal due to T_2 decay is available. Each signal has its own echo time TE_1, TE_2, ... after the 90° RF excitation.

6.3.2 Gradient Echo

The gradient echo (GRE) pulse sequence utilizes partial flips with angles below 90°, which allow for faster acquisitions compared to SE sequences. Note that the acquisition time for a single slice in a typical spin echo sequence is given by $\mathrm{TR} \cdot N_y \cdot N_{\mathrm{ex}}$, where N_y and N_{ex} are the number of phase encoding steps and excitations, respectively. As these parameters determine the result-

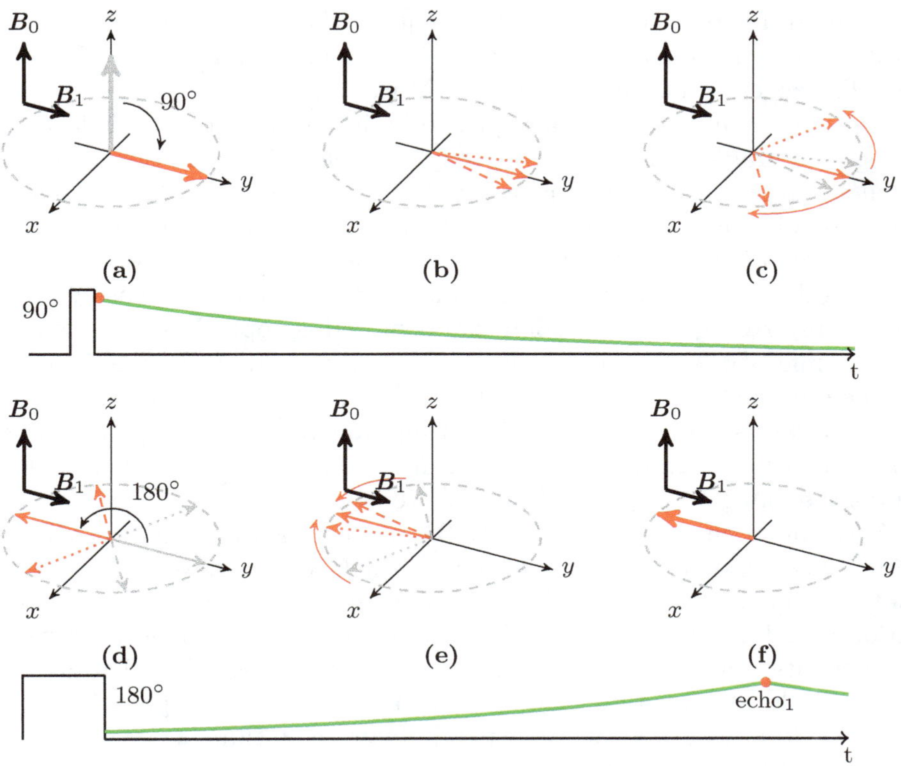

Figure 6.10: A 90° pulse tips the magnetization into the xy plane (a). Some nuclei spin slightly faster (dashed) and others slower (dotted) than the resonance frequency due to local field variations (b). This process continues and leads to a reduction of measurable signal (green line on timeline) along $\boldsymbol{B}_1$ (c). A 180° pulse inverts the magnetization vectors at $t = \frac{1}{2}\mathrm{TE}$ and the spins start to rephase again (d). The total magnetization builds up as the magnetization vectors become in phase (e) and reaches its peak at $t = \mathrm{TE}$ (f). This yields the first echo of the original signal, indicated by the red dot in the timeline.

ing resolution and SNR, one wishes to reduce the scan time by selecting a TR as small as possible that still yields enough signal. However, with a typical 90° pulse the longitudinal magnetization $\boldsymbol{M}_z$ cannot recover sufficiently for very short TR. Thus, the trick is to use low-flip angles which tip only parts of the longitudinal magnetization into the transversal plane such that enough longitudinal magnetization is available for the next repetition after a short TR. The flip angle α of the RF pulse directly controls the resulting magnitude of the transversal magnetization $\|\boldsymbol{M}_{xy}\| = \|\boldsymbol{M}_0\| \sin \alpha$, and the residual longitudinal magnetization $\|\boldsymbol{M}_z\| = \|\boldsymbol{M}_0\| \cos \alpha$, where $\boldsymbol{M}_0$ is the initial magnetization.

Another difference to the spin echo sequence is that GRE uses no 180° refocusing pulse which makes it more susceptible to field inhomogeneities leading to a T_2^* weighting instead of a T_2 weighting.

Also, as there is no 180° pulse, the echo in a GRE sequence is formed via a negative gradient in readout or frequency encoding direction which is an intended dephasing of the magnetization. The idea behind it is that since some time for preparations such as the spatial encoding is needed before the actual signal can be read out, we intentionally delay the time of the peak signal (echo) to a more convenient time. To this end, the dephasing gradient has the inverse sign of the readout gradient and is applied in advance for half of the time of the readout gradient. This ensures that the maximal signal can be obtained at the half of the readout period, since the positive readout gradient reverses the effects of dephasing and recalls the signal during the first half while it gradually dephases again during the second half. This is where the name *gradient recalled echo* stems from.

Yet another characteristic of the GRE sequence is the formation of a *steady state*. In contrast to spin echo sequences, the GRE can have such a short TR that the signal decay due to T_2^* is incomplete and some transversal magnetization remains when the next RF pulse follows. In consequence, transversal magnetization accumulates over a few cycles which is referred to as steady state. As the steady state may be unfavorable for some applications, the so called *spoiled* GRE sequence tries to eliminate the residual transverse magnetization. Otherwise its effects will manifest itself in the image contrast. More on this is subject to further reading [3].

6.4 Advanced Topics

Up to this point, the principles for morphological imaging have been introduced. We will now look at some advanced topics related to speeding up the acquisition process, suppressing signals from unwanted or enhancing signals from desired tissue classes as well as methods for functional imaging.

6.4.1 Parallel Imaging

Long acquisition times are a major drawback of MRI systems, with manifold negative consequences. Patients may experience discomfort, having to spend extended amounts of time in a narrow space. There is an impact on image quality, as patient motion during the acquisition is inevitable. And from a financial standpoint, the amount of MRI examinations per unit time is much less than for other modalities.

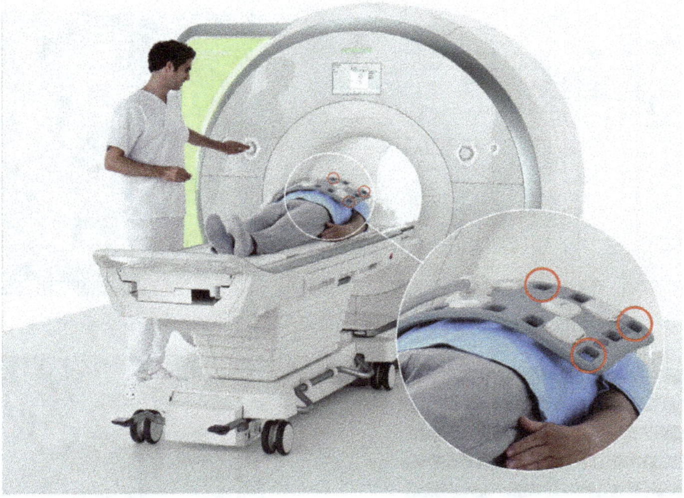

Figure 6.11: Parallel imaging uses local receiver coils placed around the patient which capture the signal from multiple positions, allowing for a reduction of acquisition time. The coils are embedded in the table as well as in the flexible coil on top of the patient's chest, in this case an 18-element body coil where individual coil elements are arranged in 6 columns and 3 rows. Three individual coil elements are exemplarily indicated by the red circles. Image courtesy of Siemens Healthineers AG.

Techniques for shortening the acquisition time are, thus, of vital importance and an active field of research. Parallel imaging is an established technique which allows a reduction of the amount of data needed to be acquired in order to reconstruct an image. The name stems from the use of multiple local receiver coils which are placed around the patient and acquire resonance signals in parallel. Modern MRI systems have coil elements which are embedded in the table as well as flexible coil elements which can be placed on the patient (see Fig. 6.11).

This enables many possibilities for undersampling in $\boldsymbol{k}$-space to reduce the acquisition time, one of which we will present here. Suppose we regularly undersample the $\boldsymbol{k}$-space by acquiring only every n-th line. The value n is referred to as the undersampling factor, indicating the reduction in acquisition time. A standard reconstruction by performing a Fourier transform is no longer possible in this case because it will introduce aliasing artifacts in the reconstructed image (see Fig. 6.12).

A reconstruction technique called sensitivity encoding (SENSE) is able to reconstruct an image without aliasing artifacts from such undersampled data by employing the information collected from the multiple receiver coils. It exploits the fact that each local receiver coil "sees" a slightly different image, namely one in which parts closer to the coil are better represented than those

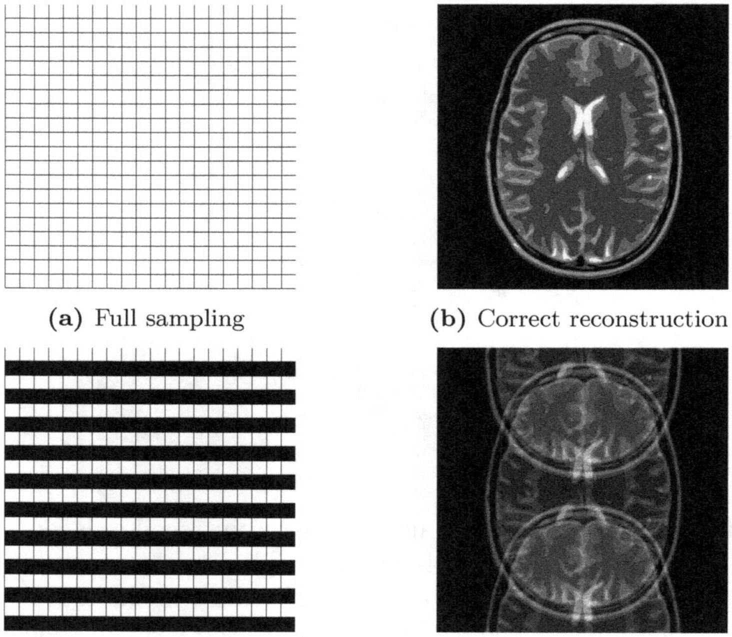

(a) Full sampling **(b)** Correct reconstruction

(c) Regular undersampling **(d)** Aliased reconstruction

Figure 6.12: A visualization of a fully sampled $\boldsymbol{k}$-space (a) with its corresponding reconstruction (b) as well as a regularly undersampled $\boldsymbol{k}$-space with every second line missing (c) with a reconstruction showing aliasing artifacts (d).

farther away. A so-called coil sensitivity map $s_\gamma(\boldsymbol{r}_\rho)$ describes how well a coil γ sees a pixel at position $\boldsymbol{r}_\rho$.

In case of regular undersampling, each pixel in the aliased image (see Fig. 6.12(d)) can be described as a weighted sum of several pixels in the unaliased image (see Fig. 6.12(b)). In the given example, 2 pixels in the unaliased image contribute to a pixel in the aliased image. Different local receiver coils "see" different aliased images, where the weights for the weighted sum of pixels are described by the coil sensitivity map of the respective coil. Geek Box 6.3 illustrates this for an idealized 2-coil setup whereas Geek Box 6.4 discusses how to calibrate the sensitivity maps online.

Geek Box 6.3: Coil Sensitivity Maps

The parallel measurement can be described by a linear system of equations:

$$\boldsymbol{a} = \boldsymbol{S}\boldsymbol{v}, \tag{6.9}$$

where $\boldsymbol{v}$ is a vector of length m of unaliased pixel values contributing to an aliased pixel, $\boldsymbol{a}$ is a vector of length c of the aliased pixel value as seen by the c different coils and $\boldsymbol{S}$ is a $c \times m$ matrix containing the coil sensitivities as

$$\boldsymbol{S}_{\gamma,\rho} = s_\gamma(\boldsymbol{r}_\rho), \tag{6.10}$$

where γ is the coil index and $\boldsymbol{r}_\rho$ are the pixel positions of the pixels contained in $\boldsymbol{v}$. The reconstruction then consists of solving Eq. (6.9) for all pixels in the unaliased image.
This process can be visualized looking at idealized coil sensitivity maps for a 2-coil setup where one coil is more sensitive in the upper part of the image and the other in the lower part of the image:

Sensitivity map of Coil 1

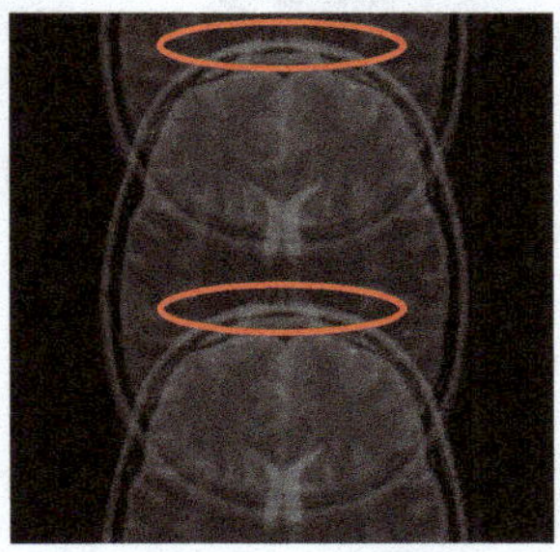

Aliased image of Coil 1

Sensitivity map of Coil 2

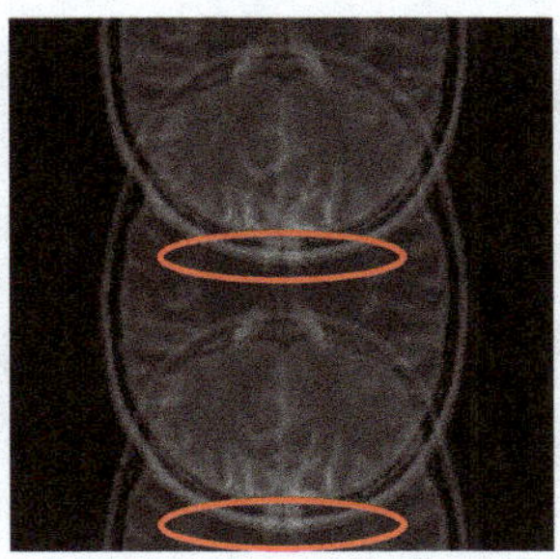

Aliased image of Coil 2

Here, brighter values represent higher weights. The aliased images seen by these coils differ, one has a better representation of the top part of the head and one a better representation of the bottom part, see the red highlights.

Geek Box 6.4: Coil Sensitivity Map Calibration

A remaining problem is how to compute the coil sensitivity maps. An a-priori calibration is infeasible as they are dependent on the imaging volume. Therefore, we describe an *auto-calibration* approach can be used to determine coil sensitivity maps during the scan.
In addition to the undersampled acquisition as shown in Fig. 6.12(c), a small, fully sampled region around the center of $\boldsymbol{k}$-space is measured. A direct Fourier transform reconstruction of this region for each coil leads to low-resolution versions of the volume as seen by the respective coil, for our two-coil example:

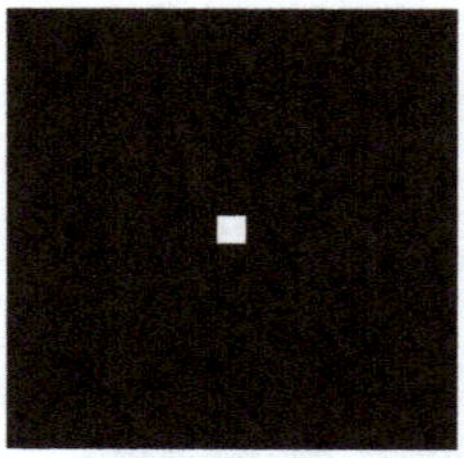
Acquisition mask

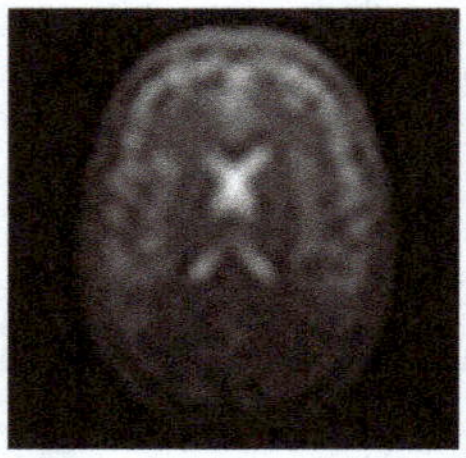
Image of Coil 1

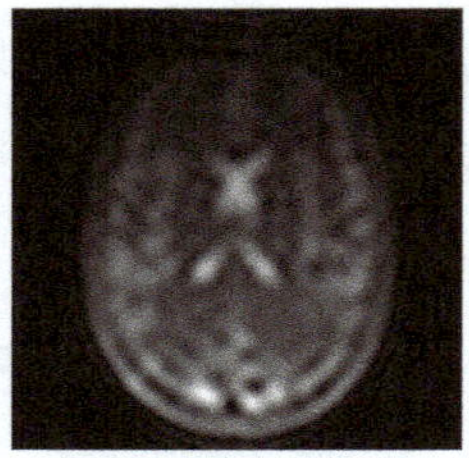
Image of Coil 2

An approximation of the coil sensitivity maps is obtained by dividing these images by a sum-of-squares combination of all coil images:

$$s_\gamma(\boldsymbol{r}_\rho) = \frac{i_\gamma(\boldsymbol{r}_\rho)}{\sqrt{\sum_{\gamma'=1}^{C} i_{\gamma'}(\boldsymbol{r}_\rho)^2}}, \tag{6.11}$$

where $i_\gamma(\boldsymbol{r}_\rho)$ is the image of coil γ and C is their total number:

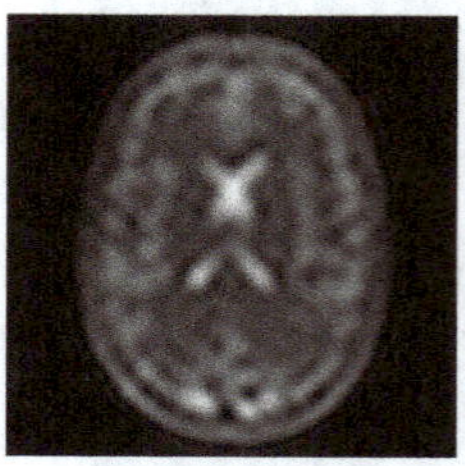
Fusion of Coil 1 and 2 $\sqrt{\sum_{\gamma'=1}^{C} i_{\gamma'}(\boldsymbol{r}_\rho)^2}$

Sensitivity Map 1 $s_1(\boldsymbol{r}_\rho)$

Sensitivity Map 2 $s_2(\boldsymbol{r}_\rho)$

The resulting coil sensitivity maps show artifacts in the regions with little to no signal as compared to the idealized maps. Reconstructions using these coil sensitivity maps will display noise amplification in air regions due to these artifacts. More advanced methods exist to deal with these issues, but they are beyond the scope of this text.

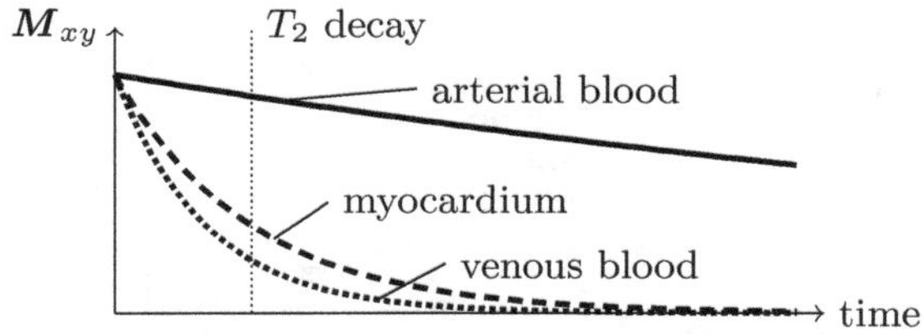

Figure 6.13: A T_2 preparation sequence can be used to increase the contrast between myocardium and arterial blood due to their large difference in T_2 constants (35 ms vs. 250 ms). Figure recreated from [6].

6.4.2 Spectrally Selective Excitation

For bright-blood coronary imaging, it is often desirable to increase contrast between the myocardium (the heart muscle) and the arterial blood within the heart chambers. This allows a better delineation of the heart walls and thus increases the diagnostic value of images. A method called T_2 preparation exploits the fact that arterial blood has a much larger T_2 constant than myocardial tissue and venous blood. This means that the decay of transversal magnetization $\boldsymbol{M}_{xy}$ is slower for arterial blood, see Fig. 6.13.

Using a sequence of pulses, we can reduce the magnetization of the myocardium and venous blood while keeping the magnetization of arterial blood virtually untouched. Fig. 6.14 illustrates the process. In the initial state, spins of all tissue types are aligned with the main magnetic field $\boldsymbol{B}_0$. A 90° pulse pushes the spins into the transversal plane, where they precess. At this point, T_1, T_2 and T_2^* relaxation (see Sec. 6.1.2) start to affect the spins:

$\boldsymbol{T_1}$ relaxation: We will ignore T_1 relaxation here because it happens on a much larger timescale than the duration of the T_2 preparation sequence.

$\boldsymbol{T_2^*}$ relaxation: Due to magnetic field inhomogeneities, spins would rapidly dephase and lose their transversal magnetization, known as T_2^* relaxation. To counteract this effect, we apply a series of 180° pulses to refocus the spins.

$\boldsymbol{T_2}$ relaxation: This is the effect we actually want to happen. While the spins remain in the transversal plane, myocardium and venous blood spins lose their transversal magnetization much faster than arterial blood.

After a set amount of time, a final −90° pulse realigns spins with the main magnetic field. At this point, arterial blood spins have a higher magnetization and subsequent imaging sequences (e. g., GRE or spin echo sequences) will show an increased contrast to myocardial tissue.

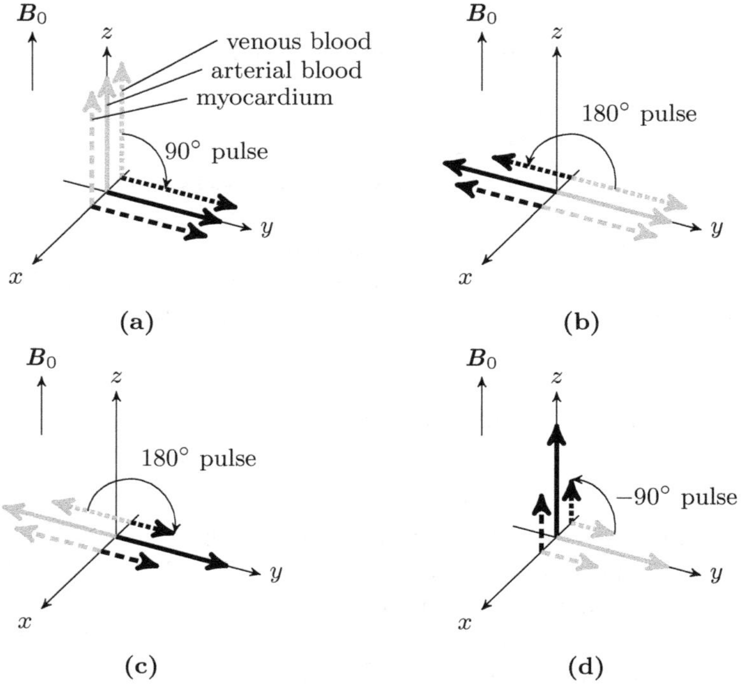

Figure 6.14: In the initial state, the spins for myocardial tissue, venous and arterial blood are all aligned along the main magnetic field. A 90° pulse pushes them into the xy plane, where they precess (a). 180° refocusing pulses are used to counteract T_2^* relaxation, so only T_2 relaxation affects the spins while they are in the xy plane (b), (c). Due to the different T_2 constants, the transversal magnetization decays faster for myocardial and venous blood spins. After a set amount of time, spins are realigned with the main magnetic field by a $-90°$ pulse (d). An imaging sequence following this preparation sequence will now display increased contrast between arterial blood and myocardial tissue. Figure recreated from [6].

6.4.3 Non-contrast Angiography

Up to this point, we have quietly assumed that all measured spins remain stationary for the duration of the imaging. This assumption is, of course, invalid if we image the human body. For many applications, we have to adapt the acquisition protocol to minimize artifacts due to motion. For example, we may ask the person being scanned to hold their breath to minimize respiratory motion artifacts. Imaging sequences with a short TR can be used to "freeze" cardiac motion. But in some cases, we can actually use non-stationary spins to our advantage.

Angiography, the imaging of blood vessels, is commonly performed by administering a contrast agent which increases the contrast of blood to sur-

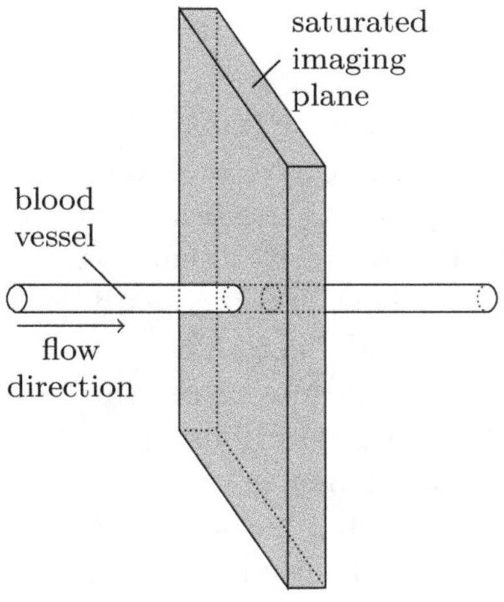

(a) Directly after saturation

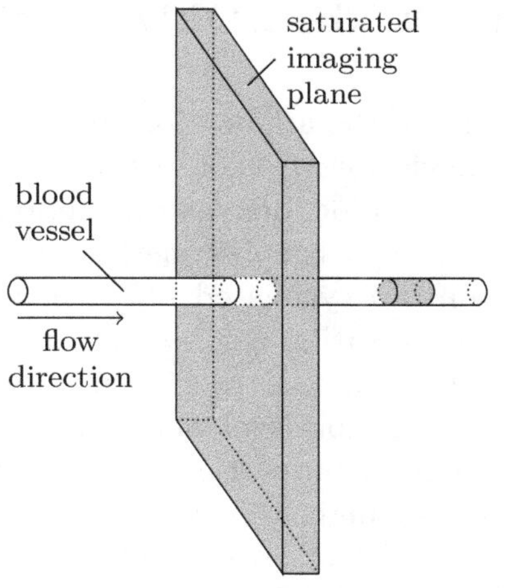

(b) Unsaturated spins enter the imaging plane due to blood flow

Figure 6.15: For non-contrast TOF angiography, all spins in the desired imaging plane are saturated, i. e., put in a state such that they cannot be excited by an RF pulse, indicated by the gray shading (a). Due to blood flow, unsaturated spins enter the imaging plane for blood vessels that are not entirely parallel to the imaging plane (b). Subsequent imaging sequences will show a high contrast between those vessels and surrounding stationary tissue.

rounding tissues. In MRI, we can use the fact that blood spins move continuously during the image acquisition to perform a non-contrast angiography. In the magnetic resonance context, the TOF effect refers to the short amount of time that flowing blood spins remain within an imaging slice.

For TOF angiography, we first saturate all spins within our imaging plane, i. e., put them in a state where they cannot be excited by an RF pulse. For the duration of their T_1 relaxation, stationary spins within the imaging plane will thus show little to no signal if we perform an imaging sequence. But due to the TOF effect, unsaturated blood spins continuously flow into the imaging plane and will appear bright in contrast to the surrounding stationary tissue if imaged.

This imaging technique works best for blood vessels perpendicular to the imaging plane. For vessels that lie within the imaging plane, the contrast becomes weaker with increasing distance to the point where unsaturated spins enter the imaging plane. Fig. 6.15 illustrates the concept of TOF angiography.

6.4.4 The BOLD Effect

One of the applications of functional magnetic resonance imaging (fMRI) is the visualization of neuronal activity in the brain. Increased neuronal activity leads to local oxygen depletion in the active regions of the brain. This lack of oxygen is subsequently overcompensated, leading to a higher concentration of oxygenated blood in the active regions. Thus, an increased oxygen concentration can be seen as an indication of neuronal activity.

Our aim is to measure this increased concentration using the blood-oxygenation-level dependent (BOLD) effect, which describes the different magnetic properties of oxygenated and deoxygenated hemoglobin. Blood containing higher concentrations of oxygenated hemoglobin has a higher T_2^* constant, i. e., less dephasing due to local magnetic field inhomogeneity (see Sec. 6.1.2). Thus, to measure the neuronal activity due to an external stimulus, we can compare images acquired in a resting state to images acquired during the application of the stimulus to see which brain regions experience a change in local oxygen concentration.

A GRE sequence (see Sec. 6.3) can be used to obtain T_2^* weighted images. However, as the T_2^* differences are very slight, the usual approach to gain robust results is to acquire multiple resting state images and multiple images while the stimulus is applied in an alternating fashion, followed by a statistical test to determine if the intensity of a given pixel significantly differs in both sets of images.

Further Reading

[1] Christoph Forman et al. "Free-Breathing Whole-Heart Coronary MRA: Motion Compensation Integrated into 3D Cartesian Compressed Sensing Reconstruction". In: *MICCAI 2013, Part II, LNCS 8150.* Ed. by K. Mori et al. Nagoya, Japan, 2013, pp. 575–582.

[2] Lars G Hanson. *Introduction to Magnetic Resonance Imaging Techniques.* Tech. rep. Danish Research Centre for Magnetic Resonance, 2009. URL: `http://eprints.drcmr.dk/37/`.

[3] R.H. Hashemi, W.G. Bradley, and C.J. Lisanti. *MRI: The Basics.* Lippincott Williams & Wilkins, 2010. ISBN: 9781608311156.

[4] Alexander Hendrix. *Magnets, Flows and Artifacts: Basics, Techniques, and Applications of Magnetic Resonance Tomography.* Siemens AG, Erlangen, 2004. URL: `http://www.healthcare.siemens.de/magnetic-resonance-imaging/magnetom-world/publications/mr-basics`.

[5] Alexander Hendrix. *Magnets, Spins and Resonances: An introduction to the basics of Magnetic Resonance.* Siemens AG, Erlangen, 2003. URL: `http://www.healthcare.siemens.de/magnetic-resonance-imaging/magnetom-world/publications/mr-basics`.

[6] Vivian S Lee. *Cardiovascular MRI: Physical Principles to Practical Protocols*. Lippincott Williams & Wilkins, Dec. 2005. ISBN: 0781779960.

[7] Dwight G Nishimura. *Principles of Magnetic Resonance Imaging*. Self-published, 2010. URL: `http://www-ee.stanford.edu/~dwight/book.html`.

[8] Klaas P Pruessmann et al. "SENSE: sensitivity encoding for fast MRI". In: *Magn Reson Med* 42.5 (Nov. 1999), pp. 952–962.

[9] G. Lawrence Zeng. *Medical Image Reconstruction: A Tutorial*. Higher Education Press, Springer, Beijing, 2009. ISBN: 978-3-642-05367-2.

7

Physical Principles of X-Ray Imaging

Authors: Martin Berger, Qiao Yang and Andreas Maier

7.1 Introduction

In this chapter, the physical principles of X-rays are introduced. We start with a general definition of X-rays compared to other well known rays, e. g., the visible light. In Sec. 7.2, we will learn how X-rays can be generated and how they can be characterized with respect to their energy. The most relevant concept to understand how X-ray imaging works is the behavior of X-rays when they interact with matter. This is outlined in detail in Sec. 7.3. In Sec. 7.4, conventional X-ray imaging is described with a focus on detector types and sources of noise. Finally, we finish this chapter with an overview of well known application areas for X-ray imaging in Sec. 7.5.

7.1.1 Definition of X-rays

X-rays belong to the group of electromagnetic rays, hence, they follow the rules of electromagnetic radiation. Electromagnetic radiation transports en-

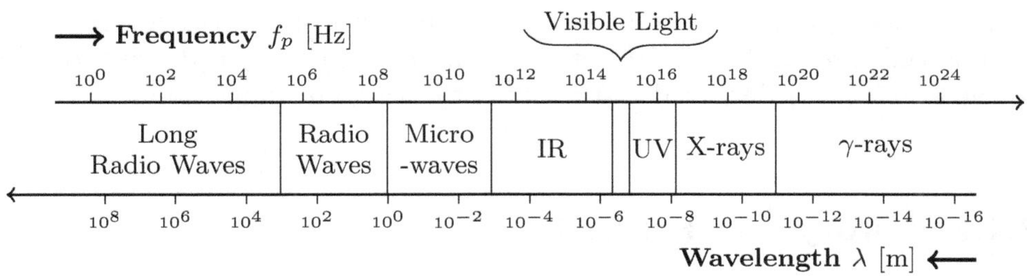

Figure 7.1: Wavelengths and frequencies of the different groups of electromagnetic radiation. X-rays lie in the range of 0.01 nm up to 10 nm.

ergy, also called radiant energy, through space by waves and photons, just as radio waves, the visible light or microwaves. It can either be represented by photons or by a wave model. We will use both representations in the process of this chapter. Radiation can be classified by its wavelength λ_p which is the length of one period of the wave. The wavelength can also be represented by frequency f_p and the waves propagation speed, i. e., the speed of light c_0.

$$\lambda_p = \frac{c_0}{f_p} \tag{7.1}$$

In Eq. (7.2) the energy of photons is given, where h denotes Planck's constant ($\approx 6.626\,069 \times 10^{-34}\,\mathrm{J\,s}$) and c_0 is the speed of light ($\approx 2.997\,92 \times 10^5\,\mathrm{m\,s^{-1}}$). The energy is directly related to the photon's wavelength λ_p or its frequency f_p and is given by the unit electron volt [eV]. We can easily obtain that the photon energy is proportional to its frequency and inverse proportional to its wavelength, that means the higher its frequency, the higher its energy.

$$E_p = \frac{h\,c_0}{\lambda_p} = f_p\,h \tag{7.2}$$

The energy is also used to characterize electromagnetic radiation into different groups, i. e., radio waves, microwaves, infrared (IR), visible light, ultraviolet (UV) light, X-rays and γ-rays. Fig. 7.1 shows these groups with respect to their characteristic ranges of frequency and wavelength. Note that the wavelength of most X-rays lies in the range of 0.01 nm up to 10 nm. This corresponds to an energy range of 100 keV down to 100 eV.

As visible light, X-rays loose a certain amount of energy when they pass through different materials. The energy loss depends on the absorption behavior of the material. For example if X-rays pass through 10cm of water, they loose less energy than if they would pass trough 10cm of bone. The reduction of energy is caused by absorption which is the main principle of traditional X-ray imaging. Generally speaking, X-ray radiography measures the amount of energy loss. Because this energy loss differs for the different materials, we can see a certain contrast in the image. For example an X-ray image shows high intensities for soft tissue and lower intensities where the X-rays passed through bones. Note that the absorbed energy is directly related to the dose that is delivered to the patient during an acquisition.

7.1.2 History and Present

Discovery of X-rays

X-rays have been discovered by Wilhelm Conrad Röntgen in Würzburg, Germany. On November 8, 1895, he conducted experiments including Crookes tubes, which are typically used to visualize streams of electrons. He further used a fluorescent screen and covered the actual tube with black cardboard. When moving the fluorescent screen away from the tubes opening he realized that there was still a glimmer visible on the fluorescent screen, which had to be the result from radiation that passes through the black cardboard. Additional experiments where he replaced the cardboard with denser materials, e. g., books led to the same observation. After that, he began a systematic study of the new radiation, which he then named "X"-rays. One of the first acquired X-ray images is shown in Fig. 7.3. It depicts the hand of Röntgen's wife, where we can clearly see the ring she was wearing on her annular finger. It is not to be confused with a similar image depicted in Fig. 7.4 which was taken later in January of 1896.

Only on December 28, 1895, about six weeks after the first discovery, Röntgen submitted the first known article on X-rays entitled "Über eine neue Art von Strahlen" (On a new type of rays) which shows first reports on the absorption properties of different materials, e. g., paper, wood and also metal. Already in January 1896, Röntgen demonstrated his discovery to the German medical-physical society. Creating an X-ray of Albert von Kölliker's hand (cf. Fig. 7.4) – a well-known anatomist at that time – in front of the audience immediately convinced Röntgen's colleagues of the utility of his invention. For his groundbreaking discovery, Röntgen received the first awarded Nobel Prize in Physics in 1901. In Fig. 7.2, we can see an image of Wilhelm Conrad Röntgen, taken for the Nobel-Prize committee. The actual commercial implementation was performed by others (cf. Geek Box 7.1).

X-rays Today

Today, X-rays are routinely used in diagnostic but also in interventional medical imaging around the globe. Also in industry, X-rays are often the method of choice, for example to test for very small cracks in metal parts in the field of non-destructive testing. In medical imaging, a variety of applications have been developed that go far beyond simple radiographic imaging. For example

Geek Box 7.1: Commercial Success of X-rays

Röntgen donated his discovery to humanity and never made any commercial profit. He also never filed a patent for his invention. The actual commercial roll-out of the technology was performed by several small companies:

- In 1877, *Erwin Moritz Reiniger*, a former employee of *Friedrich-Alexander-University Erlangen-Nuremberg*, Germany, founded a small workshop right next to the university with the aim of producing batteries and physical measurement devices. In 1886, *Max Gebbert* and *Karl Friedrich Schall* joined Reiniger's workshop founding the *Vereinigte Physikalisch-Mechanische Werkstätten Reiniger, Gebbert & Schall — Erlangen, New York, Stuttgart.* In 1896, they switched the focus of production to X-ray tubes. Over the years this small company grew and is today known under the name *Siemens Healthineers AG.*
- *Victor Electric Company* was founded in 1893 by C. F. Samms and J. B. Wantz in a basement in Chicago, United States of America, with the aim of producing physical measurement gear. In 1896, they also began with the production of X-ray tubes. Also this small company turned out to be very commercially successful and is today known as *General Electric Healhcare.*
- In 1896, *C. H. F. Müller* developed the first commercial X-ray tube in Hamburg, Germany, in cooperation with the *University Clinic Hamburg-Eppendorf.* In 1927, the company was bought and is today an integral part of *Philips Medizin Systeme GmbH.*

fluroscopy allows for real time X-ray sequences which are often inevitable in minimally invasive interventions. Further, digital subtraction angiography (DSA) provides an effective tool to visualize even small vessel structures. In the 1970s, the step to CT was done which now allows to visualize the complete human body in three dimensions. Another point of rapid development is the awareness that X-rays can also be harmful. High energies emitted to the body during an X-ray acquisition can lead to ionization. That means the radiation changes the atomic structure of the tissue which can potentially lead to an increased risk for the development of cancer. Here, deoxyribonucleic acid (DNA) becomes damaged by the radiation. In most cases, the DNA will be repaired by the cell itself. Yet, the repair process sometimes fails which in some cases leads to an unregulated division of cells that might result in cancer. X-ray-based foot scanners where still in use to measure foot sizes in shoe stores until the 1970s. Nowadays, the majority of people is aware of the risk posed by X-rays and the transmitted patient dose during X-ray scans

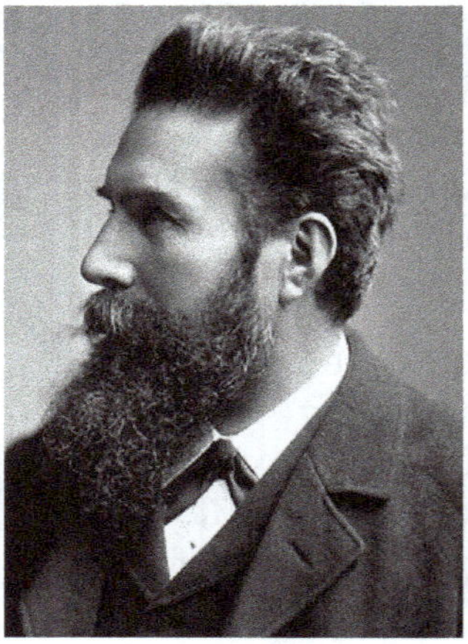

Figure 7.2: Wilhelm Conrad Röntgen

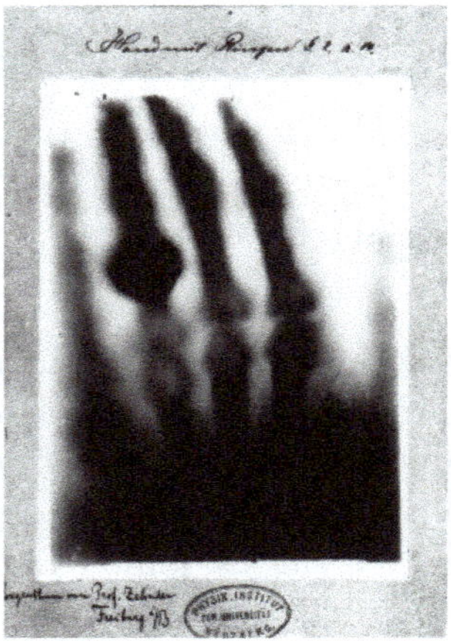

Figure 7.3: One of the first X-rays, taken from Wilhelm Röntgen of his wifes hand.

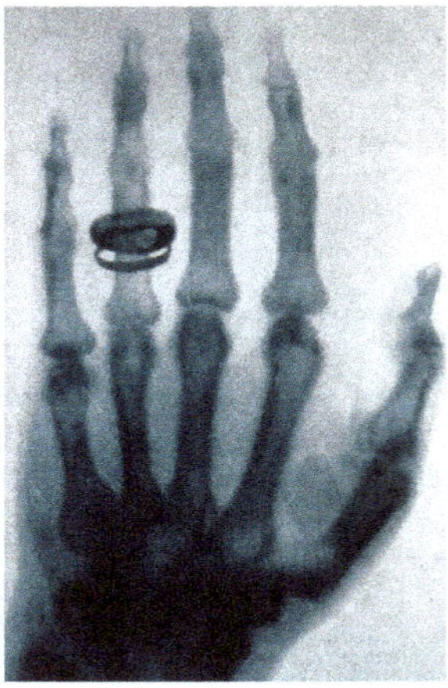

Figure 7.4: Image taken in 1896 showing Albert von Kölliker's hand.

has been significantly reduced in the past decades[1]. In Fig. 7.5, we can see an X-ray taken in mammography which typically uses low-energy X-rays to increase soft-tissue contrast. Another example is shown in Fig. 7.6, where we can see an X-ray image taken from the thorax, i. e., the chest, of a patient.

7.2 X-ray Generation

A classical X-ray tube is depicted in Fig. 7.7. An X-ray tube is basically an evacuated tube made of glass with a cathode and a solid metal anode in it. Thermionic emission occurs by the heated filament at the cathode. Heat induced electrons e^- are produced because the thermal energy applied to the filament material is larger than its binding energy. Then, the electrons are accelerated by the tube's acceleration voltage between the negative cathode and the positive anode. When those fast electrons hit the anode, they are decelerated and deflected by the electric field of the atoms of the anode material. Any acceleration of loaded particles results in electromagnetic waves. So does the slowing down, i. e., the negative acceleration, of the electrons in the metal anode. It generates X-rays.

The anode is tilted by a certain angle to direct the emerging X-rays in the right direction. Typically each electron is slowed down or deflected several times so it causes the creation of several photons. However it can also happen

[1] Although being full of mistakes (as claimed by the authors), a good overview on radiation doses is found at `https://xkcd.com/radiation/`.

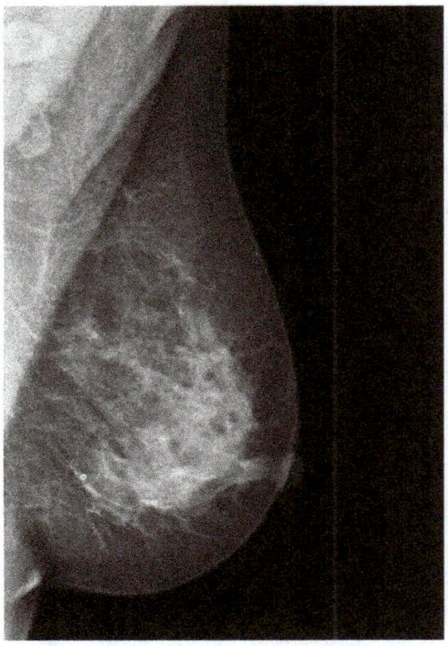

Figure 7.5: Example of a breast X-ray. Note the clearly visible structures in the soft-tissue.

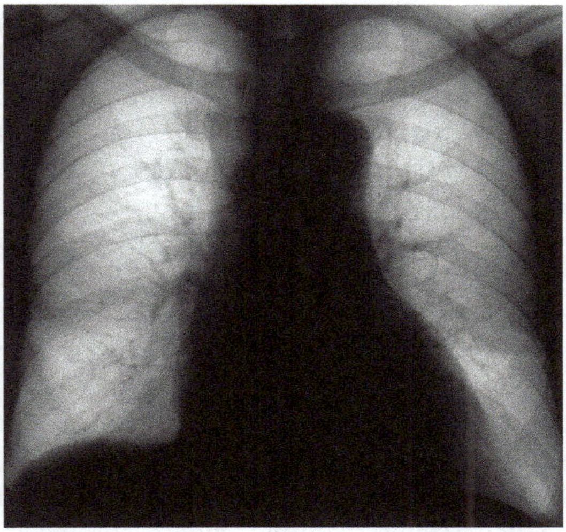

Figure 7.6: Example of an X-ray taken from the chest of a patient.

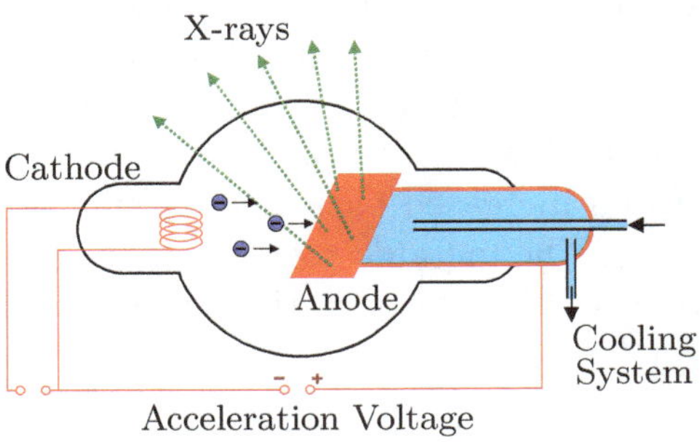

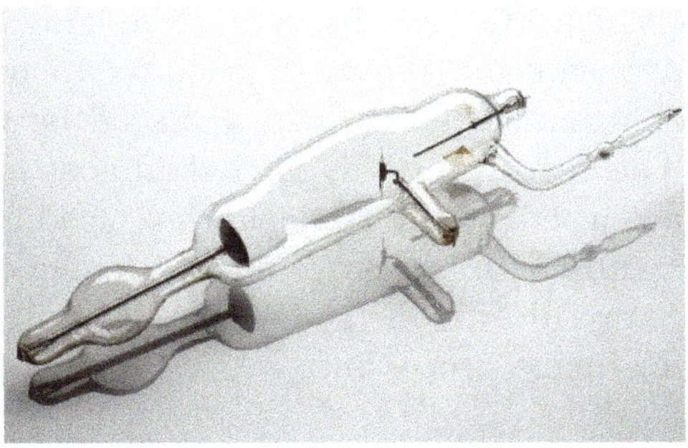

Figure 7.7: Vacuum X-ray tube: The image on the left shows a schematic how electrons are accelerated from the cathode to the anode to genereate X-ray photons. The image on the right shows a historic vacuum X-ray tube. Image provided by Science Museum, London.

that an electron loses all its velocity and thus its energy in one step. In this case, only one photon containing the complete energy of the electron is created.

The production of X-rays is caused by two different processes as shown in Fig. 7.8. First, if the electron interacts with an inner-shell electron of the target, characteristic X-radiation can be produced. This kind of X-rays results from a sufficiently strong interaction that ionizes the target atom by a total removal of the inner-shell electron. The resulting "hole" in the inner-shell is filled with an outer-shell electron. The transition of an orbital electron from an outer-shell to an inner-shell is accompanied by the emission of an X-ray photon, with an energy equal to the difference in the binding energies of the orbital electrons involved. Therefore, the characteristic radiation produces a line spectrum, or discrete spectrum. Obviously, this kind of radiation is material dependent. Both the production of characteristic X-rays as well as thermal energy involve interactions between the accelerated electrons and the electrons of the target material.

Another type of interaction in which the electron can lose its kinetic energy delivers the second process of X-ray production, caused by the interaction of the electron with the nucleus of a target atom. As the colliding electron passes by the nucleus of an anode atom, it is slowed down and deviated in its course, leaving with reduced kinetic energy in a different direction. This loss in kinetic energy reappears as an X-ray photon. This type of X-rays is called Bremsstrahlung, where "bremsen" is the German verb for slowing down. The amount of kinetic energy that is lost in this way can vary from zero to the total incident energy. While the characteristic radiation results in a discrete X-ray spectrum of characteristic peaks, the Bremsstrahlung provides a continuous spectrum. The number of X-rays emitted decreases rapidly at very low photon energies. The spectrum of a tungsten source is given in Fig. 7.8. In medical imaging, very low energies of an X-ray spectrum are typically removed prior to an interaction with the patient by using a thin metal plate which is placed between the patient and the X-ray source. The reason for this is that almost all of the low energy photons would be absorbed by the patient, thus, leading to an increased patient dose without a substantial improvement of image quality. The metallic plate is also called X-ray filter, which is not to be confused with the mathematical filters used for image processing.

7.3 X-ray Matter Interaction

X-rays have the ability to penetrate matter, yet, the amount of penetrating X-ray photons is material-dependent. Their ability to penetrate human tissue is in fact the reason why they can be used to get information on internal organs. Different tube voltages between the cathode and the anode produce higher or lower energy X-ray spectra. In the energy range that is used for medical imaging, there are three kinds of relevant interactions that can occur when X-rays pass through matter:

- interaction with atomic electrons,
- interaction with nucleons,
- interaction with electric fields associated to atomic electrons and atomic nuclei.

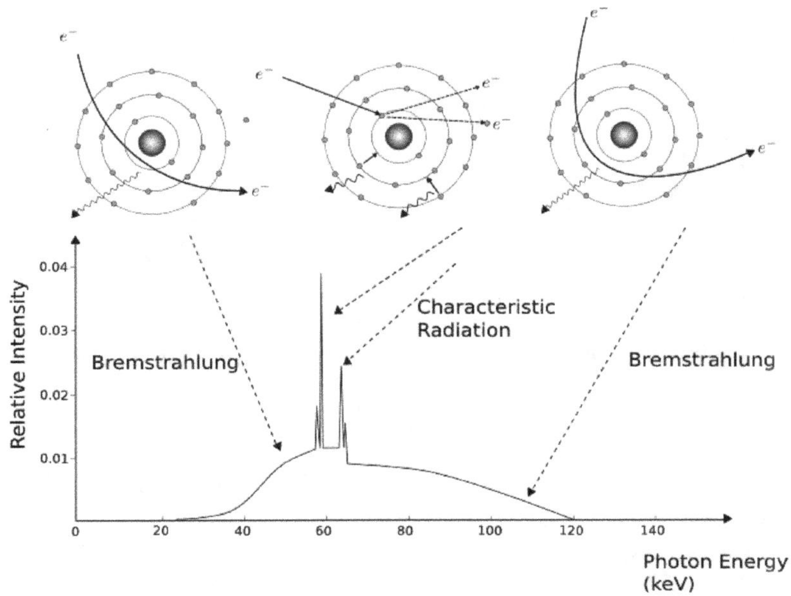

Figure 7.8: X-ray spectrum of a tungsten tube. The peaks correspond to the characteristic radiation; the continuous part of the spectrum represents the Bremsstrahlung.

Consequently, the X-ray photons either experience a complete absorption, elastic scattering or inelastic scattering.

The interaction that is used for medical imaging consists of a reduction of radiation intensity which is nothing else than a reduction of the number of photons that arrive at the detector. That process is usually referred to as attenuation. There are several different physical effects contributing to attenuation, including a change of the photon count, photon direction, or photon energy. All of these effects have in common that they are based on an interaction between single photons and the material that they are passing through and that the attenuation induced by each of them is highly energy-dependent. Sec. 7.3 shows an overview on the different relevant effects. Note that pair production is not relevant for typical diagnostic X-ray energies. To produce a positron and an electron, the photon's energy must exceed at least $2 \times 511\,\text{keV}$.

7.3.1 Absorption

When a monochromatic X-ray beam traverses a homogeneous object with absorption coefficient μ, according to Lambert-Beer's law, the observed intensity I is related to the intersection length of the object x and the ray:

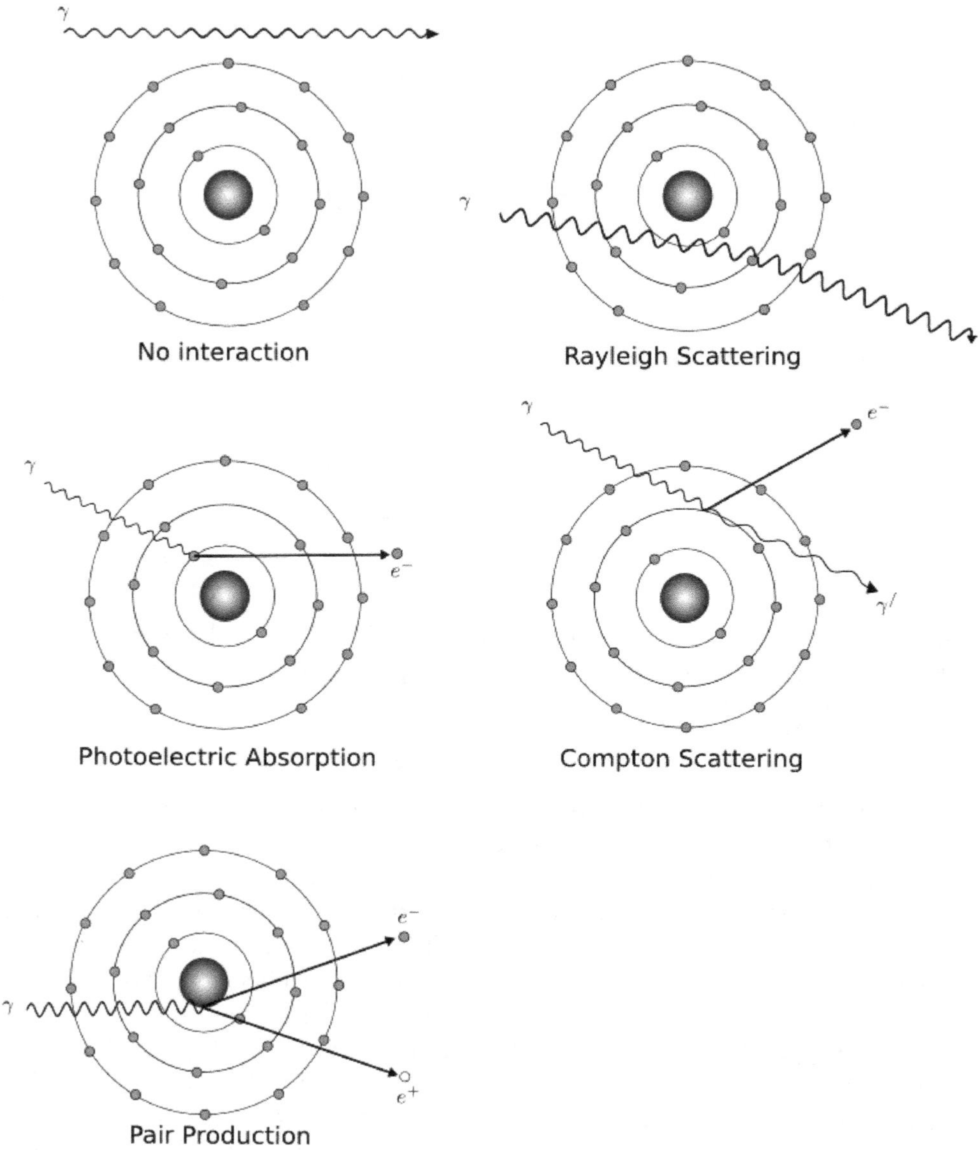

Figure 7.9: Principles of photon-matter interactions.

$$I = I_0 \cdot e^{-\mu x} \ . \tag{7.3}$$

Here, I_0 is the X-ray intensity at the X-ray source. A derivation is found in Geek Box 7.2.

In X-ray CT, the fractional transmitted intensity I/I_0 is used to measure a large number of ray paths through the object. The logarithm of this ratio is used to obtain a set of line integrals as an input to reconstruction algorithms.

Geek Box 7.2: Lambert-Beer's Law

The radiation intensity decreases which leads to an ordinary linear and homogeneous, first order differential equation with constant coefficient

$$\frac{dI}{I} = -\mu \mathrm{d}x \ .$$

I is the intensity of the incident radiation, dx is the thickness of the material and μ is the material attenuation coefficient. μ mainly consists of contributions from the photoelectric absorption effect and the Compton scattering. If we take the integral on both sides we obtain

$$\int_0^x \frac{dI(x)}{I(x)} \mathrm{d}x = -\int_0^x \mu \mathrm{d}x$$
$$\log I(x) - \log I(0) = -\mu x \ .$$

To solve the logarithms in the equation, we take exponential of both sides. Thus, the equation can be rewritten as

$$I(x) = I(0) \cdot e^{-\mu x} \ .$$

In general, we can define I_0 as the energy of the incident beam and I as the energy after the beam traversed through material with thickness x.

When the ray passes through inhomogeneous objects, factor $\mu(x)$ is the linear attenuation coefficient at each point on the ray path

$$-\ln \frac{I}{I_0} = \int \mu(x) \mathrm{d}x \ . \tag{7.4}$$

However, in practical setups, the emitted X-ray photons have various energies, resulting in polyenergetic energy spectra as shown in Fig. 7.8. The measured intensity of a polychromatic beam I on the detector can be written as the sum of monochromatic contributions for each energy E in the X-ray spectrum ($E \in [0, E_{max}]$). The attenuation coefficient μ is also energy dependent. When polychromatic X-rays are taken into account, we get

$$I = \int_0^{E_{\max}} I_0(E) \exp\left(-\int \mu(x, E) \mathrm{d}x\right) \mathrm{d}E \tag{7.5}$$

where $I_0(E)$ is the normalized energy spectrum, i. e., $\int I_0(E) \mathrm{d}E = 1$.

7.3.2 Photoelectric Effect

The photoelectric effect was originally described by Einstein under the establishment of the quantized nature of light. It describes a situation in which the incident X-ray photon energy is larger than the binding energy of an electron in the target material atom. The incident X-ray photon gives up its entire energy to liberate an electron from an inner-shell. The ejected electron is called photoelectron. The incident photon then ceases to exist. The photoelectric effect often leaves a vacancy in the inner shell of the atom, where the ejected electron was previously located. As a result, the "hole" created in the inner-shell is filled by an outer shell electron. Since the outer shell electron is at a higher energy state, a characteristic radiation occurs. Therefore, the photoelectric effect produces a positive ion, a photoelectron, and a photon of characteristic radiation. For tissue-like materials, the binding energy of the K-shell electrons is very small. Thus, the photoelectron acquires essentially the entire energy of the X-ray photon.

7.3.3 Compton Scattering

The second type of matter interaction is the Compton scattering, which is named after Arthur Holly Compton, who received the Nobel Prize in 1927 for his discovery. For high X-ray energies, Compton scattering is the most dominant interaction mechanism in tissue-like materials. The energy of the incident X-ray photon is considerable higher than the binding energy of the electron. As a result, the incident X-ray photon strikes an electron and ejects the electron from the atom. In Compton scattering, the incoming photon is deflected or scattered through an angle θ with partial loss of its initial energy. The incident photon transfers a portion of its energy to the electron, which is so called "recoil electron", or Compton electron. Therefore, the interaction produces a positive ion, a "recoil electron", and a scattered photon. The scattered photon may be deflected at any angle from 0 to 180 degree. After Compton interaction, most of the energy is retained by the scattered photon, corresponding to a small deflection angle.

7.3.4 Rayleigh scattering

Rayleigh scattering is a coherent process and is the predominant kind of scattering at low X-ray energies. It is caused by an interaction of the incident wave with several, usually outer shell electrons. A very low energy photon interacts with bounded orbital electrons of the atom. No ejection occurs, but the electrons and thus the whole atom is set to vibration with respect to the

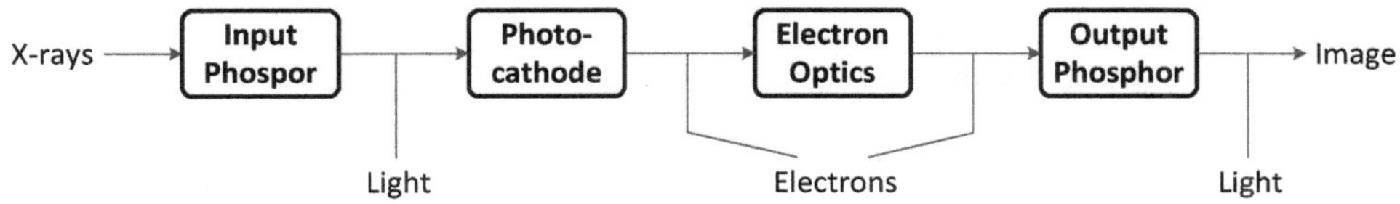

Figure 7.10: Schematic principle of an image intensifier detector. The X-rays are first converted to light, which is converted to electrons. An optic accelerates the electrons towards a fluorescent screen which converts the electrons to light, which eventually results in an image.

incident photon's wavelength. The excess energy from the vibrating electron transfers to an electromagnetic photon which has the same wavelength but possibly a different direction than the incident photon. In this interaction, electrons from the material's atom are not ejected and no energy is converted into kinetic energy, thus, no ionization occurs. Rayleigh scattered photons are mostly emitted in a forward direction with respect to the incident photon's direction. For X-rays used for imaging, the contribution of Rayleigh scattering to total attenuation is usually small compared to other contributions.

7.4 X-ray Imaging

In the previous sections, the concepts of X-ray generation and also their interaction behavior with matter has been outlined. In this section, we will now focus on different detection methods used to convert the X-rays that have passed the patient to an actual image. Unlike the old X-ray films, which use X-rays directly to change the chemical properties of the X-ray film material, the modern detection systems first convert the X-rays to light and eventually to electrons.

7.4.1 Image Intensifiers

X-ray image intensifiers are vacuum tubes that are used to convert X-rays into visible light, i. e., an image. The schematic principle of this process is shown in Fig. 7.10. First, the incoming X-ray photons are converted to light photons using a phosphorus material called the input phosphor. The produced light is further converted to electrons by exploiting the photoelectric effect inside a photocathode. These electrons are then accelerated and focused towards the output phosphor using an electron optic system. In the output phosphor, the electrons are converted back to visible light which can then be captured by film material or television camera tubes.

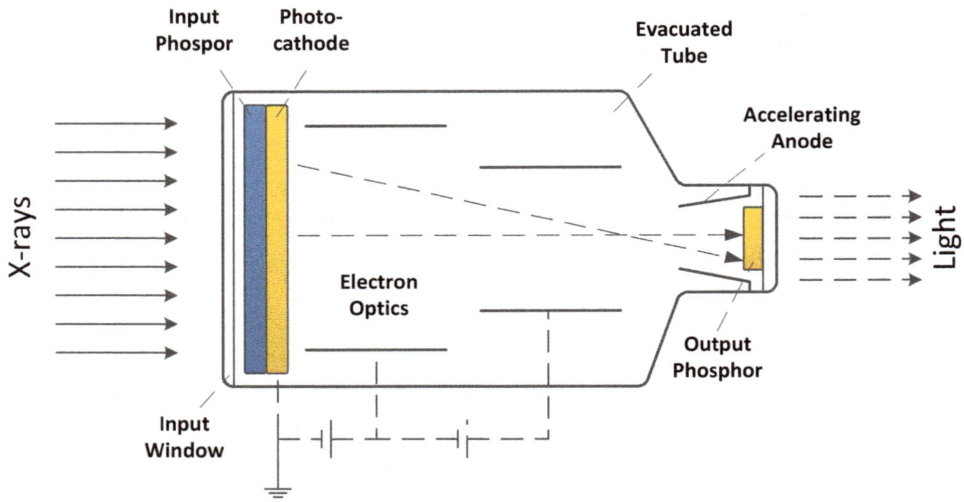

Figure 7.11: Detailed principle of an image intensifier detector. The X-rays are first converted to light, which is converted to electrons. An optic focuses the electron beam to a fluorescent screen or film material which converts the electrons to light, i. e., the image.

Before the introduction of image intensifiers in the late 1940s, fluoroscopic detection system consisted of only one phosphorus material where X-rays have been directly converted to light. However, the mismatch between the high amount of needed X-ray quanta and the low amount of emerging visible light quanta led to very dark images and high radiation exposure. Thus, the radiologists had to view the images in dark surroundings and after a certain time of dark-adaptation of their eyes. The biggest advantage of image intensifier systems is that the brightness of the output image was now adjustable by the amount of acceleration supplied by the electron optics. Modern X-ray image intensifiers have an input field diameter of about 15 to 57 cm. They are characterized by conversion factors that indicate how efficient X-rays are transformed to visible light.

7.4.1.1 Function

A more detailed overview of the individual parts of an image intensifier is given in Fig. 7.11. First the the incoming X-rays pass through the **input window** which typically consists of a convex shaped aluminum plate with a thickness of a approximately 1 mm. The convex shape is used to enhance mechanical stability but also to reduce the distance to the patient which effectively increases the useful entrance field size.

After passing through the input window, the X-rays hit the **input phosphor** used to convert X-ray photons to light photons. The generated light photons trigger a photoelectric effect in the **photocathode** which then emits (photo-)electrons. The input phosphor and the photocathode are typically layered to one piece. Starting with the input phosphor that consists of another aluminum plate coated with the phosphor layer, followed by an intermediate layer and the photocathode layer.

Let us focus on the input phosphor layer in more detail. One important property that influences the efficiency of the input phosphor layer is its thickness. The thicker the phosphor layer, the higher is its absorption, thus, more X-ray photons are absorbed and converted to light. Hence, less X-ray photons are required which reduces radiation exposure to the patient. However, with increasing thickness also more light photons become scattered within the phosphor layer which effectively reduces the spatial resolution.

Another property that is used to increase conversion factors is the chemical composition of the input phosphor material and its resulting mass attenuation coefficient. Ideally, the input phosphor's attenuation coefficient is adjusted to the residual incoming X-ray spectrum. Initially, zinc-cadmium sulfide (ZnCdS) has been used as phosphoric material, which has been replaced by cesium iodide (CsI) in modern detector systems. The advantages of CsI over ZnCdS are twofold. In Fig. 7.12 we illustrate the mass attenuation coefficient of CsI (dashed, dark blue line) and ZnCdS (dotted, light blue line) w. r. t. the photon energy. Additionally, the estimated spectral distribution of a typical X-ray spectrum after transmission through the patient is depicted as solid, orange line. The higher the overlapping area between attenuation characteristics and residual X-ray spectrum, the better its conversion efficiency. We can clearly see that the mass attenuation coefficient of CsI matches better to the expected residual X-ray spectrum and is thus favorable.

Additionally, the manufacturing process of CsI allows to build the phosphor layer as a collection of small and local cylindrical structures as indicated in Fig. 7.14. The cylindrical wires act as optical fibers which can steer the emitted light to the photocathode with a high spatial accuracy. Thus, scattering of the light photons within the phosphor material can be drastically reduced. In modern detectors, the input phosphor is about 300 µm to 500 µm thick and can absorb up to 70 % of the incoming X-ray photons. A single 60 keV X-ray photon can create up to 2600 light photons, where approximately 62 % reach the photocathode.

The **photocathode** layer typically consists of antimony-cesium ($SbCs_3$). Similar to the input photon layer, the incoming light should fit to the sensitivity spectrum given by the photocathode. Fig. 7.13 shows the sensitivity spectrum of an $SbCs_3$ photocathode, together with the characteristic light spectra emitted from a CsI as well as a ZnCdS phospor layer. We can see that also here CsI seems to produce a light spectrum that matches better to the photocathode, hence, leading to a higher conversion efficiency from light photons to electrons.

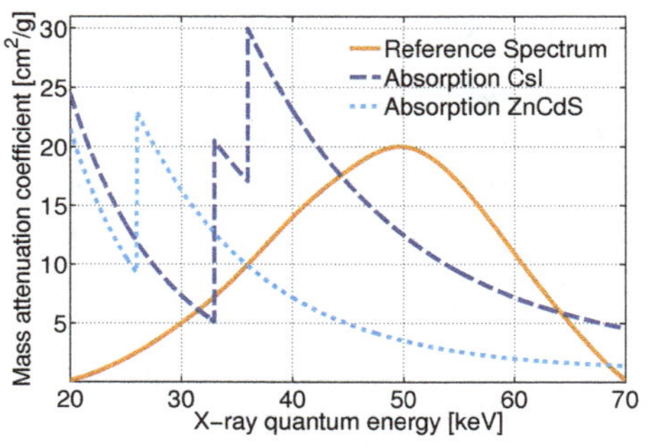

Figure 7.12: Mass attenuation coefficient of CsI and ZnCdS and the estimated X-ray spectrum after transmission through the patient.

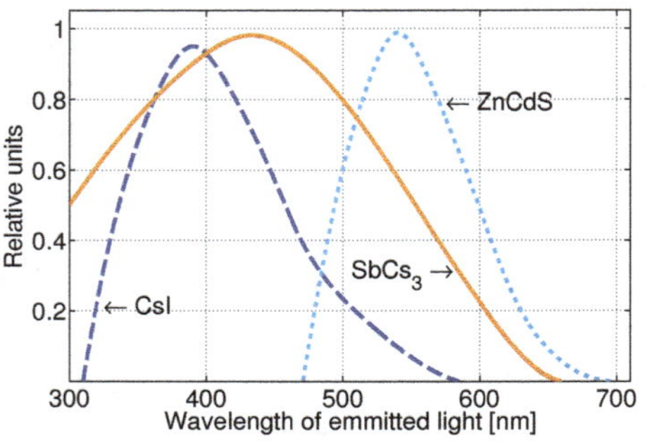

Figure 7.13: Sensitivity of an $SbCs_3$ photocathode and characteristic light spectra emitted from a CsI as well as a ZnCdS phospor layer.

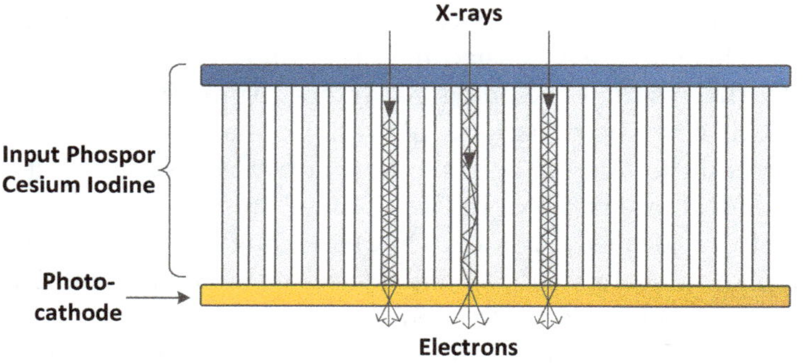

Figure 7.14: Cesium-iodine layer has cylindrical structure and acts as optical fibers. Thus, the scattering of the light photons is reduced significantly.

After the electrons leave the photocathode, they are accellerated by the **anode** as shown in Fig. 7.11. Moreover, the accelerated electrons are focused onto the output phosphor using electrostatic fields produced by the **electron optic**. No additional electrons are induced into the system by this process, the existing electrons are merely accelerated and deflected. The increase of kinetic energy that originates of the acceleration process results in a higher number of light photons that are emitted when the electrons hit the **output phosphor**. Hence, the intensity or brightness of the output phosphor can be altered by a regulation of the acceleration voltage. The output phosphor consists typically of silver-activated zinc-cadmium sulfide (ZnCdS:Ag) and is very thin (4 µm to 8 µm). About 2000 light photons are generated for a single 25 keV electron. Due to the fact that one electron is emitted by one light photon in the photocathode, this also represents an increased brightness by a factor of 2000.

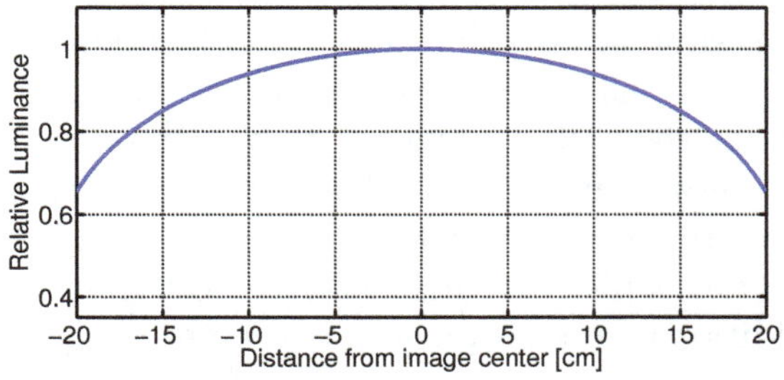

Figure 7.15: Vignetting artifact, i. e., luminescence drops at image periphery.

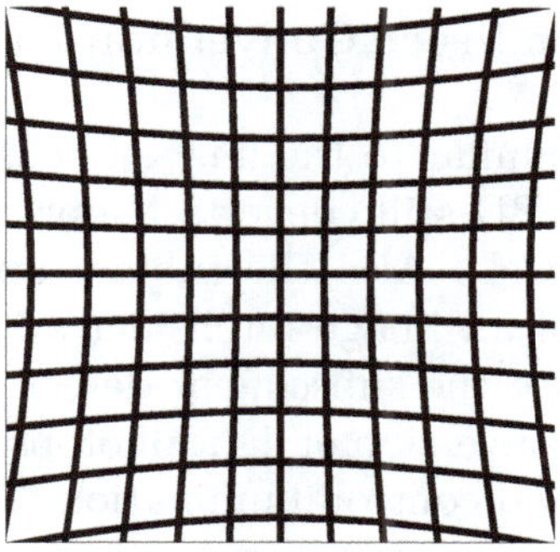

Figure 7.16: Distortion artifacts due to external electric or magnetic field.

7.4.1.2 Known Problems

Besides common limitations that all imaging systems share, e. g., spatial resolution and contrast ratio, image intensifier systems are most known for vignetting and distortion artifacts. Vignetting, as described in Fig. 7.15, describes a drop in brightness that occurs at the outer parts of the screen. It is caused by light scattering that deflects light photons in the output phosphor from the outer part of the phosphor to the inside. However, no scattering occurs from completely outside the material to the outer regions of the phosphor, yielding an increased brightness at the central regions. Another common artifact is image distortion as indicated in Fig. 7.16. It is known that the electron optics of image intensifiers is susceptible to external magnetic or electric fields. Even the earth's magnetic field causes considerable distortions in the output image. To correct for distortion artifacts, regular calibration is needed where the distortion field is estimated by measuring predefined calibration objects. The distortion can be corrected by either adjusting the electron optics accordingly or by subsequent image processing in case the images have been digitized.

7.4.2 Flat Panel Detectors

In the recent years, flat panel detector (FPD) became the state-of-the-art in X-ray detector technology for radiography, angiography, and C-arm CT applications. They were first introduced in the mid 1990s and their main advantages are a direct digital readout of the X-ray image and an increased spatial resolution. Flat panel detectors can be categorized into direct and indirectly conversion FPDs.

Indirect Conversion FPDs

Similar to the image intensifier system discussed in the previous section, the FPD still converts X-rays to light photons by using a layer of cesium iodide (CsI). Also the tubular structure of the CsI is identical to the input layer of an image intensifier system as shown in Fig. 7.14. The major difference are the subsequent detection steps. Image intensifiers make use of a further conversion of light photons to electrons which are then accelerated to increase and control illumination. This additional conversion step is not necessary for flat panel detectors. Instead a matrix of photodiodes is directly attached to the CsI layer and converts the emitted light photons to an electric charge which is then stored in capacitors for each pixel. Each pixel also contains a thin-film transistor (TFT) which acts as small "switch" used for the readout of the stored charges.

Direct Conversion FPDs

Instead of an explicit conversion to light photons, direct conversion FPDs have a homogeneous layer of X-ray sensitive photoconducters on the TFT matrix. The top layer is a high-voltage bias electrode that builds an electric field across the photoconductor. If X-rays are absorbed by the photoconductor, so called charge-carriers are released, i. e., electron-hole pairs. These pairs are then separated to negative and positive charges and transported to the pixel's electrodes by the global electric field. Positive charges travel to the bottom of the individual pixel electrodes where they are stored in capacitors.

Data Readout and Properties

For both the indirect but also the direct conversion FPDs, the readout of the pixels is done row-wise using a certain readout frequency. A row is selected by "switching on" the TFTs of this row's pixels, i. e., by applying a voltage to the gate of the TFTs. The stored charges of each pixel are directed to a charge integrating amplifier and subsequently converted to a digital representation. These digital pixel values are serialized and transferred over a bus system to the imaging computer. Common FPDs for medical imaging can have a side length of up to 40 cm and a pixel size of about 100 µm to 150 µm. They are available in quadratic but also in wide formats. The analog to digital conversion uses a quantization of 12 to 16 Bit. To increase the signal to noise ratio multiple pixels are often combined to a bigger pixel during the readout process, which is also known as binning. Typical binning modes are 2x2 or 4x4 binning, reducing the image size by a factor of 2 or 4, respectively. Because binning does not require any additional time, the frame rate increases by the binning factor. Frame rates typically vary between 7.5 and 30 frames per second, depending on the medical application, dose requirements, and binning factors.

Major advantages of flat panel detectors are a significant reduction of space and weight needed for the detection unit. This may sound trivial but the benefit becomes more clear when we consider that space is typically limited, especially in an interventional environment and that increased weight is directly related to rotation speeds of CT or C-arm CT devices. Another advantage is the robustness against (moderate) electrical and magnetic fields, which posed a huge problem for image intensifiers. Moreover, the images are directly available in digital form, which makes patient handling and data storage more efficient.

7.4.3 Sources of Noise

There are two types of undesirable effects in medical imaging systems: probabilistic noise and artifacts. Similar to noise, artifacts are image degradations that also find their source in physical effects during the scan. However, the difference to noise is that when a scan is repeated using the exact same object and scan parameters, artifacts are reproduced exactly whereas noise effects will change based on a probabilistic scheme. Some artifacts, for example, distortion and vignetting, have already been shown in the section Sec. 7.4.1 on image intensifier detectors. In the following, we focus on the sources and propagation of noise in X-ray imaging.

As illustrated in Fig. 7.17, there are different states of an X-ray photon. Each step in this chain follows either a Poisson distribution (cf. Geek Box 7.3) or a binomial distribution (cf. Geek Box 7.4). In Fig. 7.18, we show both distributions in comparison. The X-ray photon generation process (cf. Geek Box 7.5) follows a Poission distribution. The matter interaction and the detection step (cf. Geek Box 7.6) follow a binomial distribution. Both processes interact along the path of the X-ray (cf. Geek Box 7.7) resulting in yet another Poisson distribution. As such Lambert-Beer's law also has a probabilistic interpretation (cf. Geek Box 7.8) and every observation on the detector is Poisson distributed in the monochromatic case.

A common quality measure for imaging is the signal-to-noise ratio (SNR). It is not uniquely defined over different fields of applications. In X-ray imaging it makes sense to use the definition based on statistics, i. e.,

$$SNR(\mathcal{N}) = \frac{\bar{n}}{\sigma} = \frac{E(\mathcal{N})}{\sqrt{E((\mathcal{N} - \bar{n})^2)}} \ . \tag{7.6}$$

For random variables $\mathcal{N}$ that follow a normal distribution, $\bar{n}$ is the mean value and σ represents the standard deviation. More generally speaking, the two variables define the first moment ($\bar{n}$) and the second central moment (σ)

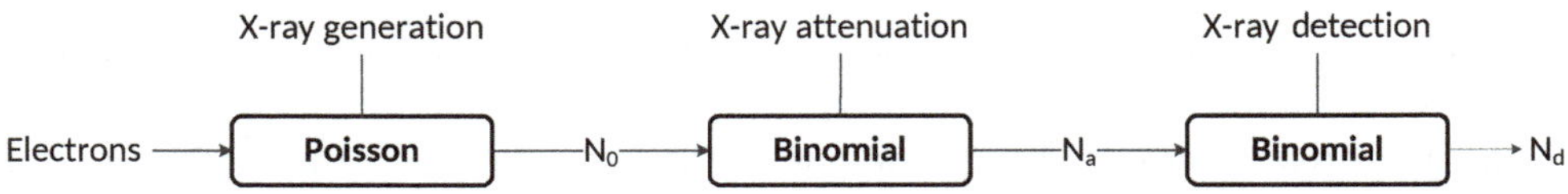

Figure 7.17: Overview of noise related processes in X-ray imaging.

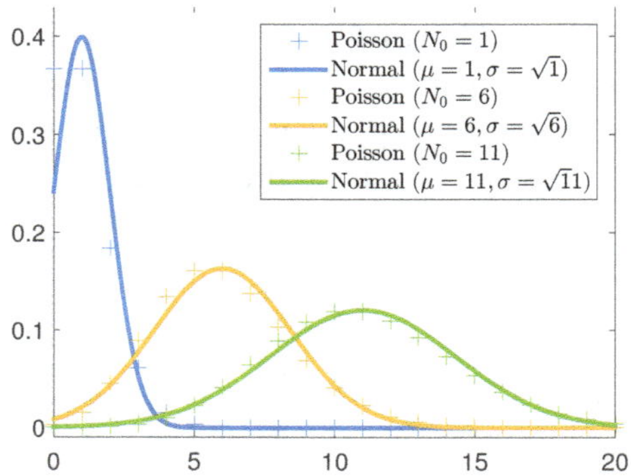

(a) Mass distribution functions of Poisson distributions with varying expectation value N_0, plus their Gaussian counterparts.

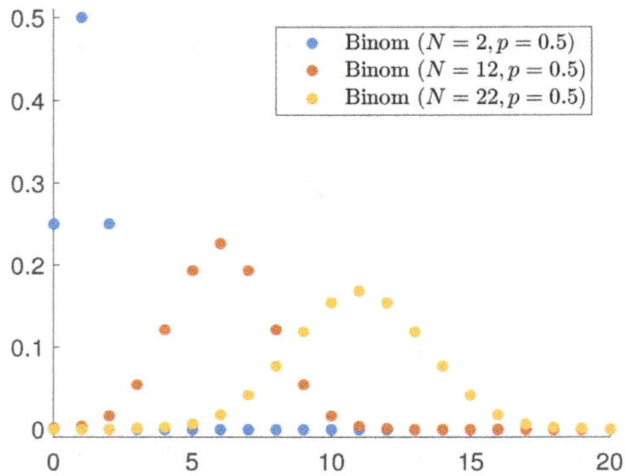

(b) Mass distribution functions of binomial distributions with varying number of trials N and fixed probability $p = 0.5$.

Figure 7.18: Mass distribution functions of Poisson and binomial distributions.

of the underlying distribution. The first moment of the Poisson distribution is given by its expectation value $\bar{n} = E(\mathcal{N})$, whereas the second central moment is the square root of the expectation value of the squared difference between the random variable and its expectation value $\sigma = \sqrt{E((\mathcal{N} - \bar{n})^2)}$. Hence, no matter what distribution, σ provides a measure of variation, i. e., a measure of noise. As a result, the SNR gives a measure for the signal quality by dividing the expectation value with the second central moment. If the measured data would not contain any noise, σ would be zero and the SNR would approach infinity. If the noise level increases, also σ increases, thus the SNR decreases. The expectation value $\bar{n}$ in the numerator makes the SNR stable to scaling, that means if we measure very high values at the detector a small amount of noise is less critical as if we measure small values that contain the same amount of noise. For X-rays, we can demonstrate that the $SNR(\mathcal{N}) \propto \sqrt{N_0}$ (cf. Geek Box 7.9). As a consequence, SNR only doubles if we use four times as many photons for N_0. Note this estimation is simplified and neglects some effects such as detector read-out noise.

Geek Box 7.3: Poisson Distribution

The Poisson distribution is a discrete probability distribution and its mass distribution function is defined by

$$\text{Poisson}(N_0) = p(\mathcal{N} = n) = \frac{(N_0)^n}{n!} e^{-N_0} \ , \qquad (7.7)$$

where N_0 is the expectation value of the observed event $E(\mathcal{N})$. We now show a simple example for the usage of the Poisson distribution. Assume a local shop records its daily number of customers for a year which results in an average of $N_0 = 15$ customers per day. The Poisson distribution can now be used to calculate the probability that on a new day there will be $n = 20$ customers in the shop, i. e., $p(\mathcal{N} = 20) = \frac{(N_0)^n}{n!} e^{-N_0} = \frac{15^{20}}{20!} e^{-15} \approx 0.0418$. In Fig. 7.18(a), the mass distribution function as defined in Eq. (7.7) is shown for three different expectation values N_0. If the number of N_0 becomes high, the Poisson distribution approaches a normal distribution with mean $\bar{n} = N_0$ and standard deviation $\sigma = \sqrt{N_0}$. This is based on the so called "central limit theorem". In Fig. 7.18(a), we have also added the corresponding mass distribution functions for each Poisson distribution. You can clearly see that the higher N_0, the closer the discrete Poisson distribution gets to a normal distribution.

7.5 X-ray Applications

7.5.1 Radiography

Radiography describes the process of creating two dimensional projection images by exposing an anatomy of interest to X-rays and measuring the attenuation they undergo when passing through the object. It is a very common form of X-ray imaging and is used in clinics around the globe.

The main application area is the examination of fractures and changes of the skeletal system. Here, the high attenuation coefficient of bones compared to the surrounding tissue delivers a good contrast and allows for distinct detection and classification of fractures. Moreover, radiography can be used to detect changes of a bone's consistency or density, e. g., in case of osteoporosis or bone cancer. In Fig. 7.19, two X-ray images of an arm with fractures of Ulna and Radius bones are shown on the left. Furthermore, the figure shows a color image taken from the arm after intervention and also two further X-ray images of the treated arm where the bones have been internally fixated using metal plates.

Geek Box 7.4: Binomial Distribution

The binomial distribution is also a discrete distribution and can be used to model a series of Bernoulli trials, i. e., a series of random experiments with binary outcome. The mass distribution function is given by

$$p(\mathcal{N}=n) = \binom{N}{n} p^n \, (1-p)^{N-n} = \frac{N!}{n! \, (N-n)!} \, p^n \, (1-p)^{N-n} \ . \quad (7.8)$$

It describes the probability that exactly n positive outcomes occur in a series of N independent trials, where p denotes the probability for an individual trial having a positive outcome. The most intuitive example for a binomial distribution is coin tossing. From coin tossing we know that the probability of getting head or tails in a single toss is "fifty-fifty", i. e., $p = 0.5$. If we now want to know the probability to get exactly $n = 20$ times heads when you toss the coin $N = 30$ times, $p(\mathcal{N} = 20) = \binom{N}{n} p^n \, (1-p)^{N-n} = \frac{30!}{20! \, (30-20)!} \, (0.5)^{20} \, (1-0.5)^{30-20} \approx 0.028$. In Fig. 7.18(b), three cases of a binomial mass distribution function are shown for a varying number of trials N. The probability of a single trial being true was fixed with $p = 0.5$.

Geek Box 7.5: Statistics of the X-ray Generation Process

How is the Poisson distribution related to X-ray imaging? It can be shown that the number of generated X-ray photons at the anode is Poisson distributed. As input parameters we have the number of accelerated fast electrons N_e and the probability for one fast electron being converted to an X-ray photon p_{ex}. The distribution is then given by

$$\begin{aligned} N_0 &= N_e \, p_{ex} \\ P(\mathcal{N}=n) &= \frac{(N_e \, p_{ex})^n}{n!} \, e^{-N_e \, p_{ex}} \ , \end{aligned} \quad (7.9)$$

where N_0 denotes the expected value for the number of electrons that trigger an X-ray photon, which is also known as a measure for the radiation intensity. We use $P(N_x)$ as the probability that an X-ray source produces exactly N_x X-ray photons. $P(N_x)$ is then given by above equation, where n has been replaced by N_x.

Geek Box 7.6: Statistics of the X-ray Matter Interaction

The generated X-ray photons are now traveling through space towards the detector and interact with the matter they pass through according to Beer's law as introduced in Eq. (7.3). Whether the photons interact with the matter or pass through it unaffected can be interpreted as Bernoulli trial, i. e., an experiment with random binary outcome. If a single photon encounters an interaction depends on the material properties along the photons path, i. e., the attenuation $\mu(x)$. The probability p_a for the photon passing unaffected is again given by Beer's law:

$$p_a = e^{-\int \mu(x) \mathrm{d}x} \quad . \tag{7.10}$$

As the individual X-ray photons are independent from each other in terms of interacting or not, the process can be described as a binomial distribution. Furthermore, it can be shown that when we have a Poisson distributed variable (N_x) that represents the number of samples in a binomial distribution, the outcome is again Poisson distributed. We refer to Geek Box 7.7 for further information.

Geek Box 7.7: Combining Poisson and Binomial Distribution

As the individual X-ray photons are independent from each other in terms of interacting or not, the process can be described as a binomial distribution

$$\begin{aligned} P(\mathcal{N} = n_s) &= \sum_{N_x = n_s}^{\infty} P(N_x) \cdot P(n_s | N_x) \\ &= \sum_{N_x = n_s}^{\infty} \frac{(N_0)^{N_x}}{N_x!} e^{-N_0} \cdot \binom{N_x}{n_s} p_a^{n_s} (1 - p_a)^{N_x - n_s} \quad , \\ &= \frac{(N_0 \, p_a)^{n_s}}{n_s!} e^{-N_0 p_a} \end{aligned}$$

where N_x is the number of X-ray photons, n_s is the number of photons that pass through the object unaffected, $P(N_x)$ is the probability that the X-ray generation produces N_x photons and $P(n_s|N_x)$ is the conditional probability that models the number of unaffected photons, given the number of input photons. The sum comes from the "Law of Total Probability" and is necessary to eliminate the conditional probability. $P(\mathcal{N} = n_s)$ now gives the overall probability that n_s photons will arrive at the detector after having passed the object. We refer to [1, p. 65] for a detailed derivation.

Geek Box 7.8: Probabilistic Lambert-Beer Law

The resulting distribution for the number of photons after matter interaction is thus given by

$$P(\mathcal{N} = n_s) = \frac{(N_0\, p_a)^{n_s}}{n_s!}\, e^{-N_0 p_a} \quad , \tag{7.11}$$

where n_s is the number of photons that pass through the matter unaffected. We can also determine the expectation value of this Poisson distribution, i. e.,

$$E[n_s] = N_0\, p_a = N_0\, e^{-\int \mu(x)\mathrm{d}x} \quad . \tag{7.12}$$

Hence, the expectation value as given by Eq. (7.12) is again Lambert-Beer's law which was introduced in Sec. 7.3.
Note that each process that now follows in the X-ray detection step can also be modeled or at least approximated by a binomial distribution. This holds for the conversion of X-ray photons to light photons in scintillator based detectors, for the subsequent conversion of light photons to electrons but also for the conversion of X-ray's to electrical charges in direct conversion flat panel detectors. Each of these steps yields another Poisson distribution for the number of outgoing photons or electrons, hence also the final value at the end of the detection step follows a Poisson distribution. This observation is crucial, as it tells us that all of the measurements that we get from our detection system follow Poisson distributions including its behavior regarding noise which will be discussed next.

7.5.2 Fluoroscopy

Conventional radiography typically refers to the acquisition of a single or small number of X-ray projection images for a specified view. In contrast, fluoroscopy describes a sequence of radiographic images acquired periodically at a certain frame rate. The X-ray source can either be triggered for each frame or simply provide a constant radiation exposure to the region of interest. Potential X-ray detectors can be image intensifiers (see Sec. 7.4.1) or the newer FPDs (see Sec. 7.4.2). The frame rate is typically limited by the acquisition speed of the detection system. For image intensifiers, it is given by the inertia of the final fluorescent screen, whereas for FPDs it is determined by the speed of the electronic detector readout step. In practice, frame rates of 30 frames per second are possible. However, rates are often reduced for dose reasons.

Geek Box 7.9: Signal to Noise Ratio for X-rays

Let us focus on the distribution for the number of photons that arrive at the detector, i. e., n_s. The distribution is given by Eq. (7.11). From Poisson statistics we know that the expectation value is the only parameter of the mass distribution function, which was already computed in Eq. (7.12), hence, $\bar{n} = N_0\, p_a$. Further, it can be shown that the variance (σ^2) of a Poisson distribution is equal to the expectation value, i. e., $\sigma^2 = N_0\, p_a$. The SNR after photon interaction with the object can then be computed by

$$\begin{aligned} SNR(\mathcal{N}) &= \frac{N_0\, p_a}{\sqrt{N_0\, p_a}} \\ &= \sqrt{N_0\, p_a} \qquad (7.13) \\ &= \sqrt{N_0}\; e^{-\frac{1}{2}\int \mu(x)\mathrm{d}x} \;. \end{aligned}$$

Above equation shows us that the SNR of an X-ray imaging system of course depends on the object, represented by $e^{-\frac{1}{2}\int \mu(x)\mathrm{d}x}$ and also on the number of generated photons at the source N_0. The SNR is proportional to the square root of the number of emitted X-ray photons, hence increasing the number of photons also increases the SNR. However, a higher number of photons also means a higher dose level for the patient which is often the limiting factor and gives an upper bound for the SNR.

Fluoroscopy is of special importance in minimally invasive interventions, where catheters, endoscopes, and other tools need to be guided and operated without direct visual contact to the region where the actual intervention takes place. It is also the key technology for visualizing vessels such as arteries or veins by the use of contrast agent, as described in the following section. In Fig. 7.20(a), an example image from a fluoroscopy sequence is depicted that shows the placement of the two electrodes and wires of a heart pacemaker. A typical clinical setup for a minimally invasive surgery is shown in Fig. 7.20(b), where the X-ray imaging unit is given by a C-arm scanner that can be freely positioned around the patient.

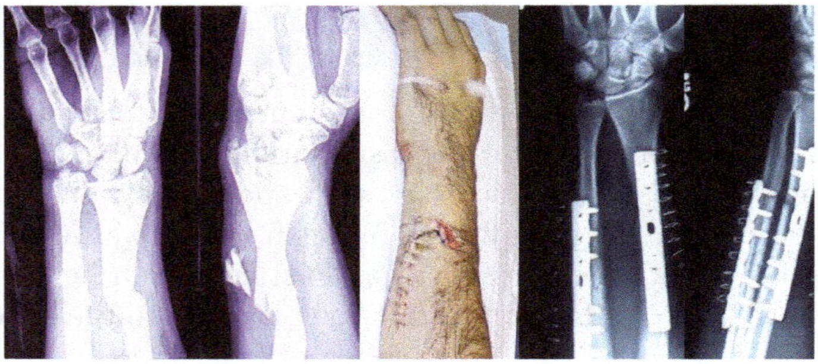

Figure 7.19: Arm showing fractures in radiographic images, the corresponding color image after surgery and the radiographic images after fixation of the bones using metal rods. Image is in public domain and was taken from [11].

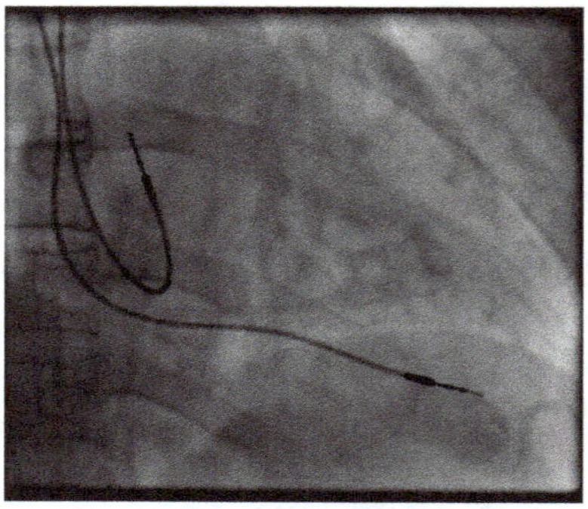

(a) Pacemaker Fluroscopy. Image taken from [5].

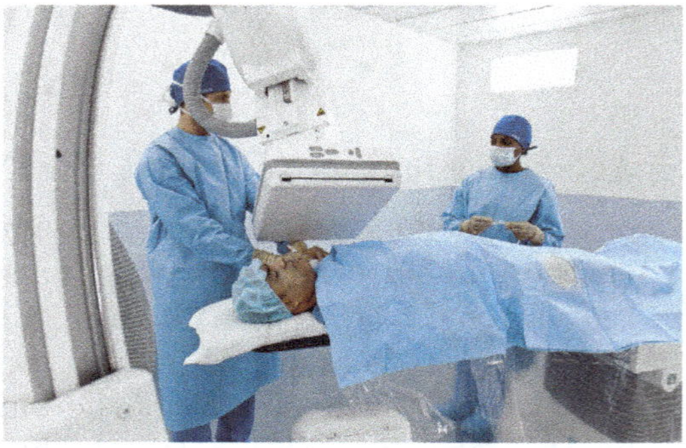

(b) Clinical Setup. Image courtesy of Siemens Healthineers AG.

Figure 7.20: Left: Image from a fluoroscopy sequence showing the placement of two electrodes of a pacemaker. Right: Typical clinical setup of a minimally invasive surgery. The fluoroscopy is acquired using a freely positionable C-arm device. The image shows the X-ray source at the bottom and the FPD is right above the patient.

7.5.3 Digital Subtraction Angiography

Angiography refers to the imaging of arteries (venography for veins) to analyze properties such as shape, size, lumen, or flow rate. Usually, the attenuation properties of vessels do not substantially differ from that of the surrounding tissue which makes X-ray-based imaging hard and yields poor contrast.

To increase image quality and contrast often contrast agent is injected into the blood circulation. Contrast agent is a liquid that provides an increased attenuation coefficient compared to normal soft tissue. Typical contrast media

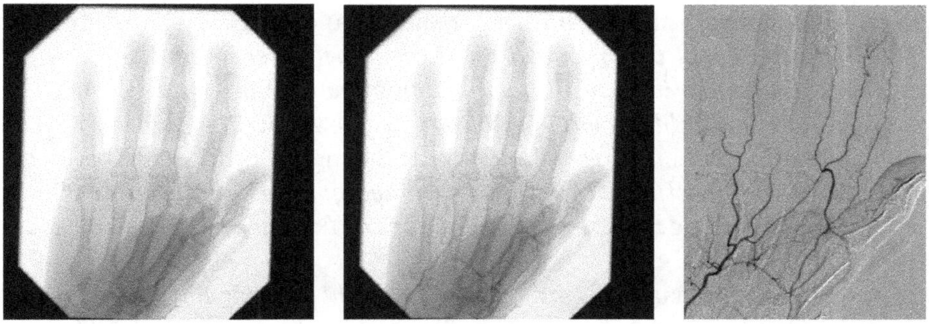

(a) Mask Image (b) Fill Image (c) Angiogram

Figure 7.21: Process of creating a DSA. In (a) the hand was imaged and no contrast agent has been injected (mask image). In (b) the same hand has been imaged but including injected contrast agent. The difference of (b) and (a) represents the angiogram as shown in Figure (c). Images provided by Adam Galant, Siemens Healthineers AG.

are iodine and barium, where the first is used for intravascular and the latter for gastrointestinal examinations. Thus, iodine is injected into the blood circulation whereas barium can be swallowed to investigate, e. g., the stomach or colon.

In DSA, a fluroscopic sequence of a fixed anatomy is acquired. At the same time contrast agent is injected in regular intervals into the vessel system. X-ray images that have acquired the scene without contrast agent are assumed to show the background tissue that is typically not of interest. If we now subtract the initially acquired background image from an X-ray image with contrast and assume that no patient motion has taken place, we can measure the attenuation caused only by the injected contrast agent. As the contrast agent is limited to the vessel system, it has been injected to, the outcome of such a subtraction will be a visualization of the vessels only. In Fig. 7.21, an example for a DSA acquisition is presented. First the contrast agent free image, i. e., the mask image, is acquired as shown in Fig. 7.21(a). Then contrast is injected into the vascular system and after some waiting a further image, i. e., the fill image, is acquired. The difference of both images is then the so called angiogram that shows only the contributions given by the contrast agent and thus the vessels are visualized (cf. Fig. 7.21(c)).

Further Readings

[1] Thorsten M. Buzug. *Computed Tomography: From Photon Statistics to Modern Cone-Beam CT.* Berlin, Germany: Springer, 2008, p. 536. ISBN: 3642072577.

[2] PM De Groot. "Image intensifier design and specifications". In: *Proc. Summer School on Specification, Acceptance Testing and Quality Control of Diagnostic X-ray Imaging Equipment* (1994), pp. 429–60.

[3] Olaf Dössel. *Bildgebende Verfahren in der Medizin - Von der Technik zur medizinischen Anwendung*. Vol. 1. Springer Berlin Heidelberg, 2000.

[4] Jeff Fessler. *Lecture Notes / X-ray imaging: noise and SNR*. 2009. URL: http://web.eecs.umich.edu/~fessler/course/516/l/c6-noise.pdf.

[5] Steven Fruitsmaak. *Right atrial and right ventricular leads as visualized under X-ray during a pacemaker implant procedure. The atrial lead is the curved one making a U shape in the upper left part of the figure.* 2008. URL: http://commons.wikimedia.org/wiki/File:Fluoroscopy_pacemaker_leads_right_atrium_ventricle.png (visited on 11/04/2014).

[6] Erich Krestel. "Imaging systems for medical diagnostics". In: (1980).

[7] Benedikt Lorch et al. "Projection and Reconstruction-Based Noise Filtering Methods in Cone Beam CT". In: *Bildverarbeitung für die Medizin 2015*. Ed. by H. Handels. Lübeck, 2015, pp. 59–64.

[8] Andreas Maier and Rebecca Fahrig. "GPU Denoising for Computed Tomography". In: *Graphics Processing Unit-Based High Performance Computing in Radiation Therapy*. Ed. by Xun Jia and Jiang Steve. 1st ed. Vol. 1. Boca Raton, Florida, USA, 2015. ISBN: 978-1-4822-4478-6. DOI: 10.1201/b18968-9.

[9] Andreas Maier et al. "Three-dimensional anisotropic adaptive filtering of projection data for noise reduction in cone beam CT". In: *Medical Physics* 38.11 (2011), pp. 5896–5909. DOI: 10.1118/1.3633901.

[10] Jihong Wang and Timothy J. Blackburn. "The AAPM/RSNA Physics Tutorial for Residents". In: *RadioGraphics* 20.5 (2000), pp. 1471–1477.

[11] Wikimedia. *Broken fixed arm*. 2006. URL: http://en.wikipedia.org/wiki/Bone_fracture#mediaviewer/File:Broken_fixed_arm.jpg (visited on 11/04/2014).

[12] Wei Zhao and JA Rowlands. "X-ray imaging using amorphous selenium: Feasibility of a flat panel self-scanned detector for digital radiology". In: *Medical Physics* 22.10 (1995), pp. 1595–1604.

8

Medical Imaging: CT

Authors: Oliver Taubmann, Martin Berger, Marco B¨ogel,
Yan Xia, Michael Balda and Andreas Maier

8.1 Introduction

CT is doubtlessly one of the most important technologies in medical imaging and offers us views inside the human body that are as valuable to physicians as they are fascinating (cf. Fig. 8.1).

8.1.1 Motivation

In the previous chapter, we have seen how X-rays can be used to acquire 2-D projection images. However, a single projection image does not retain all spatial information, as it merely shows something akin to "shadows" of the imaged objects. An example is given in Fig. 8.3(a), which shows an X-ray projection image of a luggage bag. Two arrows indicate objects that cannot easily be identified. Using multiple projection images from different angles, we

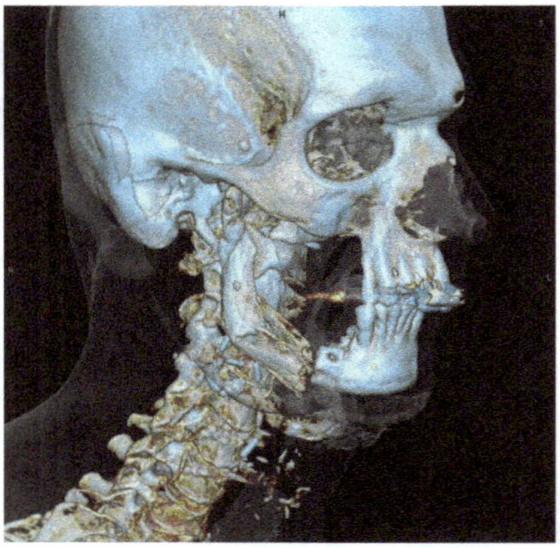

Figure 8.1: Volume rendering of a CT head scan. Image courtesy of Siemens Healthineers AG.

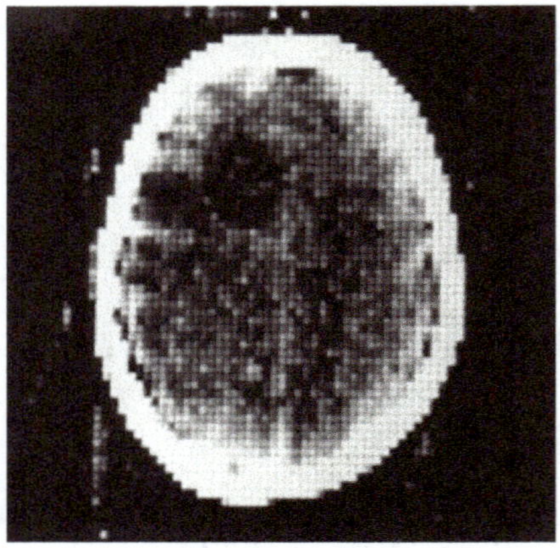

Figure 8.2: The first clinical CT scan, acquired October 1971 at Atkinson Morley's Hospital in London.

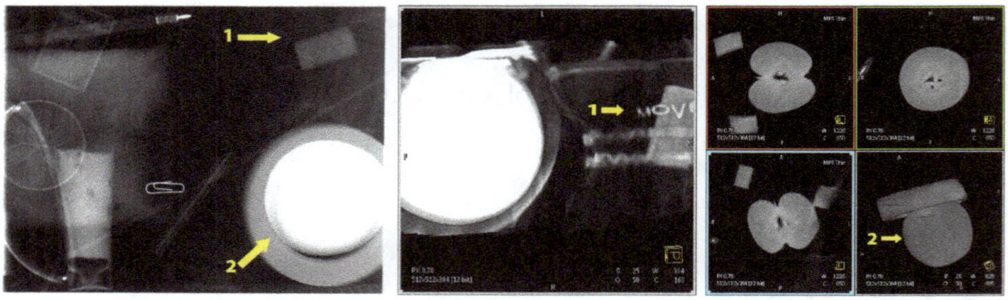

(a) (b) (c)

Figure 8.3: 2-D X-ray projection image of a luggage bag **(a)** and a corresponding 3-D reconstruction, visualized with a volume rendering technique and **(b, c)** and as orthogonal cross-sectional slices **(c)**. 1) Indicates a hidden text revealed in **(b)** and 2) an apple that is virtually sliced in **(c)**. Images courtesy of Chris Schwemmer.

are able to perform a 3-D reconstruction and obtain cross-sectional views of the objects. Looking at the reconstructed volume, we can read the letters on the bag (Fig. 8.3(b)) and recognize the bright object as an apple (Fig. 8.3(c)).

8.1.2 Brief History

In 1917, Johann Radon published an article about "the determination of functions by their integrals along certain manifolds," which would not find a practical application for the following 50 years. The main concepts introduced in his article will be outlined in Sec. 8.2 and used in Sec. 8.3 to explain how CT image reconstruction works.

Only in 1971, the first CT system was built by Sir Godfrey Newbold Hounsfield and Allan McLeod Cormack[1]. Fig. 8.2 shows the result of the first clinical scan of a patient's head performed in the same year. For their seminal invention, they received the Nobel prize in medicine in 1979.

A major advance in the field was the introduction of spiral (or, more accurately, helical) CT by Willi Kalender et al. in 1990. Its name is derived from the novel aspect of its acquisition trajectory describing a helix. Amongst others, this geometry and its advantages will be described in Sec. 8.3.3.

In the early days of CT imaging, data acquisition was fairly slow, taking approximately 4 minutes per rotation. The reconstruction of a single 2-D slice with a low spatial resolution of 80×80 pixels and 3 bit quantization took several hours. By 2002, rotation speed had improved drastically with one rotation performed in only 0.4 seconds. Up to 16 slices in parallel could be reconstructed on-the-fly, at a higher resolution of 512×512 pixels and a quantization depth of 16 bit.

In recent years, this trend continued with temporal and spatial resolutions constantly improving. In this context, the development of dual source CT in 2005 was another significant milestone, featuring two X-ray sources and detectors in a single scanner. In addition to offering additional information when both employed X-ray tubes are operated at different voltages (dual energy scan), it can also be used to speed up the acquisition significantly. The amount of slices acquired in parallel had also increased further, covering a field of view measuring up to 16 cm in axial direction at voxel sizes below one millimeter. This allows imaging of complete organs such as the heart in a single rotation, thus reducing motion artifacts.

In 2014, a modern CT system (cf. Fig. 8.4) was able to acquire up to 128 slices in parallel at a temporal resolution as low as 195 ms with a single X-ray source.

8.2 Mathematical Principles

In this section, we will first introduce the Radon transform as the underlying mathematical principle of the image formation process in CT imaging. Inverting this transform is the fundamental problem solved by image reconstruction methods. Subsequently, we will detail the Fourier slice theorem, a

[1] Both researchers were working for EMI at the time, a British music recording and publishing company well known for housing the Beatles' label. This has spawned a widespread belief that the Beatles' success contributed to financing the initial development of CT.

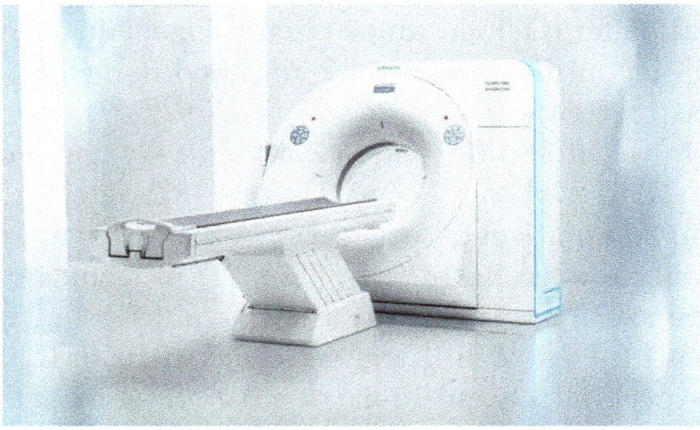

Figure 8.4: At the time of writing, a modern CT scanner can acquire up to 128 image slices in parallel. Image courtesy of Siemens Healthineers AG.

property related to the Radon transform that constitutes the core idea of an important class of reconstruction algorithms.

8.2.1 Radon Transform

Radon's key insight was that any integrable function $f(x, y)$ can be uniquely represented by – and therefore recovered from – all straight line integrals over its domain,

$$p(\ell) = \int_{-\infty}^{+\infty} f(x(l), y(l)) \, \mathrm{d}l, \quad \forall l : (x(l), y(l))^\top \in \text{line } \ell \tag{8.1}$$

In order to write down all of these integrals without duplicates, a representation of the lines is needed that describes each one uniquely. For this purpose, we can formulate Eq. (8.1) in terms of polar coordinates,

$$p(\theta, s) = \iint_{-\infty}^{+\infty} f(x, y) \delta(x \cos\theta + y \sin\theta - s) \, \mathrm{d}x\mathrm{d}y, \tag{8.2}$$

with θ the angle between the line's normal vector and the x-axis and s the orthogonal distance between line and origin (cf. Fig. 8.5). Implicitly, this line is described by the equation $x \cos\theta + y \sin\theta = s$. Only those points that satisfy it, i. e., those that fall on the line, are selected by the Dirac function δ in Eq. (8.2), as it vanishes everywhere else (cf. Eq. (2.10)). In that way, the integration of $f(x, y)$ is only performed along the respective line.

The complete set of line integrals $p(\theta, s)$ can now be obtained by going through the angles $\theta \in [0°, 180°]$ and distances $s \in [-\infty, +\infty]$. Apart from orientation which has no influence on the integration, any other line would be

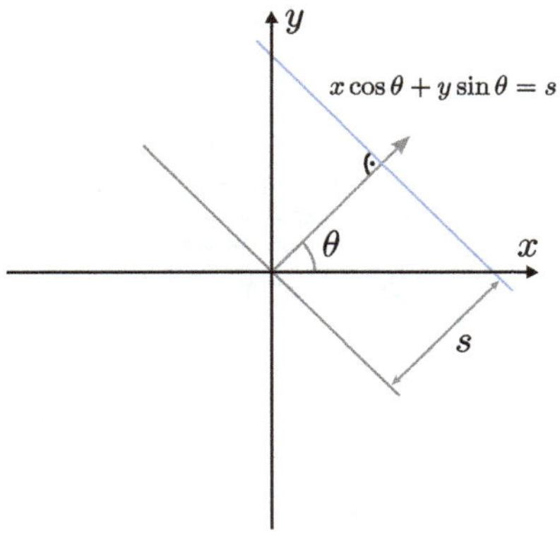

Figure 8.5: The blue line is uniquely described by its distance s to the origin and the angle θ which defines its normal vector $(\cos\theta, \sin\theta)^\top$. This representation immediately gives rise to the implicit line equation.

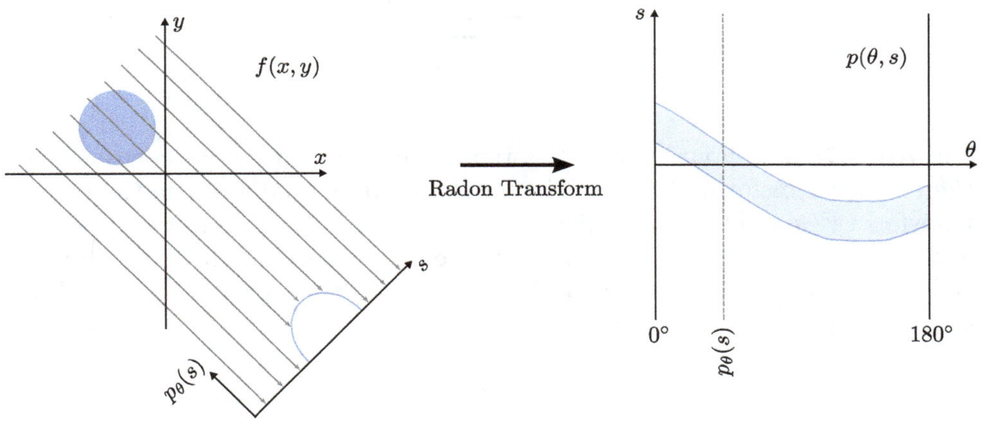

Figure 8.6: $f(x,y)$ has a constant non-zero value inside the blue circle and vanishes everywhere else. We see a single projection on the left and where it fits into the whole sinogram on the right.

equivalent to one of these. For a fixed angle θ, the 1-D function $p_\theta(s) = p(\theta, s)$ is called a projection. It contains all line integrals over $f(x,y)$ with a constant angle θ and variable distance s to the origin. Arranging all projections side-by-side as a 2-D image yields the sinogram. It owes its name to the sinusoidal curves emerging from the underlying geometry. We can see that every point in 2-D except for the origin is found at different distances along the s-axis depending on the angle θ. An example of a sinogram is given in Fig. 8.6.

Turning the function values $f(x,y)$ into line integral values $p(\theta, s)$ is known as the Radon transform in 2-D. The aim of CT reconstruction is the computation of the original function values from measured line integral values, i. e., the inverse Radon transform.

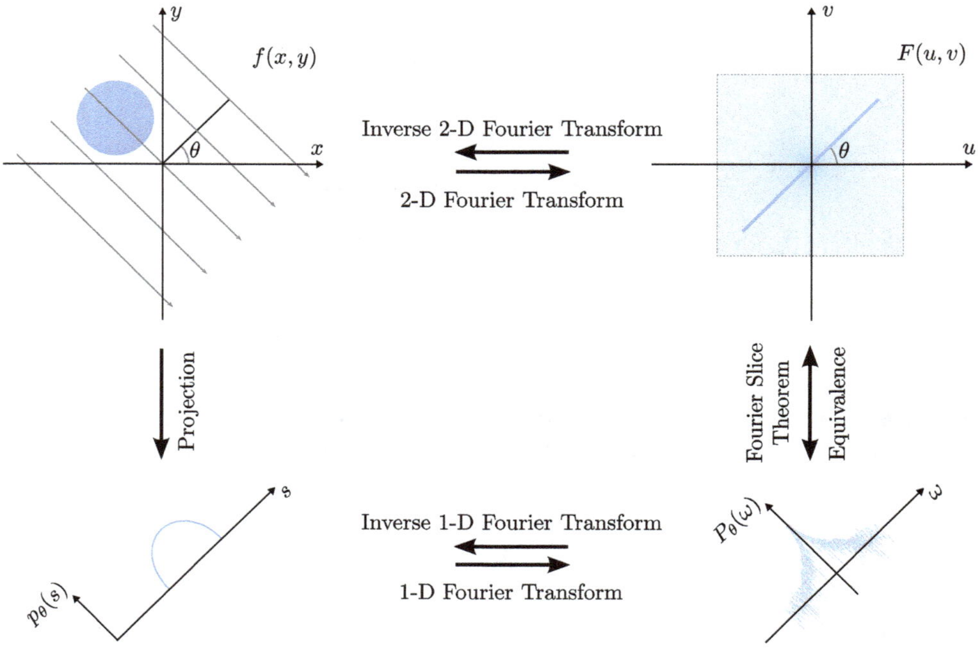

Figure 8.7: The Fourier slice theorem establishes an equivalence between the Fourier transform $P(\xi, \theta)$ of the projection $p_\theta(s)$ and a line in the Fourier transform $F(u, v)$ of $f(x, y)$ which runs through the origin and forms the angle θ with the u-axis. Please note that in the frequency domain images on the right, the magnitudes of the complex numbers were plotted on a logarithmic scale for improved readability.

8.2.2 Fourier Slice Theorem

While it is not immediately clear how to invert the process of projection, we can take a detour through frequency domain. Fig. 8.7 depicts the principle behind the Fourier slice theorem by establishing relationships between the relevant domains. We start by computing the 1-D Fourier transform $P(\xi, \theta)$ of the projection $p_\theta(s)$. The Fourier slice theorem establishes an equivalence that exists between $P(\xi, \theta)$ of the projection $p_\theta(s)$ and a line in the Fourier transform $F(u, v)$ of $f(x, y)$ which runs through the origin and forms the angle θ with the u-axis. A proof of this property can be found in Geek Box 8.1. An intuitive visualization of this relation is displayed in Fig. 8.8. Computation of one 2-D Fourier coefficient is equivalent to projecting the image first, followed by a correlation with the respective 1-D frequency. This is possible as Fourier transform and projection operate in orthogonal direction and are therefore separable as shown in Fig. 8.9. With the complete set of projections, we get many such lines and therefore obtain a good estimate of $F(u, v)$. An inverse 2-D Fourier transform then leads us back to the desired function $f(x, y)$.

Geek Box 8.1: Fourier Slice Theorem

An essential relationship between the projections $p_\theta(s)$ and the function $f(x,y)$ can be established by looking at the frequency domain representations

$$F(u,v) = \mathcal{F}\{f(x,y)\}, \quad (8.3)$$
$$P(\xi,\theta) = \mathcal{F}\{p_\theta(s)\}, \quad (8.4)$$

using the Fourier transform $\mathcal{F}$ (cf. Sec. 2.3 (p. 22)). As illustrated in Fig. 8.7, $P(\xi,\theta)$ is equivalent to the part of $F(u,v)$ that falls on a radial line with angle θ. To see why this is the case, we start with the 1-D Fourier transform $P(\xi,\theta)$ of $p_\theta(s)$,

$$P(\xi,\theta) = \int_{-\infty}^{+\infty} p_\theta(s) e^{-2\pi i \xi s} \, \mathrm{d}s. \quad (8.5)$$

Using the definition of the projection $p_\theta(s)$ from the previous section, we obtain

$$P(\xi,\theta) = \int_{-\infty}^{+\infty} \iint_{-\infty}^{+\infty} f(x,y)\delta(x\cos\theta + y\sin\theta - s) \, \mathrm{d}x\mathrm{d}y \; e^{-2\pi i \xi s} \, \mathrm{d}s. \quad (8.6)$$

Rearranging the order of the integrals yields

$$P(\xi,\theta) = \iint_{-\infty}^{+\infty} f(x,y) \int_{-\infty}^{+\infty} \delta(x\cos\theta + y\sin\theta - s) e^{-2\pi i \xi s} \, \mathrm{d}s\mathrm{d}x\mathrm{d}y. \quad (8.7)$$

Eliminating the delta function reads as

$$P(\xi,\theta) = \iint_{-\infty}^{+\infty} f(x,y) e^{-2\pi i (x\cos\theta + y\sin\theta)\xi} \, \mathrm{d}x\mathrm{d}y. \quad (8.8)$$

Variable substitution yields the definition of the 2-D Fourier transform,

$$P(\xi,\theta) = \iint_{-\infty}^{+\infty} f(x,y) e^{-2\pi i (xu + yv)} |_{u=\xi\cos\theta,\; v=\xi\sin\theta} \, \mathrm{d}x\mathrm{d}y, \quad (8.9)$$

which finally results in the proposed theorem,

$$P(\xi,\theta) = F(\xi\cos\theta, \xi\sin\theta) = F_{\text{polar}}(\xi,\theta). \quad (8.10)$$

In effect, we can get the complete Fourier transform $F_{\text{polar}}(\xi,\theta)$ of the unknown function $f(x,y)$ in polar coordinates (ξ,θ) by varying θ.

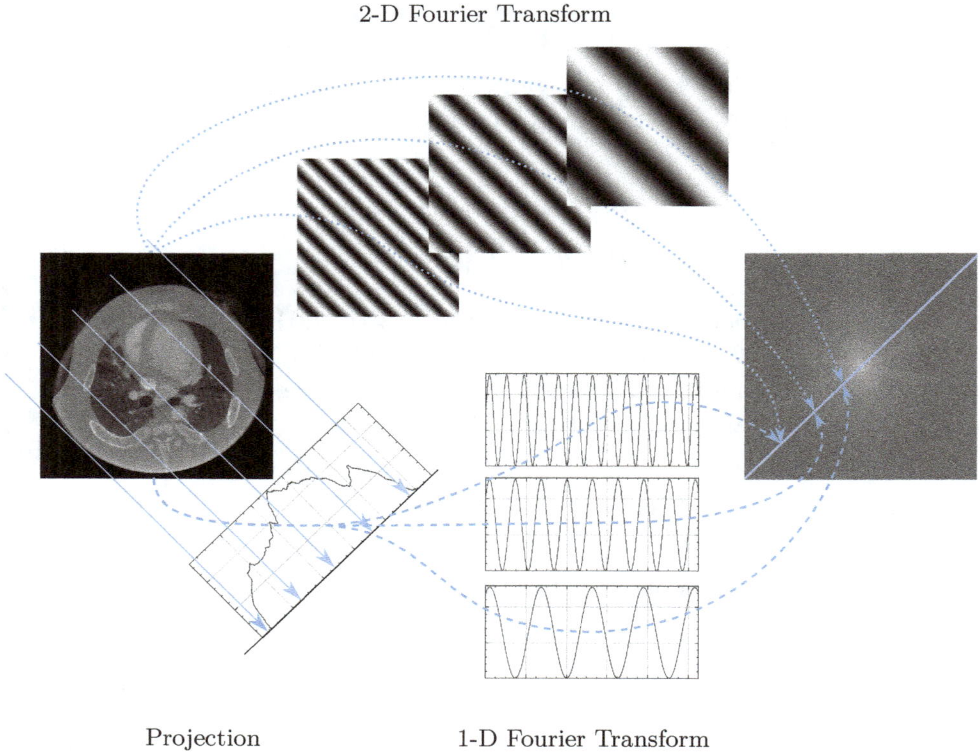

Figure 8.8: Graphical visualization of the Fourier slice theorem. In fact, computation of the projection and correlation with a sinusoidal function (dashed lines) is equivalent to a 2-D correlation with the respective Fourier base function (dotted lines, cf. Fig. 6.9).

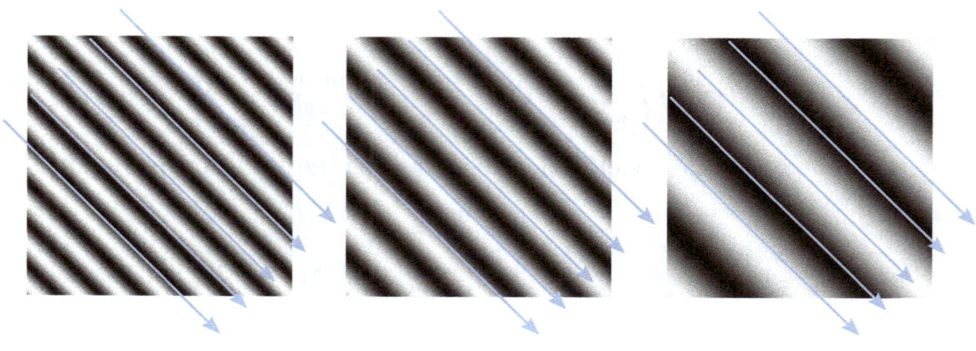

Figure 8.9: A close look at the Fourier base functions reveals that they are actually computing an integration along the wave front. As such projection and convolution operate in orthogonal domains and can therefore be separated into a projection and a 1-D correlation, i. e., a 1-D Fourier transform.

Material / Tissue	HU
Air	−1000
Lung	−600 to −400
Fat	−100 to −60
Water	0
Muscle	10 to 40
Blood	30 to 45
Soft tissue	40 to 80
Bone	400 to 3000

Table 8.1: HUs observed in several materials and tissue classes found in the human body. In general, denser structures exhibit larger HUs.

8.3 Image Reconstruction

As described in Sec. 7.3 (p. 125), X-ray projections can be converted to line integrals using Beer's law, which enables us to apply Radon's ideas to CT reconstruction. A single slice of our imaged object corresponds to the bivariate function $f(x, y)$. More precisely, the function values reconstructed in CT are the linear attenuation coefficients of the imaged material. Typically, they are linearly transformed to the Hounsfield scale, which is normalized such that the absorption of water equals 0 HU,

$$\mu^* = \left(\frac{\mu}{\mu_{\text{Water}}} - 1\right) \cdot 1000, \tag{8.11}$$

where μ and μ^* denote the coefficients before and after Hounsfield scaling, respectively. Tab. 8.1 lists the HU ranges of several tissue classes found in the human body.

Below, we will discuss the two main methods for 2-D image reconstruction from parallel-beam projections as they have been introduced above. In conventional CT imaging, a 3-D image volume is then obtained simply by acquiring and reconstructing multiple axial slices at slightly offset locations such that they can be stacked on top of each other (Fig. 8.10).

8.3.1 Analytic Reconstruction

Using the Fourier slice theorem, we can derive an analytic reconstruction method known as filtered back-projection.

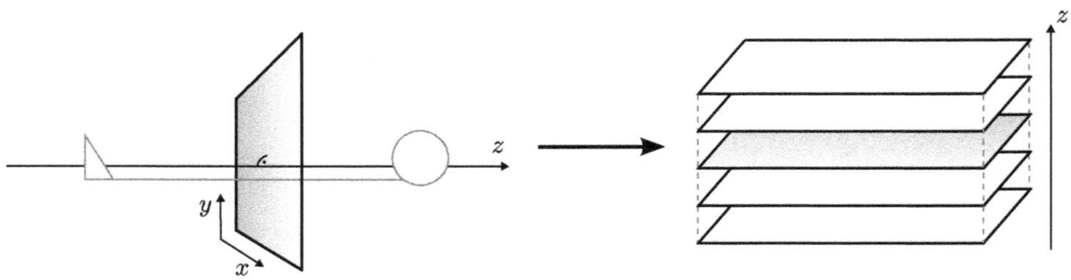

Figure 8.10: In conventional CT, a 3-D image of the body is formed by acquiring, reconstructing, and subsequently stacking 2-D image slices in axial direction. For each slice, all projection rays lie in a plane, which is why we only deal with bivariate functions $f(x, y)$. However, be aware that there are other geometries where this assumption is no longer valid (cf. Sec. 8.3.3).

8.3.1.1 Filtered Back-Projection

It is possible to invert the process of projection directly, without explicitly computing the computations in frequency space suggested by Fig. 8.7. In Geek Box 8.2, it is shown that the required calculations reduce to

$$f(x, y) = \int_0^{\pi} p_\theta(s) * h(s)|_{s=x\cos\theta+y\sin\theta}\, \mathrm{d}\theta, \qquad (8.12)$$

where $h(s)$ corresponds to the inverse Fourier transform of $|\xi|$. This amounts to the back-projection of $p_\theta(s)$ convolved with $h(s)$. As a consequence, this method is called filtered back-projection.

Unfiltered back-projection, i. e., just "smearing" line integrals in a projection $p_\theta(s)$ back along their corresponding lines without filtering (cf. Fig. 8.12), is equivalent to adding $P(\xi, \theta)$ to $F(u, v)$, as suggested by the Fourier slice theorem, without considering the factor $|\xi|$. In fact, this is not the inverse, but the dual or adjoint of the Radon transform.

8.3.1.2 Filters

Due to the shape of $|\xi|$, the filter $h(s)$ is typically called ramp filter. Sampling in polar coordinates leads to an oversampling in the center of the Fourier space (cf. Fig. 8.11). Using a ramp filter, this oversampling is corrected by enhancing the high frequency components while dampening the low frequencies in the center of the Fourier space.

According to the sampling theorem, as described in Sec. 2.4.2 (p. 32), with a detector spacing of Δs, the largest frequency that can be detected in $p_\theta(s)$ is $\xi_{\max} = \frac{1}{2\Delta s}$. Additionally, noise in the projections is amplified when using an unlimited ramp filter $|\xi|$. Therefore, high frequencies should be limited in the

Geek Box 8.2: Filtered Back-Projection

To derive the filtered back-projection algorithm, we start with the inverse Fourier transform of $F(u,v)$,

$$f(x,y) = \int_{-\infty}^{+\infty} \int_{-\infty}^{+\infty} F(u,v) e^{2\pi i(ux+vy)} \, \mathrm{d}u\mathrm{d}v.$$

We can rewrite this equation in polar coordinates $F_{\text{polar}}(\xi,\theta)$ by substituting $u = \xi \cos\theta$ and $v = \xi \sin\theta$. A change in integration variables requires an additional "correction" factor in the integral. This factor is the absolute value of the determinant of the transformation's Jacobian matrix $\boldsymbol{J}$:

$$|\det \boldsymbol{J}| = \left|\det \begin{pmatrix} \frac{\mathrm{d}u}{\mathrm{d}\xi} & \frac{\mathrm{d}u}{\mathrm{d}\theta} \\ \frac{\mathrm{d}v}{\mathrm{d}\xi} & \frac{\mathrm{d}v}{\mathrm{d}\theta} \end{pmatrix}\right| = \left|\det \begin{pmatrix} \cos(\theta) & -\xi\sin(\theta) \\ \sin(\theta) & \xi\cos(\theta) \end{pmatrix}\right| =$$

$$= |\xi \cos^2(\theta) + \xi \sin^2(\theta)| = |\xi|.$$

Therefore, performing the change in coordinates, we obtain

$$f(x,y) = \int_{0}^{\pi} \int_{-\infty}^{+\infty} F_{\text{polar}}(\xi,\theta)|\xi| e^{2\pi i\xi(x\cos\theta + y\sin\theta)} \, \mathrm{d}\xi\mathrm{d}\theta.$$

From the Fourier slice theorem, we know $F(\xi,\theta) = P(\xi,\theta)$, thus

$$f(x,y) = \int_{0}^{\pi} \int_{-\infty}^{+\infty} P(\xi,\theta)|\xi| e^{2\pi i\xi(x\cos\theta + y\sin\theta)} \, \mathrm{d}\xi\mathrm{d}\theta.$$

Replacing $x\cos\theta + y\sin\theta$ with s, this reads as

$$f(x,y) = \int_{0}^{\pi} \int_{-\infty}^{+\infty} P(\xi,\theta)|\xi| e^{2\pi i\xi s} \, \mathrm{d}\xi\mathrm{d}\theta,$$

which contains a product of $P(\xi,\theta)$ and $|\xi|$. A product in Fourier space corresponds to a convolution in spatial domain (cf. Sec. 2.3.2 (p. 25)). If we denote the inverse Fourier transform of $|\xi|$ with $h(s)$, we find the following spatial domain representation:

$$f(x,y) = \int_{0}^{\pi} p_\theta(s) * h(s)|_{s=x\cos\theta+y\sin\theta} \, \mathrm{d}\theta. \tag{8.13}$$

This amounts to the back-projection of $p_\theta(s)$ convolved with the filter kernel $h(s)$.

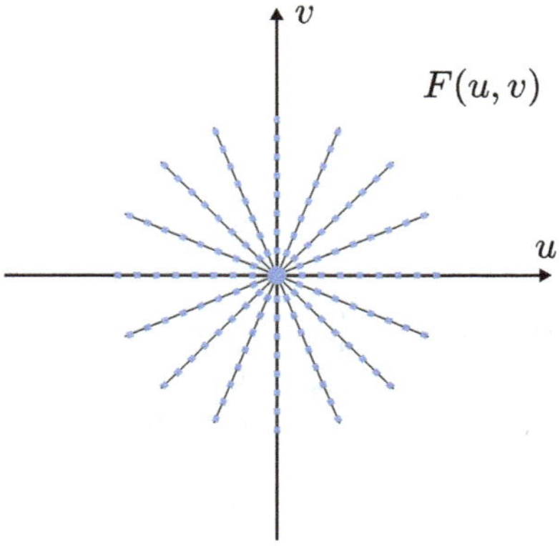

Figure 8.11: Sampling in polar coordinates causes the density of samples to increase with proximity to the origin, whereas the more distant areas are under-represented.

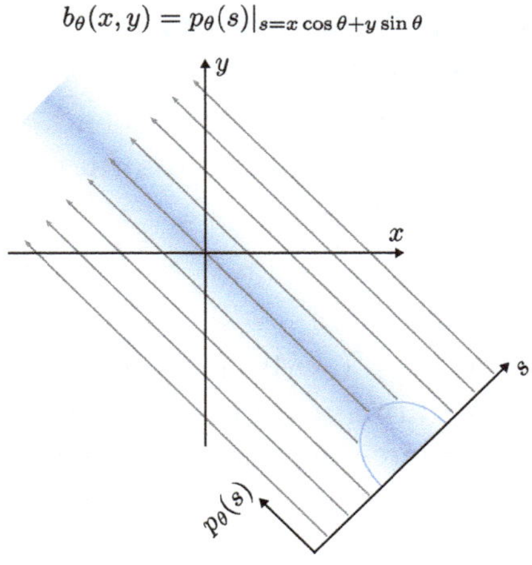

Figure 8.12: The back-projection $b_\theta(x, y)$ of a single projection $p_\theta(s)$ hardly gives us an idea of the original function $f(x, y)$. However, we can reconstruct it by back-projecting a sufficient set of appropriately filtered projections.

filtered projections $\tilde{p}_\theta(s)$. For this purpose, we can generalize the following equation

$$\tilde{p}_\theta(s) = \int_{-\infty}^{+\infty} P(\xi, \theta)|\xi| e^{2\pi i \xi s} \, \mathrm{d}\xi, \tag{8.14}$$

by replacing $|\xi|$ with an arbitrary filter $H(\xi)$:

$$\tilde{p}_\theta(s) = \int_{-\infty}^{+\infty} P(\xi, \theta) H(\xi) e^{2\pi i \xi s} \, \mathrm{d}\xi, \tag{8.15}$$

In practice, various ramp-like filters are used depending on the desired image characteristics, typically involving a trade-off between a smoother image appearance and a higher spatial resolution.

One of the most widely known filters was described by Ramachandran and Lakshminarayanan, in short known as the "Ram-Lak" filter. It corresponds to $|\xi|$ cut off at $\xi_{\max}$ on both sides. In the spatial domain, this results in a filter kernel that reads

$$h(s) = \frac{\operatorname{sinc}\left(\frac{s}{\Delta s}\right)}{2(\Delta s)^2} - \frac{\operatorname{sinc}^2\left(\frac{s}{2\Delta s}\right)}{4(\Delta s)^2}, \tag{8.16}$$

a discretized version of which can be convolved with the discrete projection. A derivation of the Ram-Lak filter is given in Geek Box 8.3.

Geek Box 8.3: Ram-Lak Filter

In order to derive the Ram-Lak filter, we need to start with the inverse Fourier transform of $|\xi|$

$$h(s) = \int_{-\infty}^{+\infty} |\xi| e^{2\pi i \xi s} \, \mathrm{d}\xi.$$

Now, we introduce a band limitation that only allows frequencies $|\xi| \leq B$:

$$h(s) = \int_{-B}^{B} |\xi| e^{2\pi i \xi s} \, \mathrm{d}\xi = \int_{-\infty}^{+\infty} |\xi| e^{2\pi i \xi s} \, \mathrm{rect}\left(\frac{\xi}{2B}\right) \mathrm{d}\xi$$

Note the we use the rectangular function (cf. Tab. 2.2) to express the band limitation above. Furthermore, we can also use this function to express $|\xi|$ as the convolution of two rectangular functions yields a triangular function (cf. Tab. 2.2):

$$|\xi| = B - \mathrm{rect}\left(\frac{\xi}{B}\right) * \mathrm{rect}\left(\frac{\xi}{B}\right)$$

Now the band-limited inverse Fourier transform of $|\xi|$ takes the following form:

$$\begin{aligned}
h(s) =& \mathcal{F}^{-1}\left[\left(B - \mathrm{rect}\left(\tfrac{\xi}{B}\right) * \mathrm{rect}\left(\tfrac{\xi}{B}\right)\right) \mathrm{rect}\left(\tfrac{\xi}{2B}\right)\right] \\
=& \mathcal{F}^{-1}\left[B \, \mathrm{rect}\left(\tfrac{\xi}{2B}\right)\right] - \mathcal{F}^{-1}\left[\underbrace{\left(\mathrm{rect}\left(\tfrac{\xi}{B}\right) * \mathrm{rect}\left(\tfrac{\xi}{B}\right)\right)}_{\text{support on } [-B,B]} \underbrace{\mathrm{rect}\left(\tfrac{\xi}{2B}\right)}_{=1 \text{ on } [-B,B]}\right] \\
=& \mathcal{F}^{-1}\left[B \, \mathrm{rect}\left(\tfrac{\xi}{2B}\right)\right] - \mathcal{F}^{-1}\left[\left(\mathrm{rect}\left(\tfrac{\xi}{B}\right)\right] \cdot \mathcal{F}^{-1}\left[\mathrm{rect}\left(\tfrac{\xi}{B}\right)\right)\right] \\
=& 2B^2 \, \mathrm{sinc}(2Bs) - B^2 \, \mathrm{sinc}^2(Bs)
\end{aligned}$$

With $B = \xi_{\max} = \frac{1}{2\Delta s}$, we arrive exactly at Eq. (8.16). In the discrete case, s needs to be an integer number. Thus, we can simplify above equation even further to:

$$h_s = \begin{cases} \frac{1}{2\Delta s^2} & s = 0 \\ 0 & s \text{ even} \\ \frac{1}{\pi^2 (s\Delta s)^2} & s \text{ odd} \end{cases}$$

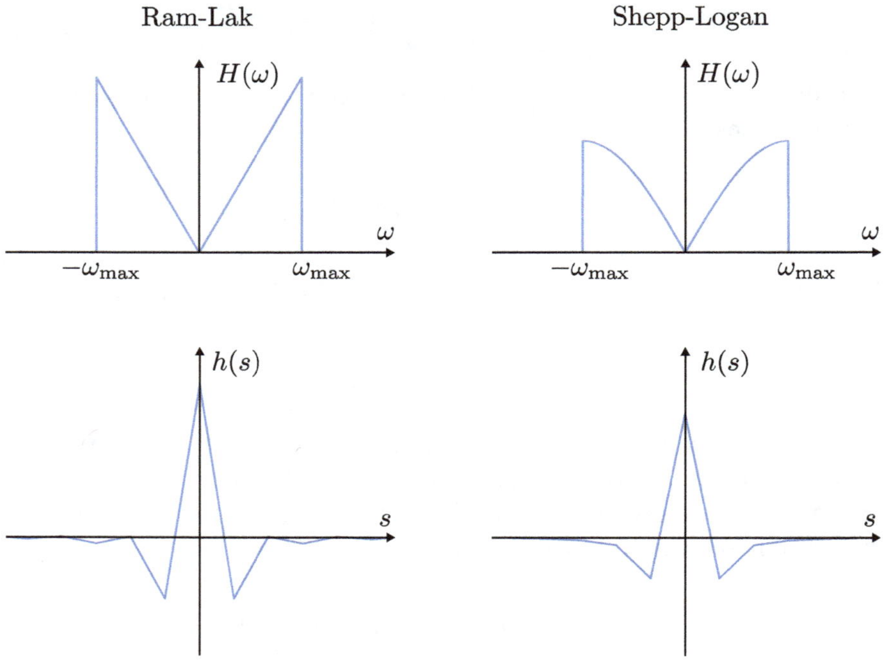

Figure 8.13: The responses in frequency domain (top row) as well as the discretized spatial domain kernels (bottom row) of the Ram-Lak and Shepp-Logan filters.

To suppress noise, a windowing function can be multiplied with the filter in frequency domain which lowers its response for frequencies close to $\xi_{\max}$. In the case of the commonly used filter proposed by Shepp and Logan, this windowing function is

$$\left|\operatorname{sinc}\left(\frac{\xi}{2\,\xi_{\max}}\right)\right|. \tag{8.17}$$

This leads to a slightly different function $h(s)$ which can be discretized in the same manner. Fig. 8.13 shows plots of the Ram-Lak and Shepp-Logan filters.

8.3.1.3 Discretization

Through discretization, the convolution

$$\tilde{p}_\theta(s) = \int_{-\infty}^{+\infty} p_\theta(s) \cdot h(s-s')\,\mathrm{d}s' \tag{8.18}$$

becomes

$$\tilde{p}_{\theta,s} = \sum_{s'} p_{\theta,s} \cdot h_{s-s'}\ \Delta s. \tag{8.19}$$

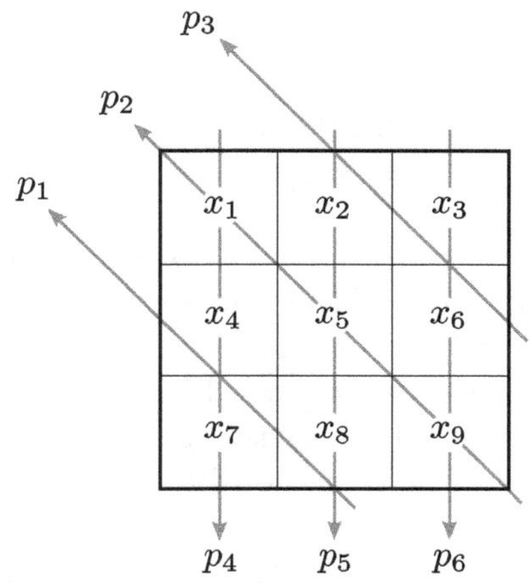

Figure 8.14: Example for an image grid and some projection rays.

An example for a discrete filter h_s is given in Geek Box 8.3.

With an angle increment of $\mathrm{d}\theta = \frac{\pi}{N}$, where N is the number of acquired projections, the final back-projection step in Eq. (8.13) can be written as

$$f(x,y) = \frac{\pi}{N} \sum_i \tilde{p}_{\theta_i}(s)|_{s=x\cos\theta_i + y\sin\theta_i}, \tag{8.20}$$

where θ_i denotes the ith angle. Note that the value $\tilde{p}_{\theta_i}(s)$ will generally have to be interpolated from the $\tilde{p}_{\theta_i,s}$ since s is not necessarily an integer number. For each position (x, y), we can find $f(x, y)$ by summing over corresponding (interpolated) values of each filtered projection $\tilde{p}_{\theta_i}$. As a rule of thumb, it is recommended to avoid interpolation in the output space, i. e., in our case, we should sample f directly. This comes naturally with the formulation given in Eq. (8.20). In contrast, back-projecting one $\tilde{p}_{\theta_i}$ at a time to the whole volume would require interpolation on grid points in the domain of f in each step.

8.3.2 Algebraic Reconstruction

A second approach to CT image reconstruction defines the problem as a system of linear equations. Each projection ray corresponds to a linear equation that sums up the image pixels the ray passes through, i. e., computes its discrete line integral, and demands it to equal the measured line integral value. Fig. 8.14 shows an exemplary image grid and a set of projections rays.

Accordingly, we can define the image reconstruction problem as

$$\boldsymbol{A}\boldsymbol{x} = \boldsymbol{p}, \tag{8.21}$$

where

$$\boldsymbol{x} = (x_1, x_2, ..., x_N)^\top \tag{8.22}$$

$$\boldsymbol{p} = (p_1, p_2, ..., p_M)^\top \tag{8.23}$$

are the sequentially numbered unknown pixels and measured line integrals, respectively. Each element a_{ij} of the system matrix $\boldsymbol{A}$ describes the contribution of a particular pixel to a particular ray. There are many possibilities to model $\boldsymbol{A}$. In the simplest case, a_{ij} is a binary value that is 1 when the ray passed through the pixel and 0 otherwise. The length of intersection can also be used, or even the area of intersection in case we assume the rays to have a non-zero thickness.

Solving this system of linear equations for the solution $\boldsymbol{x}$ directly using matrix inversion (Gaussian elimination, singular value decomposition, etc.) is not feasible in practice as the problems are typically large, ill-conditioned and over-determined. Instead, an iterative solution to this system of linear equations is sought.[2]

The algebraic reconstruction technique (ART) aims to find such an iterative solution using the Kaczmarz method. The basic idea behind this method is that each linear equation defines a line (2-D) or, generally speaking, a hyper plane (higher dimensions) in the solution space, the dimensionality of which equals the number of unknowns. All points on a hyper plane fulfill its corresponding equation. Consequently, the point of intersection of all hyper planes forms the correct solution to the problem. Thus, by repeatedly projecting the current estimate orthogonally onto a different equation's plane, we iteratively improve the solution (Fig. 8.15). A simple mathematical intuition for the ART algorithm is given in Geek Box 8.4.

Using Kaczmarz' method, we can now find an iterative solution for Eq. (8.21). For each line integral measurement p_i and each *row* $\boldsymbol{a}_i$ of the system matrix $\boldsymbol{A}$ we perform the following update step,

$$\boldsymbol{x}^{k+1} = \boldsymbol{x}^k + \frac{p_i - \boldsymbol{a}_i \boldsymbol{x}^k}{\boldsymbol{a}_i \boldsymbol{a}_i^\top} \boldsymbol{a}_i^\top, \tag{8.29}$$

and repeat until convergence.

It has been shown by Tanabe in 1971 that if a unique solution exists, this iterative scheme converges to the solution. However, in over-determined systems and in presence of noise, no unique solution might be found and the method might oscillate around the ideal solution. The rate of convergence depends on the angle between the lines. If two lines are orthogonal to each other, the method converges very quickly as the orthogonal projection immediately finds the intersection. Thus, orthogonalization methods can be applied

[2] It is worthwhile to note that while $\boldsymbol{A}^{-1}\boldsymbol{p}$ corresponds to the ideal solution, which in the previous section we would obtain by filtered back-projection, $\boldsymbol{A}^\top \boldsymbol{p}$ amounts to an *unfiltered* back-projection.

Geek Box 8.4: 2-D Algebraic Reconstruction Technique Example

In the 2-D case, consider a point $\boldsymbol{x}$ and a line $\boldsymbol{n}^\top \boldsymbol{c} = d$, where $\boldsymbol{n}$ is the normal vector, $\boldsymbol{c}$ a point on the line and d the distance to the origin. Note that $\boldsymbol{n}^\top \boldsymbol{c}$ describes the scalar vector product. The orthogonal projection $\boldsymbol{x}'$ of $\boldsymbol{x}$ on this line must be in the direction of the normal vector $\boldsymbol{n}$:

$$\boldsymbol{x}' = \boldsymbol{x} + \lambda \boldsymbol{n} \tag{8.24}$$

The projected point $\boldsymbol{x}'$ is part of the line and therefore fulfills

$$\boldsymbol{n}^\top \boldsymbol{x}' = d. \tag{8.25}$$

Plugging Eq. (8.24) into this equation we get

$$\boldsymbol{n}^\top (\boldsymbol{x} + \lambda \boldsymbol{n}) = d, \tag{8.26}$$

which can be rewritten as

$$\lambda = \frac{d - \boldsymbol{n}^\top \boldsymbol{x}}{\boldsymbol{n}^\top \boldsymbol{n}}. \tag{8.27}$$

Substituting λ in Eq. (8.24), we arrive at

$$\boldsymbol{x}' = \boldsymbol{x} + \frac{d - \boldsymbol{n}^\top \boldsymbol{x}}{\boldsymbol{n}^\top \boldsymbol{n}} \boldsymbol{n}. \tag{8.28}$$

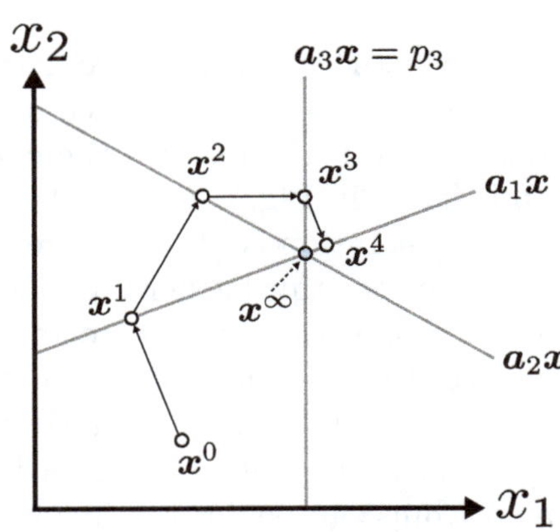

Figure 8.15: Kaczmarz iterations in 2-D space.

in advance in order to improve convergence. However, using such methods is computationally demanding and amplifies noise in the measurements.

Several extensions of this algorithm aim to improve convergence speed. Instead of orthogonalization, for instance, one can also use ordered subsets of the equations to select a better order of the performed projections. Another extension, Simultaneous ART (SART), achieves a speed-up by doing multiple updates at the same time and then combining the results. In each step, the current estimate is orthogonally projected on all lines. The centroid of all projected points is then used for the next iteration. This results in the following update rule:

$$\boldsymbol{x}^{k+1} = \boldsymbol{x}^k + \lambda_k \sum_i u_{k,i} \frac{p_i - \boldsymbol{a}_i \boldsymbol{x}^k}{\boldsymbol{a}_i \boldsymbol{a}_i^\top} \boldsymbol{a}_i^\top , \tag{8.30}$$

with

$$\sum_i u_{k,i} = 1, \tag{8.31}$$

where λ_k controls the step size in each iteration.

Other than the presented method by Kaczmarz, there are a multitude of optimization approaches to solve this problem that are not covered here, e. g., Gradient Descent, Maximum-Likelihood Expectation-Maximization, or regularized reconstruction methods. There is also an immediate relation to analytical methods as described in Geek Box 8.5.

8.3.3 Acquisition Geometries

Fig. 8.16 illustrates several important acquisition geometries in CT imaging. Different types of CT scanners have been categorized into generations. CT scanners of the first generation practically realized the parallel beam geometry as introduced above and shown in Fig. 8.16(a) (left). By introducing an array of detectors, the second generation could measure beams from several directions simultaneously. Only by the third generation, however, was this fan of directions (cf. Fig. 8.16(a), right) wide enough to remove the need for a translational motion during acquisition. The projections acquired using a fan beam geometry can be transformed ("rebinned") such that the reconstruction methods described earlier can still be applied. Alternatively, corresponding fan beam versions of the algorithms can be derived in a similar fashion to the ones presented.

Another essential development is the addition of multiple detector rows (Fig. 8.16(b), left), leading to a dramatically increased imaging speed as many slices can be acquired in parallel (multi-slice CT). Another, newer kind of CT systems expands on this notion: by acquiring full 2-D projection images with an image intensifier or – more recently – a flat panel detector, cone beam

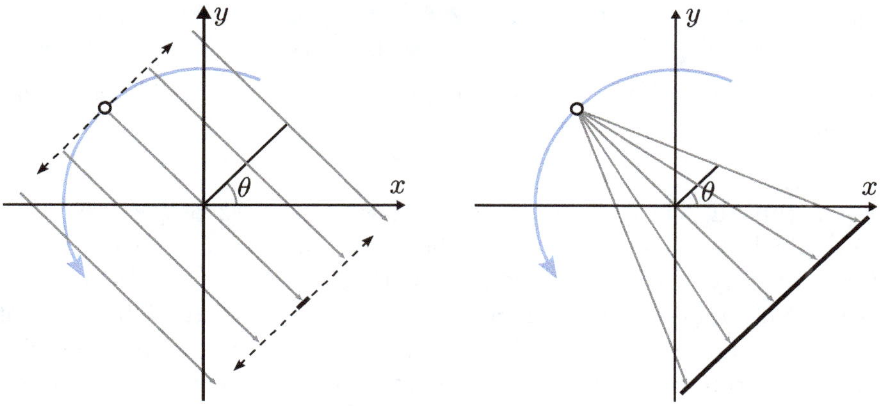

(a) For a parallel beam geometry as introduced in the previous sections (shown on the left), the X-ray source needs to be shifted perpendicularly (dotted line) to the direction of projection, casting pencil beams through the object. If all beams instead emanate from a single position for each angle, we obtain a fan of no longer parallel rays (fan beam geometry; on the right), increasing acquisition efficiency at the cost of a slightly more complicated reconstruction problem. Apart from the flat shape shown here, there also exist curved detectors with an equiangular spacing.

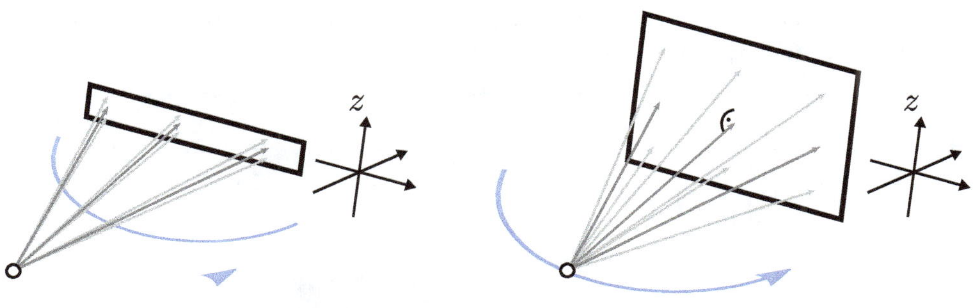

(b) Multiple detector arrays allow for simultaneous acquisition of multiple image slices from one X-ray source position (multi-slice CT; shown on the left). However, in this setup, the beams no longer all lie within the rotation plane. This issue becomes much more important in the case of cone beam CT (shown on the right): Here, the small stack of detector rows gives way to a larger detector matrix, with the beams now forming a cone in 3-D.

Figure 8.16: Basic acquisition geometries in CT imaging. Blue arrows indicate the trajectory of the X-ray source. The detector is depicted by thick black lines.

Geek Box 8.5: ART and its Relation to Filtered Back-Projection

ART formulates the reconstruction problem as a system of linear equations.

$$\boldsymbol{A}\boldsymbol{x} = \boldsymbol{p}$$

For a typical 3-D reconstruction problem with 512 projections with 512^2 pixels each, $\boldsymbol{p} \in \mathbb{R}^{512^3}$ while the corresponding volume $\boldsymbol{x} \in \mathbb{R}^{512^3}$. Consequently, the operator is huge with $\boldsymbol{A} \in \mathbb{R}^{512^3 \times 512^3}$. In order to store such a matrix in floating point precision about 65,000 TB of memory would be required. However, $\boldsymbol{A}$ is very sparse as most entries are equal to 0. In computer implementations, it is typically computed on the fly using *ray-casting*. Thus, general inversion of $\boldsymbol{A}$ is infeasible, even when using the pseudo inverse with

$$\boldsymbol{x} = \boldsymbol{A}^{\dagger}\boldsymbol{p} = \boldsymbol{A}^{\top}(\boldsymbol{A}\boldsymbol{A}^{\top})^{-1}\boldsymbol{p}.$$

However, there are certain geometries for which $(\boldsymbol{A}\boldsymbol{A}^{\top})^{-1}$ can be determined analytically. For the case of parallel-beam geometries, we know that $(\boldsymbol{A}\boldsymbol{A}^{\top})^{-1}$ takes the form of a convolution with the ramp filter. $\boldsymbol{A}^{\top}$ is the adjoint operation of the projection operator. In continuous form, we introduced this operation already as back-projection (cf. Geek Box 8.2). Thus, filtered back-projection is a direct solution for the above system of linear equations.

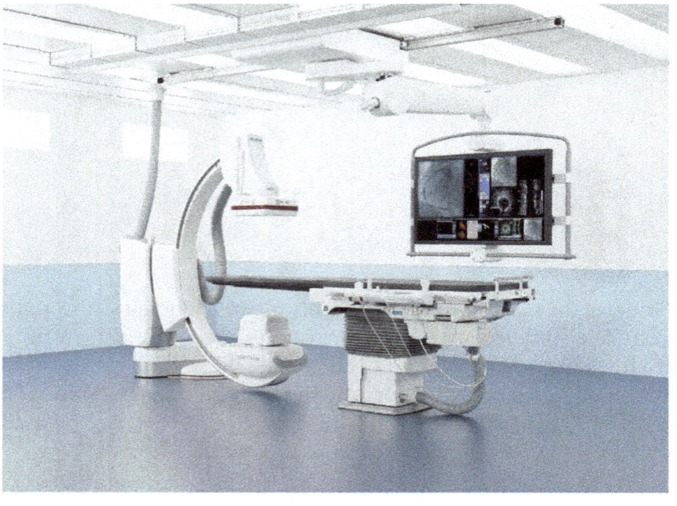

Figure 8.17: A C-arm system for interventional X-ray imaging. Image courtesy of Siemens Healthineers AG.

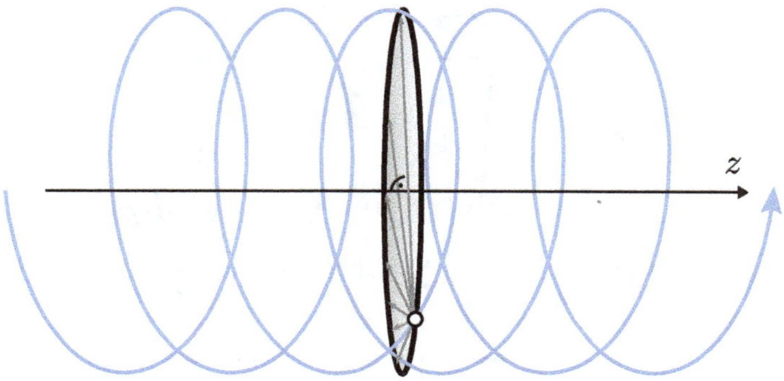

Figure 8.18: In spiral CT, although the X-ray source still conveniently rotates in the x-y plane, the trajectory it describes in relation to the imaged object is a helix due to the patient table being slowly moved through the gantry. This enables the acquisition of a large object region while rotating continuously. Projections for an ideal circular trajectory can be interpolated along z from neighboring helical segments.

CT is able to capture a large field of view containing all of the object in a single rotation (Fig. 8.16(b), right). One of the main fields of use for this technology lies in interventional imaging where the X-ray source and detector are mounted on a C-arm device (Fig. 8.17). It has to be noted, though, that for arbitrary objects, an exact reconstruction is only possible in the plane of rotation. The more the beam diverges from this plane, the more artifacts are likely to appear: due to the incomplete data obtained from oblique rays, the reconstruction problem is underdetermined.

For imaging larger parts of the body with few detector rows, it used to be necessary to perform a rotation, then halt and move the table such that the next slice to be acquired is lined up with the detector before starting anew. With the invention of helical CT, a continuous motion of both the rotating gantry and the table became possible. From the point of view of the imaged object, the X-ray source rotates in the x-y plane and moves in the axial direction at the same time, thus following a helix (Fig. 8.18). From the helical rotation, projections for all angles in an axial plane can be interpolated, enabling the use of standard reconstruction methods.

8.4 Practical Considerations

So far, we have described the theoretical background and principles for CT image reconstruction. However, in practice there are several aspects that have to be considered.

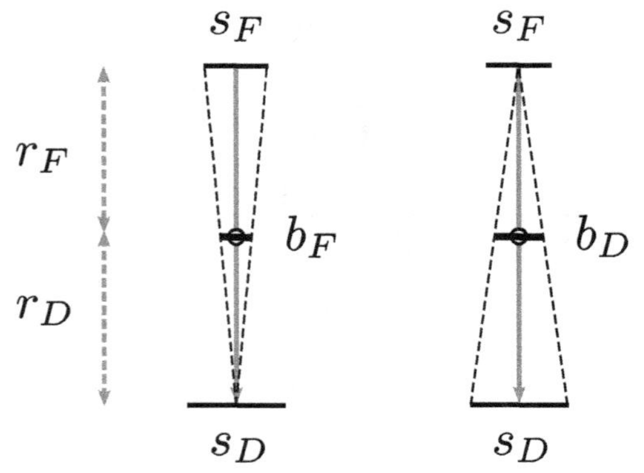

Figure 8.19: The effective sizes b_F of the focus and b_D of the detector in the isocenter can be calculated from the distances to the isocenter r_F and r_D.

8.4.1 Spatial Resolution

In many medical applications, we are not only interested in visualizing large organs, but also smaller structures, such as small blood vessels or calcifications. Visualization of these small structures requires a high spatial resolution. In the following subsection, we will discuss what affects resolution in the x-y scan plane. Resolution in the z-direction typically needs to be considered separately as it depends on different factors.

In the scan plane, resolution depends on several geometrical properties. Focus size, scan geometry, detector element spacing and aperture, and movement of the focus during image acquisition all influence the resolution.

The focus size s_F as well as the detector aperture s_D contribute to image blurring, which can be modeled by

$$b_F = \frac{r_D}{r_F + r_D} \cdot s_F \quad \text{and} \tag{8.32}$$

$$b_D = \frac{r_F}{r_F + r_D} \cdot s_D, \tag{8.33}$$

where r_F represents the distance of the isocenter, i. e., the center of rotation, to the X-ray focus and r_D the distance of the isocenter to the detector center. Effectively, b_F and b_D are the sizes of the focus and detector in the isocenter (cf. Fig. 8.19). Furthermore, the continuous movement of focus and detector during the image acquisition results in additional image blur, which we denote as b_M. The blur that occurs during image acquisition is then described by

$$b_{\text{acq}} = \sqrt{b_F^2 + b_D^2 + b_M^2}. \tag{8.34}$$

However, sampling and image reconstruction also introduce additional blur,

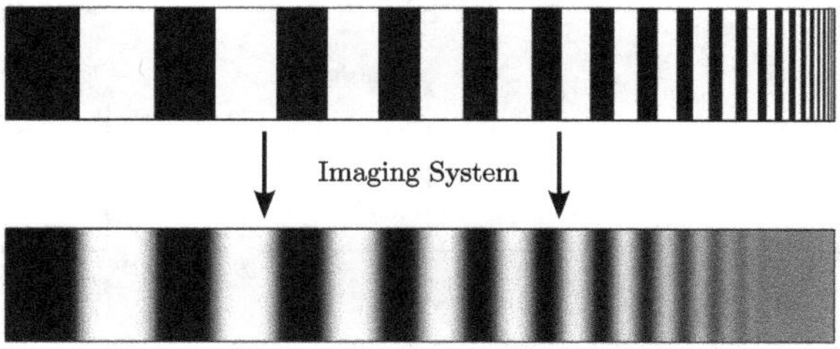

Figure 8.20: A bar phantom can be used to evaluate the spatial resolution of an imaging system. At sufficiently high spatial frequencies, individual lines can no longer be separated after imaging, i. e., we have determined the system's resolution limit.

$$b_A = c_A \cdot \Delta s, \tag{8.35}$$

with Δs the sampling distance and c_A a constant factor which represents the reconstruction algorithm characteristics[3]. Finally, the total blur is modeled by

$$b_{\text{total}} = \sqrt{b_F^2 + b_D^2 + b_M^2 + b_A^2}, \tag{8.36}$$

whereas b_{acq} represents the maximum spatial resolution given by the geometric setup, which could be achieved if we were to use a very fine sampling and a reconstruction algorithm with a sharp kernel. It becomes obvious that as a user, we only have limited influence on spatial resolution. We can decide which convolution kernel we want to use, but the geometrical parameters are defined by the system's scan modes.

Spatial resolution can be measured directly and indirectly. For direct measurement, a bar phantom can be used. Such phantoms consist of alternating black and white bars of varying thickness. The resolution is determined by evaluating whether bars of a certain thickness are still distinguishable after acquisition and reconstruction (cf. Fig. 8.20). A more reliable and objective evaluation is the indirect approach. For this purpose, we scan a thin wire phantom[4], thereby obtaining the system's so called point spread function (PSF). The Fourier transform of the PSF yields the modulation transfer function (MTF) (cf. Fig. 8.21). Frequency is typically measured in line pairs per cm (lp/cm), a unit that can be intuitively understood if we recall the bar phantoms of the direct approach mentioned before. The spatial resolution of a system is often given by the 10% value of the MTF, which represents the

[3] E. g., in filtered back-projection, a smooth convolution kernel reduces noise but also spatial resolution, whereas a sharp kernel leads to more noise but yields a high spatial resolution (cf. Sec. 8.3.1).

[4] Essentially, this mimics a point object for each 2-D slice.

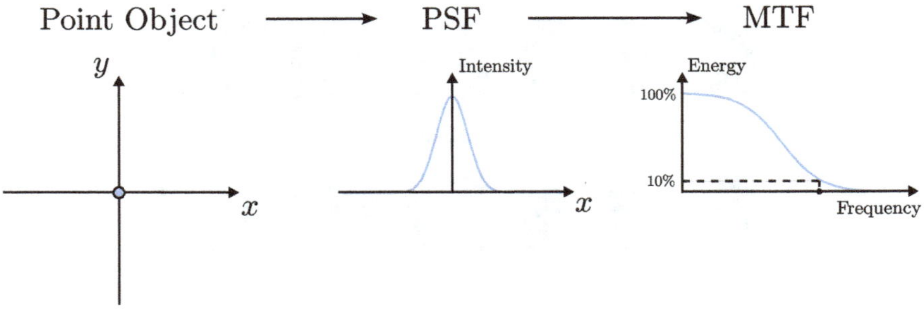

Figure 8.21: If we could scan an ideal point object, the resulting reconstructed image would be the PSF of the system. The Fourier transform of the PSF is the MTF, which shows the relative contrasts achievable for varying object frequencies. In practice, this measurement is typically performed using thin wire phantoms.

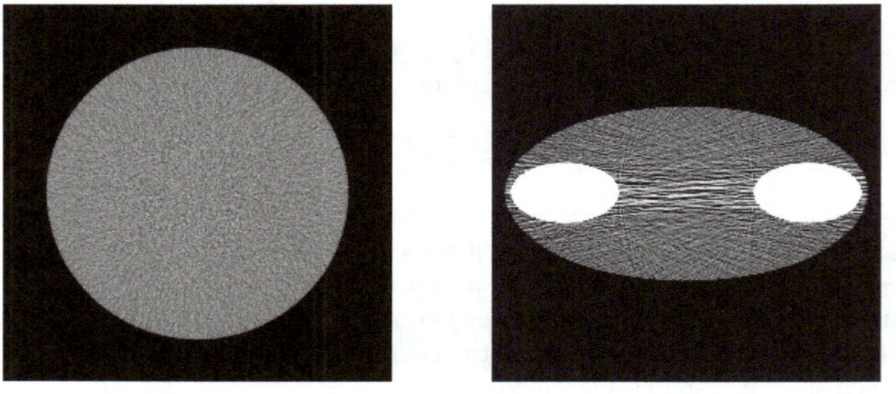

Figure 8.22: The left image shows the reconstruction of a water cylinder phantom. The noise is stronger in the center than in the peripheral regions. On the right side, an elliptic phantom with two high intensity insets is depicted. In its center, streak noise emerges that is caused by the strongly attenuating structures. For both phantom simulations, 90,000 photons per pixel with an energy of 75 keV were used.

frequency at which the contrast has dropped to 10% of the maximum value at 0 lp/cm.

8.4.2 Noise

From the considerations regarding noise in X-ray projections (cf. Sec. 7.4.3 (p. 136)), we know that the number of photons n_s measured by our detector can be modeled by a Poisson distribution with an expected value of $E[n_s] = N_0 p_a$, where N_0 is the expected value of the number of photons generated by the X-ray tube, and p_a is the probability of a photon passing through the imaged object unaffected. The Poisson process can be approximated by a Gaussian distribution with mean value $\mu = E[n_s]$ and standard deviation $\sigma = \sqrt{E[n_s]}$, if we are dealing with a high number of events, i. e., photons.

For reconstruction, we convert the measured projection images to line integral images by taking the negative logarithm (cf. Sec. 7.3.1 (p. 126)),

$$\int \mu(s)\mathrm{d}s = -\ln \frac{I}{I_0}, \tag{8.37}$$

where $\frac{I}{I_0} = \frac{N_0 p_a}{N_0} = p_a$.

Using the first order Taylor expansion, it can be shown that this transform leads to a new approximate Gaussian distribution with $\mu = -\ln p_a$ and $\sigma = \frac{1}{\sqrt{N_0 p_a}}$. Note that the noise variance increases with object thickness.

During reconstruction, the back-projection step computes a weighted sum of the (filtered) projection values. Hence, the object dependence of the noise statistics is propagated into 3-D. This can be seen in Fig. 8.22, where most of the noise is found in the center of the objects. Additionally, in a non-circular object, streak structures appear in the noise. Therefore, denoising in the reconstructed domain needs to take the directional nature of the noise generation into account.

8.4.3 Image Artifacts

An ideal image reconstruction is only possible in theory. In reality we have to deal with different physical phenomena which are detrimental to image quality and can result in image artifacts. In the following paragraphs, the most common types of image artifacts and ways to reduce their influence will be discussed.

8.4.3.1 Beam Hardening

In practice, CT uses polychromatic X-ray sources, which leads to the attenuation of a homogeneous object being not proportional to the thickness of the object along the ray. A polychromatic X-ray source produces a wide, continuous spectrum of energies and X-ray attenuation coefficients are dependent on the energy. A detailed mathematical description of the spectrum is provided in Sec. 8.5.

When an X-ray passes through an object, lower energy photons are more easily absorbed than higher energy photons. This effect is called “beam hard-

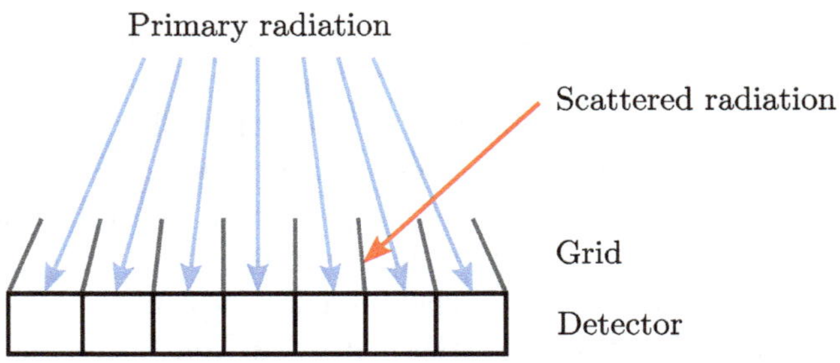

Figure 8.23: Anti-scatter grids can be placed in front of the detector to reject scattered radiation.

ening". Beam hardening results in streak and cupping artifacts. A common approach to deal with beam hardening is to physically pre-filter the X-rays using thin metallic plates, which absorb the low energy photons. An in-detail discussion of beam hardening, including examples, is provided in Sec. 8.5.3.

8.4.3.2 Scatter Artifacts

Scatter, or more specifically Compton scatter, causes X-ray photons to change direction and energy. A scattered photon can therefore be measured in a different detector element than intended. This has an especially large effect when the scattered photon is measured in a detector element that normally would have only few photons, e. g., if a high density object like a metal implant blocks all incoming photons, the corresponding detector element only detects scattered photons. Scatter artifacts are noticeable as cupping and streak artifacts especially between high density structures. Most scanners use anti-scatter grids in front of the detector to reduce scatter. This grid consists of thin lead strips, separated by a X-ray transparent spacer material. It is placed on the detector and aligned towards the focal spot. Thus, a photon that was not scattered can pass through the grid, while most scattered photons will be absorbed by the lead, cf. Fig. 8.23.

8.4.3.3 Partial Volume Effect

Partial volume artifacts appear mostly in low resolution images, especially in thick slice images. With low resolution, it is possible that one pixel consists of two regions with different absorption coefficients μ_1 and μ_2, cf. Fig. 8.24, which leads to streak artifacts in the reconstruction. Geek Box 8.6 describes the problem in more detail. This type of artifact is not often seen with state-of-the-art CT systems as the image resolution and especially slice resolution has improved drastically.

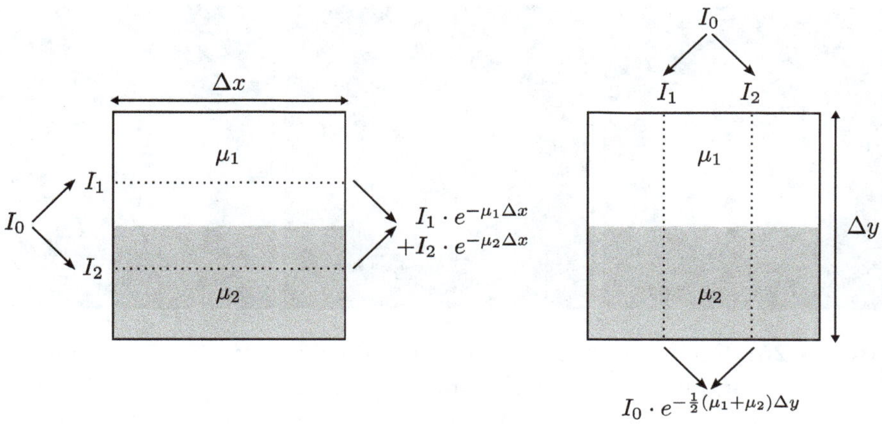

Figure 8.24: Two regions within a pixel with different absorption coefficients result in different measured intensities I for different projection angles.

Geek Box 8.6: Partial Volume Effect

In the first case, we observe two separate regions with the corresponding absorption equations

$$I_1 \cdot e^{-\mu_1 \Delta x}, \tag{8.38}$$
$$I_2 \cdot e^{-\mu_2 \Delta x}, \tag{8.39}$$

where $I_1 + I_2 = I_0$. Thus, the total measured intensity in this pixel is

$$I_x = I_1 \cdot e^{-\mu_1 \Delta x} + I_2 \cdot e^{-\mu_2 \Delta x}, \tag{8.40}$$

which is not equivalent to the average absorption we would expect,

$$I = I_0 \cdot e^{-\frac{1}{2}(\mu_1+\mu_2)\Delta x} = \tag{8.41}$$
$$= I_1 \cdot e^{-\frac{1}{2}(\mu_1+\mu_2)\Delta x} + I_2 \cdot e^{-\frac{1}{2}(\mu_1+\mu_2)\Delta x} \neq I_x. \tag{8.42}$$

However, in the case of the orthogonal direction, we do arrive at the average absorption,

$$I_y = I_1 \cdot e^{-\mu_1 \Delta \frac{y}{2} - \mu_2 \Delta \frac{y}{2}} + I_2 \cdot e^{-\mu_1 \Delta \frac{y}{2} - \mu_2 \Delta \frac{y}{2}} = \tag{8.43}$$
$$= (I_1 + I_2) \cdot e^{-\mu_1 \Delta \frac{y}{2} - \mu_2 \Delta \frac{y}{2}} = \tag{8.44}$$
$$= I_0 \cdot e^{-\frac{1}{2}(\mu_1+\mu_2)\Delta y} \neq I_x, \tag{8.45}$$

which is not equivalent to Eq. (8.40).

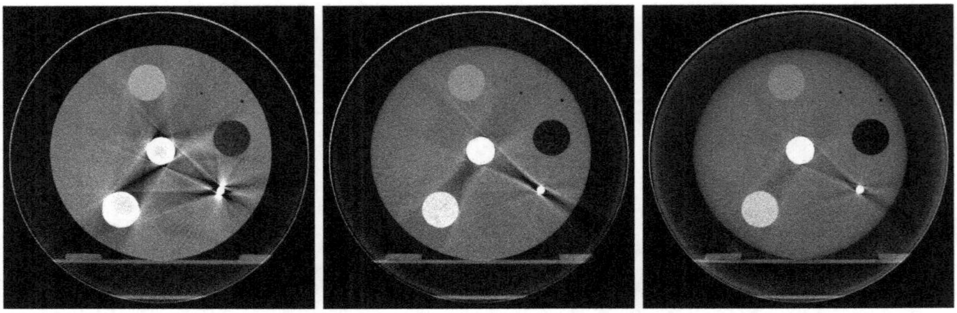

Figure 8.25: Reconstructions of an electron density phantom acquired at tube voltages of 50 kV (left), 80 kV (middle) and 125 kV (right). Photon starvation caused by the titanium rod at around 4 o'clock leads to pronounced streak artifacts. This effect decreases at higher tube voltages as more photons are produced and comparatively fewer of them are absorbed. Images courtesy of Jang-Hwan Choi.

8.4.3.4 Metal Artifacts

Metal artifacts are among the most common image artifacts in CT imaging. This term covers many different types of artifacts that we already discussed. There are various reasons why metal artifacts can occur. Metal causes beam hardening and scatter, which results in dark streaks between the metal objects. Additionally, its very large attenuation coefficient leads to photon starvation behind the metal object; as most photons are absorbed, only an insufficient number of them can be measured, leading to noisy projections. The noise is amplified in the reconstruction and will lead to streak artifacts in these regions, cf. Fig. 8.25.

Metal artifacts can be reduced by increasing the X-ray tube current or with automatic tube current modulation. Alternatively, there are metal artifact reduction algorithms that try to solve this problem without additional dose. Some algorithms aim to remove the metal objects in the reconstructed image and iteratively interpolate the holes in the forward-projected images.

8.4.3.5 Motion Artifacts

If motion, e. g., cardiac, respiratory, or patient motion, is present during an image acquisition, we end up with an inconsistent set of projection images. This can lead to blurring or streak artifacts in the reconstructed images. This type of artifact is especially prevalent with C-arm cone beam CT systems. Due to the slow rotation speed of the C-arm, a typical abdominal or heart scan takes approximately 4 – 5 s, during which significant respiratory or cardiac motion can occur. These artifacts can be reduced by estimating

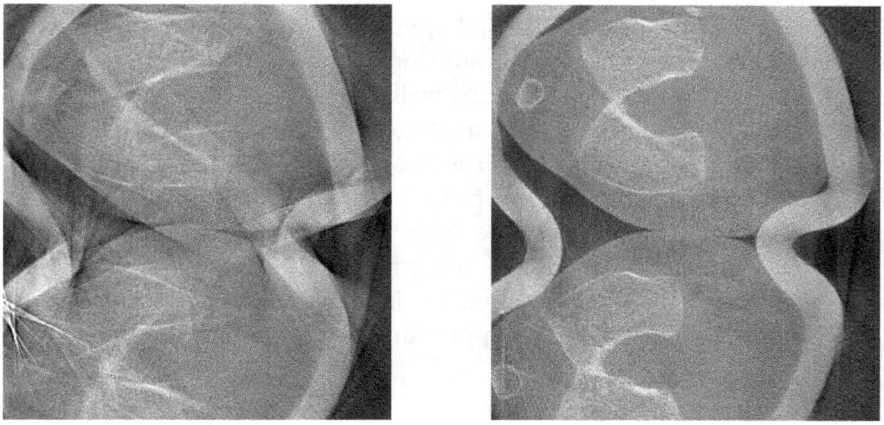

Figure 8.26: An image of human legs reconstructed from motion-corrupted projections using regular filtered back-projection (left) and with an additonal marker-based correction (right). By compensating for motion during reconstruction, structures that were originally blurred due to the movement become visible and streak artifacts caused by misalignments are reduced considerably.

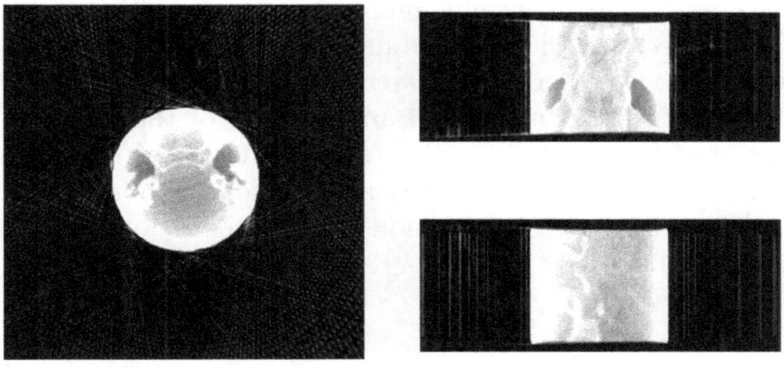

Figure 8.27: Illustration of truncation artifacts in the reconstructed slices.

the motion field and correcting it during image reconstruction. An example is shown in Fig. 8.26.

8.4.3.6 Truncation Artifacts

Truncation occurs when a scanned object is larger than the detector area or X-ray beams are intentionally collimated to a diagnostic region of interest for saving dose. Both cases will result in laterally truncated data. Due to the non-local property of the ramp filter, filtered back-projection reconstruction requires information of the whole projections for each point in the object. This requirement, however, is not satisfied anymore if projection data are laterally truncated. Thus, a noticeable degradation of image quality manifesting as a cupping-like low-frequency artifact as well as incorrect absorption values will be observed in the reconstruction, as illustrated in Fig. 8.27.

A popular truncation correction is based on estimating the missing data using a heuristic extrapolation procedure. For instance, a symmetric mirroring extrapolation scheme could be used to reduce the truncation artifacts from objects extending outside the measured field of view. Also, the missing measurements can be approximated by integrals along rays through a 2-D water cylinder since it is able to approximately describe a human body.

8.5 X-ray Attenuation with Polychromatic Attenuation

Traditional CT measures the spatial distribution of the X-ray attenuation of an object. The X-ray attenuation of a material is energy dependent, at specific energies it is governed by the composition of the material, more precisely on its mass density and the atomic number and composition of its elements. As described in Sec. 8.3, the common measure for X-ray attenuation in medical CT is the HU. However, for a material other than water and air, the HU value depends on the system design and settings of the CT device as well as the characteristics of the complete scanned object. Fig. 8.28 exemplarily shows the energy dependent X-ray attenuation for bone and soft tissue. This dependency is caused by the non-linear attenuation characteristics of polychromatic radiation.

8.5.1 Mono- vs. Polychromatic Attenuation

When a monochromatic X-ray beam at energy E_0 passes through an object, the measured intensity I_{mono} follows Lambert-Beer's law:

$$I_{\text{mono}}\left(E_0\right) = I_0\left(E_0\right) \cdot e^{-\int \mu(s,E_0)\mathrm{d}s}, \tag{8.46}$$

where $I_0\left(E_0\right)$ refers to the intensity of the incident X-ray at energy E_0, s denotes the path of the X-ray traversing the object, $\mu\left(s, E_0\right)$ denotes the spatial distribution of energy-dependent linear attenuation coefficients.

The attenuation could be obtained by rewriting Equation (8.46) as:

$$q_{\text{mono}}\left(E_0\right) = -\ln\frac{I_{\text{mono}}\left(E_0\right)}{I_0\left(E_0\right)} = \int \mu\left(s, E_0\right)\mathrm{d}s. \tag{8.47}$$

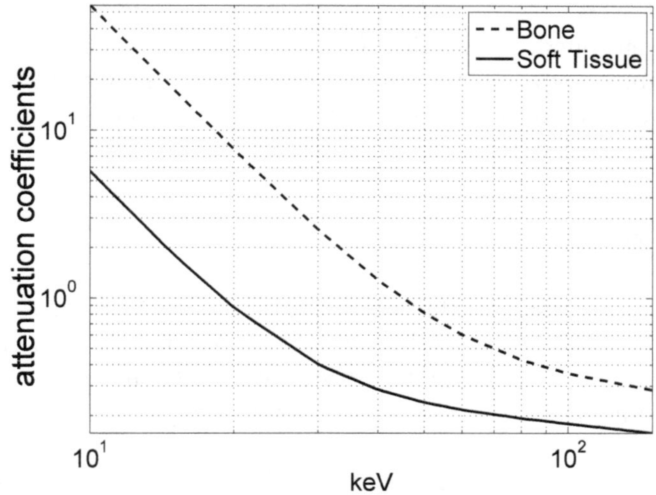

Figure 8.28: Illustration of energy dependent X-ray attenuation for bone and soft tissue.

Thus, for the monochromatic case, there is a linear relationship between the monochromatic attenuation $q_{\text{mono}}(E_0)$ and the intersection length of X-ray and the object.

However, the X-ray sources in typical clinical scanners are polychromatic sources. In addition, monochromatic measurements cannot provide real quantitative information as HUs are energy-dependent, i. e., different spectra and filters will result in different HUs. Although there exist physical ways to create monochromatic X-rays at sufficient intensity to perform X-ray CT, e. g., using a monochromator or inserting thick absorption filters to narrow the spectrum, these methods are very expensive and the usage is restricted to research experiments at few institutions. As detailed in Geek Box 8.7, in contrast to the monochromatic X-ray situation, there is no linear relationship between the polychromatic attenuation q_{poly} and the intersection length of X-ray and the object.

Fig. 8.30 depicts the relationship between the intersection length p and the attenuation q when a polychromatic X-ray beam, which is emitted at a tube voltage of 110 kV, penetrates a homogenous aluminium object, and the relationship between the intersection length p and the attenuation q when a monochromatic X-ray beam, which is emitted at the effective energy 45.56 keV of the aforementioned polychromatic X-ray beam, traverses the same object.

Geek Box 8.7: Polychromatic Line Integrals

As aforementioned, in practical setups, rather than a monochromatic X-ray beam, only a polychromatic X-ray beam is available. By summing the monochromatic contributions for each energy bin E in the X-ray spectrum gives ($E \in [0, E_{\max}]$):

$$I_{\text{poly}}(E) = \int_0^{E_{\max}} S(E)\, D(E) \cdot e^{-\int \mu(s,E)\mathrm{d}s} \mathrm{d}E, \tag{8.48}$$

where $I_{\text{poly}}(E)$ denotes the measured detector signal of a polychromatic X-ray, $S(E)$ denotes the spectral energy distribution and $D(E)$ denotes the detector energy sensitivity. Fig. 8.29 shows an example of spectrum and the integral under it for the explanation of Equation (8.48).

Consequently, adapting Equation (8.47) to polychromatic situation yields

$$q_{\text{poly}} = -\ln \frac{I_{\text{poly}}(E)}{I_0} = -\ln \int_0^{E_{\max}} N(E) \cdot e^{-\int \mu(s,E)\mathrm{d}s} \mathrm{d}E, \tag{8.49}$$

where

$$N(E) = \frac{S(E)\, D(E)}{I_0} \tag{8.50}$$

refers to the normalized energy spectrum with the effective detected intensity (system weighting function) I_0 defined by

$$I_0 = \int_0^{E_{max}} S(E')\, D(E')\, \mathrm{d}E'. \tag{8.51}$$

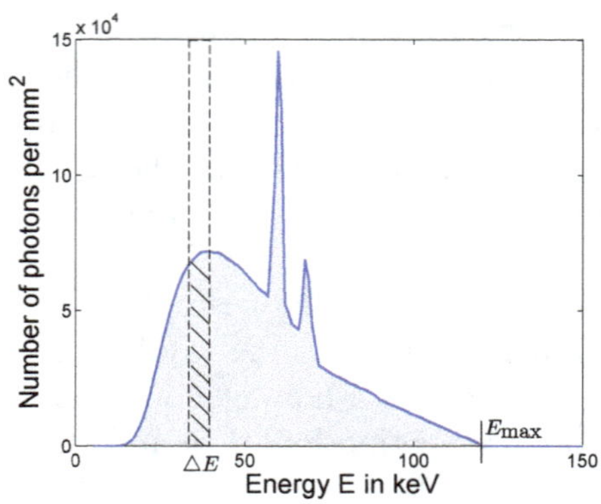

Figure 8.29: A spectrum and the integral under it.

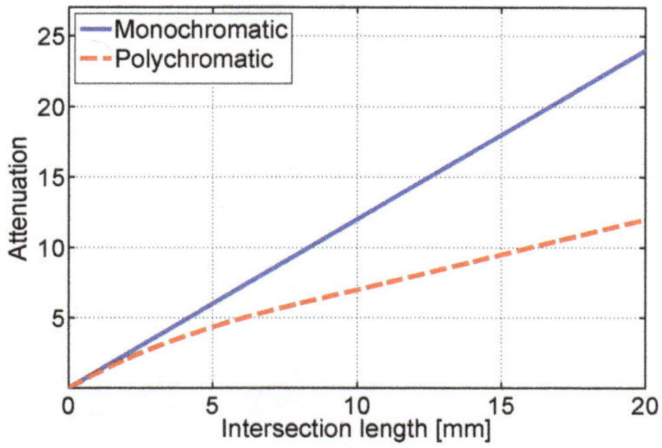

Figure 8.30: Relationship between intersection length and attenuation.

8.5.2 Single, Dual, and Spectral CT

As mentioned in the previous section, standard single energy CT reconstruction assumes mono-energetic radiation, however, common X-ray sources for medical CT are polychromatic. The fact is that in single energy CT, the energy information of the spectral attenuation coefficient is lost due to the measurement process. Therefore, the polychromatic characteristics of the input spectrum are neglected in single energy CT. Instead of an input spectrum $S(E)$ and a detection sensitivity $D(E)$, an effective detected intensity I_0 is measured in a calibration step, to recover the corresponding effective attenuation. In this manner, single energy CT is unable to provide quantitative information on tissue composition.

On the other hand, if spectral input data is acquired, i. e., multiple measurements with different spectral characteristics are made for each projection ray, real quantitative information on scanned anatomy becomes possible. For instance, dual energy CT measures two image sets at different energy weightings, e. g., by performing two scans with tube voltages set to 80 kVp [5] and 140 kVp, respectively. Fig. 8.31 shows an example of such dual energy CT scanner – Siemens Definition Flash (Siemens Healthineers AG, Forchheim, Germany). It employs two tube-detector pairs and produces two measurements simultaneously at different tube voltages. For spectral CT applications with dual source data, it is desirable to use two spectra with as little overlap as possible in order to ensure the maximal spectral separation between the two acquired datasets. For this task, usually the two tubes are operated at two different kVp settings. Additionally, a special filter can be used to attenuate the lower energy components in the high energy tube spectrum.

Although most spectral CT scanners require two spectral measurements, for some certain scenarios, more measurements are needed. The output quan-

[5] The peak acceleration voltage of X-ray tubes is usually given in kVp (kilovolt peak). An acceleration voltage of 120 kVp results in a X-ray spectrum where the individual photon energies are distributed in the range from 0 to 120 keV.

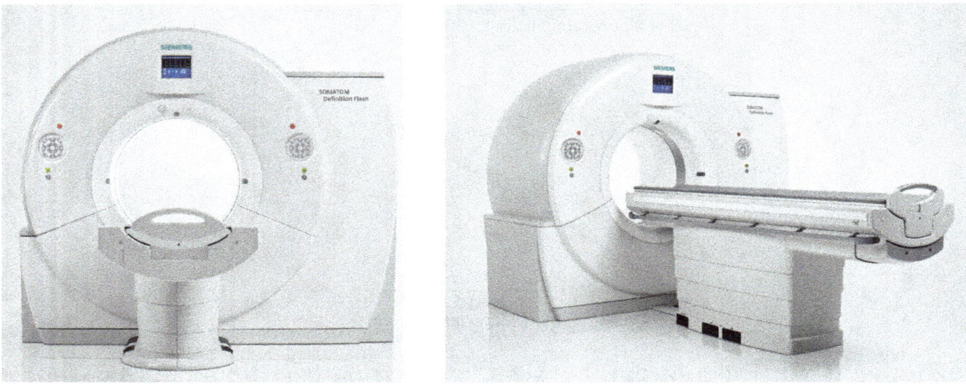

Figure 8.31: A dual energy CT scanner — Siemens Definition Flash. Image courtesy of Siemens Healthineers AG.

tities of these algorithms differ with respect to the diagnostic demands: they range from energy-normalized attenuation values over physically motivated quantities like density and effective atomic number to spatial distributions of whole attenuation spectra. The most popular current diagnostic applications are bone removal, PET/SPECT attenuation correction, lung perfusion diagnosis, or quantification of contrast agent concentrations, for instance in the myocardium.

8.5.3 Beam Hardening

When a polychromatic X-ray beam penetrates an object, photons with lower energies are easier absorbed by the object than photons with higher energies. Consequently, the average energy of an X-ray spectrum shifts toward higher energies while traversing the object, namely, the spectrum of the X-ray beam "hardens". The spectrum becomes harder with increasing intersection length of the X-ray with the object. This effect is called beam hardening.

Now we use an example to illustrate this effect in Fig. 8.32. We assume an X-ray beam is emitted at 120 kVp acceleration voltage and the material of the anode is tungsten. Now, we add additional layers of aluminum filtration to the spectrum. We can see that the corresponding effective energies E_{eff} shifts from 56.57 keV to 74.18 keV with increasing thickness of the aluminum wedge filter.

If beam hardening is not taken into consideration while doing reconstruction, the reconstructed image will be contaminated by beam hardening artifacts, which typically manifest as cupping and streak artifacts. As aforementioned, a spectrum is becoming harder when the intersection length is increasing. Hence, in reconstructed images, the inner part of the object is

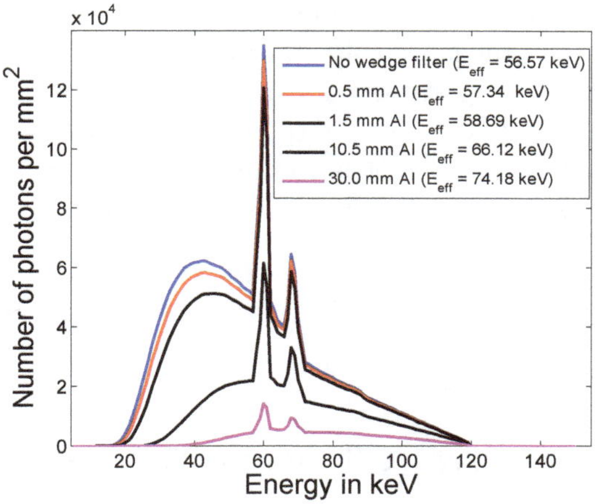

Figure 8.32: Tube spectra with different amount of filtration.

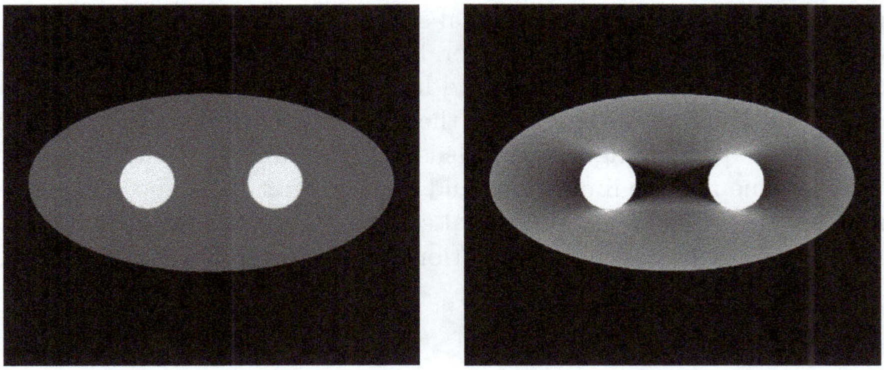

(a) (b)

Figure 8.33: Beam hardening example: (a) A simple phantom set-up consisting of water (gray), bone (white) and air (black). (b) Reconstruction of the phantom with visible beam hardening artifacts.

darker than the outer part, and a corresponding cupping appears in the reconstruction. Streak artifacts appear as dark bands or streaks in the reconstructed image. The occurrence of such artifacts is due to the fact that X-rays, which pass through only one dense object, are less hardened than those passing through both dense objects. Fig. 8.33 shows a simulated example of an elliptical water phantom with two dense bone insets.

Various beam hardening correction algorithms exist. For a soft-tissue calibration, projection measurements through soft-tissue like materials of variable known thicknesses are performed. For these, the equivalent water thicknesses are known. A simple function is fit through the pairs of measured and expected values. This function is inverted and then used as a look-up table:

for each measured attenuation, the equivalent water thickness is looked up, which then replaces the measured attenuation. If bone-induced beam hardening is also corrected, a separation into bone and water components can be performed. For dual energy CT, special quantitative correction methods exist. These take advantage of the two measurements at different energy weightings and special properties of the attenuation functions of body tissues.

8.6 Spectral CT

8.6.1 Different Spectral CT Measurements

Spectral CT detection refers to producing multiple measurements of the same object with different spectral weightings. The spectral weighting is defined by the tube spectrum and the spectral sensitivity of the detector. In spectral detection techniques, one of these or both are changed between measurements. The spectral weightings should have as little overlap as possible. This enhances the discrimination between the spectral measurements which is beneficial for spectral CT algorithms. Usually, only two spectral measurements are created due to dose limitations and the fact that most spectral CT algorithms do not benefit from additional spectral measurements. This fact can be attributed to the specific attenuation properties of body materials in the CT energy range.

8.6.1.1 Dual KVp

The easiest method for producing spectral measurements is called Dual kVp. For this method, two subsequent CT scans are performed at different tube voltages, e. g., 80 kVp and 140 kVp; see Fig. 8.34(a) for spectra of these two voltages. As mentioned before, it is desirable to use two spectra with as little overlap as possible in order to ensure the maximal spectral separation between the two acquired datasets. To this end, usually a special filter can be used to attenuate the lower energy components in the high energy tube spectrum (140 kVp); see Fig. 8.34(b).

The main advantage is that no special equipment is needed for this method. In medical CT, this method is prone to motion artifacts as the alignment of the two datasets cannot be ensured due to patient motion in between the two scans. However, this is a valid method for evaluating spectral CT algorithms on phantom data.

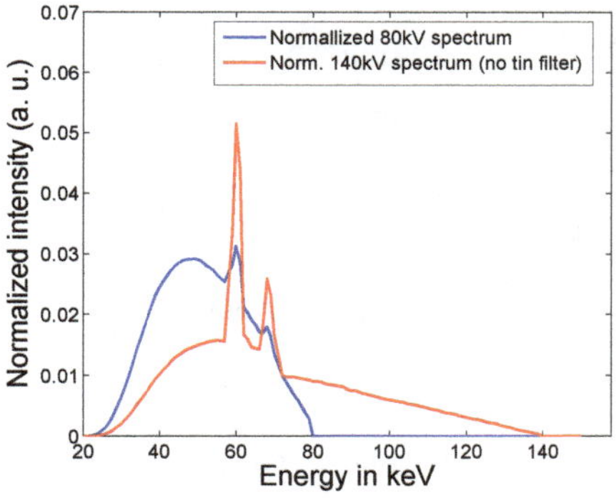

(a)

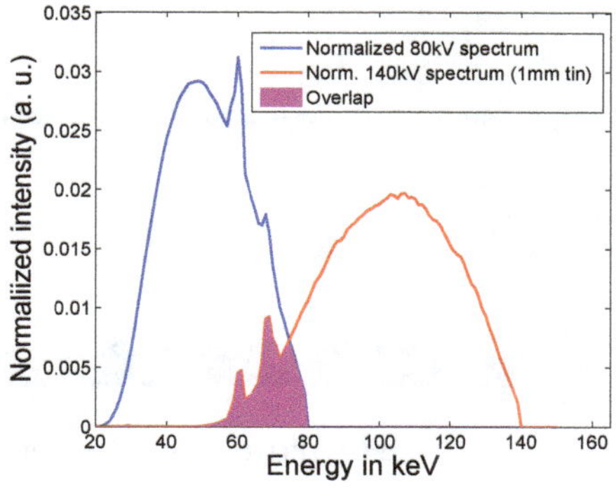

(b)

Figure 8.34: (a) Spectral measurements with different tube voltages, e. g. 80 kVp and 140 kVp. (b) A special filter was applied to high energy tube spectrum to ensure two spectra with as little overlap as possible.

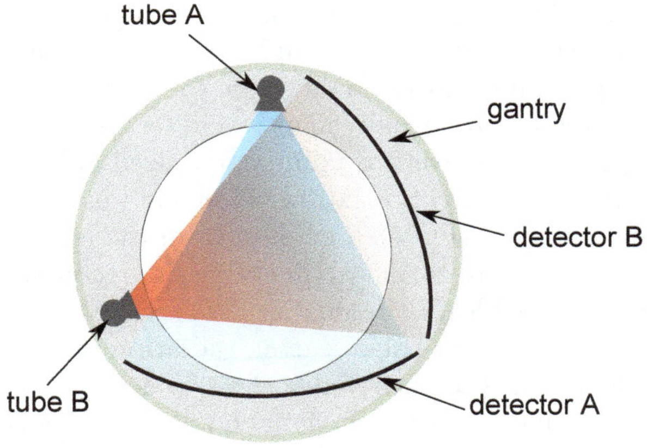

Figure 8.35: Concept of dual source CT.

8.6.1.2 KVp-switching

KVp-switching is another tube-based approach that switches the tube voltage between two readings. As read-out times are typically in the range of hundreds of micro-seconds, a special tube capable of changing the tube voltage very quickly is required. Due to dose efficiency, the tube current should also be adjusted for different kVp-settings as the attenuation properties of human body tissue are very different for different X-ray energies. The projections acquired with this approach are not perfectly aligned as the projections are interleaved. Missing projections may have to be interpolated.

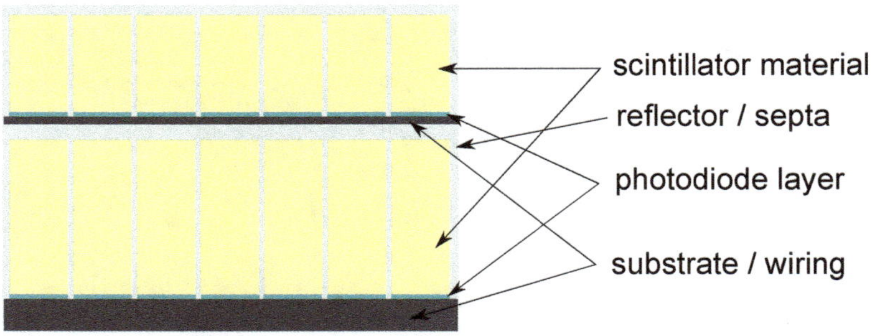

Figure 8.36: Concept of dual layer detector.

8.6.1.3 Dual Source

Dual Source CT is similar to dual kVp with the two CT scans being performed simultaneously by a special CT system. In this system, the gantry houses two tube-detector pairs A and B with a fixed angular offset (see Fig. 8.35). The two X-ray tubes are operated at different tube voltages. More recent systems offer an optional tin filter on one tube to increase spectral separation whereas the two detectors are usually identical in terms of spectral sensitivity. Most available systems, however, use differently sized detectors due to space restrictions within the gantry. So the measurements of the smaller detector offer a limited field of view (FOV). The data from the larger detector can be used to compensate for truncation artifacts in the reconstruction but Dual Energy data is only available for the smaller FOV. Since the two tube-detector pairs are operated simultaneously, scatter radiation from tube A impairs the signal of detector B and vice versa. This is a major drawback of this technology, as this property decreases signal quality and leads to an increased patient dose.

8.6.1.4 Dual Layer Detectors

This technology uses a variation of the detector spectral sensitivity to produce measurements at different energy weightings. Two scintillation detector layers are stacked upon each other and the top detector layer is a pre-filter for the lower one. This technology is also referred to as sandwich detector. Fig. 8.36 shows a possible realization of this concept. The detector efficiency is lowered, as the top layer photodiodes and wiring absorb parts of the X-rays and escape photons may enter the other layer and impair the energy separation of the layers.

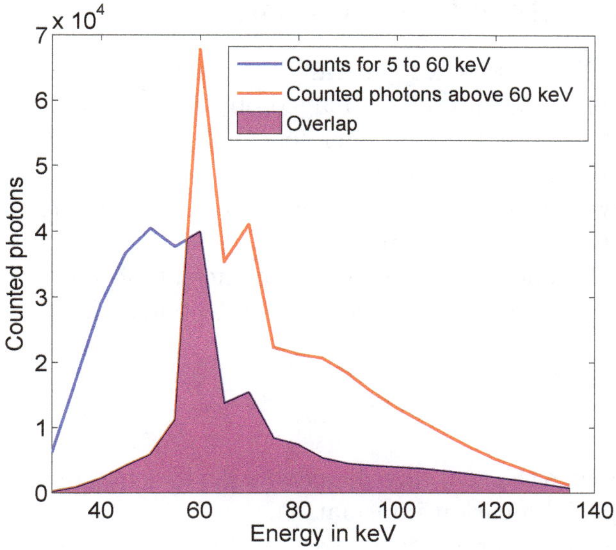

Figure 8.37: Spectral sensitivity example for a counting semiconductor detector with thresholds set to 5 keV and 60 keV. Due to several effects like cross talk, escape photons and signal pile-up, the spectral separation is reduced by a considerable overlap of the sensitivity curves.

8.6.1.5 Counting Detectors

Spectral measurements can be conducted with counting detectors by using multiple energy-thresholded photon counts. Theoretically, X-ray counting for medical CT can be performed with scintillators and semiconductor detectors. As semiconductor detectors have the advantage of being very fast and having very limited cross-talk between channels, a lot of effort has been put in evaluating the suitability of these detectors for medical CT. However, still some issues have to be resolved before this technology becomes commercially available in medical CT scanners. Counting detectors perform especially good at low X-ray flux. At high flux levels, which typically appear in medical CT, several problems arise: Signal saturation prevents distinction of individual detection events and polarization of the semiconductor material affects the signal quality. Due to physical effects, material defects, and technical limitations, the discrimination of X-ray quanta cannot be perfect. This leads to a limited spectral separation between the spectral sensitivities for each threshold signal which is dependent of the incoming X-ray flux. Fig. 8.37 shows spectral sensitivities for thresholds producing photons counts below and above 60 keV at low X-ray flux and their overlap for a 140 kVp tube spectrum.

8.6.2 Basis Material Decomposition

Fully Spectral CT approaches generally yield measures that are directly related to physical properties of the imaged object or tissue. Unlike HUs, these measures should not be system-dependent or be influenced by the surrounding object. The following section introduces basis material decomposition, which yields two or more effective basis material densities to characterize underlying material compositions.

In general, the spectral attenuation coefficient of a material can be expressed as a linear combination of M energy-dependent basis functions $f_j(E)$:

$$\mu(\mathbf{r}, E) = \sum_{j=1}^{M} c_j(\mathbf{r}) f_j(E), \tag{8.52}$$

where $c_j(\mathbf{r})$ denotes the spatially-dependent coefficients, in which $\mathbf{r} = (x, y, z)$ refers to the spatial location information.

The principle of material decomposition is based on the fact that the spectral attenuation coefficients of body materials are dominated by two effects in the energy range of medical CT: photoelectric absorption and Compton scattering, as described in Sec. 7.3 (p. 125). Since two basis materials are sufficient to express $\mu(\mathbf{r}, E)$ for body materials with very small errors, a separation of the the energy-dependent basis functions $f_j(E)$ from the spatially-dependent coefficients $c_j(\mathbf{r})$ is possible. The typical choice for basis functions in medical CT is a set of water and bone mass attenuation functions. We denote the basis functions $f_\mathrm{W}(E)$ and $f_\mathrm{B}(E)$, with $f_\mathrm{W}(E)$-component corresponding to the mass attenuation coefficient of water and $f_\mathrm{B}(E)$ to femur bone. The corresponding basis material coefficients are denoted $c_\mathrm{W}(\mathbf{r})$ and $c_\mathrm{B}(\mathbf{r})$. For this basis material set, Equation (8.52) reads:

$$\mu(\mathbf{r}, E) = c_\mathrm{W}(\mathbf{r}) \cdot f_\mathrm{W}(E) + c_\mathrm{B}(\mathbf{r}) \cdot f_\mathrm{B}(E). \tag{8.53}$$

Two methods to recover $c_\mathrm{W}(\mathbf{r})$ and $c_\mathrm{B}(\mathbf{r})$ are presented in Geek Boxes 8.8 and 8.9.

Further Reading

[1] M. Balda. *Quantitative Computed Tomography.* PhD thesis, Friedrich-Alexander-Universität Erlangen-Nürnberg, 2011.

[2] Martin Berger et al. "Marker-free motion correction in weight-bearing cone-beam CT of the knee joint". In: *Medical Physics* 43.3 (2016), pp. 1235–1248. DOI: 10.1118/1.4941012.

[3] T. M. Buzug. *Computed Tomography: From Photon Statistics to Modern Cone-Beam CT.* Springer, 2008. ISBN: 9783540394082.

[4] Frank Dennerlein and Andreas Maier. "Approximate truncation robust computed tomography - ATRACT". In: *Physics in Medicine and Biology* 58.17 (2013), pp. 6133–6148. DOI: 10.1088/0031-9155/58/17/6133.

Geek Box 8.8: Projection-Based Basis Material Decomposition

Inserting Equation (8.53) into the line integral of the spectral attenuation law yields:

$$\int \mu(\mathbf{r}, E)\,\mathrm{d}s = f_\mathrm{W}(E)\int c_\mathrm{W}(\mathbf{r})\,\mathrm{d}s + f_\mathrm{B}(E)\int c_\mathrm{B}(\mathbf{r})\,\mathrm{d}s. \quad (8.54)$$

We denote the line integral over the water coefficients $A_\mathrm{W} = \int c_\mathrm{W}(\mathbf{r})\,\mathrm{d}s$. The integral A_B over the bone coefficients is defined along the same line.
Conducting a dual energy measurement at two energy weightings $S_1(E)\,D_1(E)$ and $S_2(E)\,D_2(E)$ gives the following system of non-linear equations:

$$I_1 = \int_0^\infty S_1(E)\,D_1(E)\,e^{-f_\mathrm{W}(E)A_\mathrm{W} - f_\mathrm{B}(E)A_\mathrm{B}}\mathrm{d}E \quad (8.55)$$

$$I_2 = \int_0^\infty S_2(E)\,D_2(E)\,e^{-f_\mathrm{W}(E)A_\mathrm{W} - f_\mathrm{B}(E)A_\mathrm{B}}\mathrm{d}E \quad (8.56)$$

This system has to be solved for A_W and A_B, which is the scope of current research. Then, the basis material coefficients $c_\mathrm{W}(\mathbf{r})$ and $c_\mathrm{B}(\mathbf{r})$ can be recovered from A_W and A_B with a plain inverse Radon transform as used for standard CT reconstruction.
A general drawback of projection data-based methods is the requirement of perfectly matched projections and not all dual-energy detection techniques are able to measure line integrals at exactly the same positions for each spectrum.

[5] Joachim Hornegger, Andreas Maier, and Markus Kowarschik. "CT Image Reconstruction Basics". In: *MR and CT Perfusion and Pharmacokinetic Imaging: Clinical Applications and Theoretical Principles*. Ed. by Roland Bammer. 1st ed. Alphen aan den Rijn, Netherlands, 2016, pp. 01–09. ISBN: 9781451147155.

[6] W. A. Kalender. *Computed Tomography: Fundamentals, System Technology, Image Quality, Applications*. Wiley, 2011. ISBN: 9783895786440.

[7] B. Keck. *High Performance Iterative X-Ray CT with Application in 3-D Mammography and Interventional C-arm Imaging Systems*. PhD thesis, Friedrich-Alexander-Universität Erlangen-Nürnberg, 2014.

[8] Yanye Lu et al. "Material Decomposition Using Ensemble Learning for Spectral X-ray Imaging". In: *IEEE Transactions on Radiation and Plasma Medical Sciences* (2018). to appear.

[9] Andreas Maier and Rebecca Fahrig. "GPU Denoising for Computed Tomography". In: *Graphics Processing Unit-Based High Performance Computing in Radiation Therapy*. Ed. by Xun Jia and Jiang Steve. 1st ed. Vol. 1. 2015. ISBN: 978-1-4822-4478-6. DOI: 10.1201/b18968-9.

Geek Box 8.9: Image-Based Basis Material Decomposition

Image-based basis material decomposition avoids the matched projection problem by performing the decomposition in the reconstruction domain. For this purpose, the reconstructed attenuation values need to correspond to a constant, known energy weighting throughout the CT volume. For data measured with a polychromatic source, this can be achieved by a quantitative beam hardening correction. It homogenizes the energy weighting throughout the reconstructed CT volume. The homogenized energy weighting is denoted $\tilde{w}_i(E)$. Here, i numbers the N_i spectral measurements. As for projection data-based basis material decomposition, multiple measurements at different energy weightings are required. The relation between spectral attenuation coefficient and measured attenuation coefficient after beam hardening correction $\tilde{\mu}_i(\mathbf{r})$ is defined by the energy weighting:

$$\tilde{\mu}_i(\mathbf{r}) = \int_0^\infty \tilde{w}_i(E)\,\mu(\mathbf{r},E)\,\mathrm{d}E \tag{8.57}$$

With two basis material decomposition of $\mu(E,\mathbf{r})$ (8.53), we get

$$\tilde{\mu}_i(\mathbf{r}) = \int_0^\infty \tilde{w}_i(E)\left(c_\mathrm{W}(\mathbf{r})\,f_\mathrm{W}(E) + c_\mathrm{B}(\mathbf{r})\,f_\mathrm{B}(E)\right)\mathrm{d}E \tag{8.58}$$

Here, we can exchange summation and integration,

$$\tilde{\mu}_i(\mathbf{r}) = c_\mathrm{W}(\mathbf{r})\int_0^\infty \tilde{w}_i(E)\,f_\mathrm{W}(E)\,\mathrm{d}E + c_\mathrm{B}(\mathbf{r})\int_0^\infty \tilde{w}_i(E)\,f_\mathrm{B}(E)\,\mathrm{d}E. \tag{8.59}$$

The complete basis material decomposition with all measurements then leads to the following linear system of equations:

$$\tilde{\mu}(\mathbf{r}) = \tilde{\mathbf{K}}\cdot\mathbf{c}(\mathbf{r}) \tag{8.60}$$

with $\tilde{\mu}(r) = \left(\tilde{\mu}_1(\mathbf{r}), \tilde{\mu}_2(\mathbf{r}), ..., \tilde{\mu}_{N_i}(\mathbf{r})\right)^\top$, $\mathbf{c}(\mathbf{r}) = \left(c_\mathrm{W}(\mathbf{r}), c_\mathrm{B}(\mathbf{r})\right)^\top$ and

$$\tilde{\mathbf{K}} = \left[\int_0^\infty \tilde{w}_i(E)\,f_\mathrm{W}(E)\,\mathrm{d}E \;\; \int_0^\infty \tilde{w}_i(E)\,f_\mathrm{B}(E)\,\mathrm{d}E\right].$$

The quantitative accuracy of the image-based basis material decomposition approach depends on the accuracy of the beam-hardening correction and the image quality of the resulting basis-material images is reduced since the solution of Equation (8.60) is very sensitive to noise in the input data. So far, more advanced image-based material decomposition methods have been developed to overcome these drawbacks.

[10] Andreas Maier et al. “Fast Simulation of X-ray Projections of Spline-based Surfaces using an Append Buffer”. In: *Physics in Medicine and Biology* 57.19 (2012), pp. 6193–6210.

[11] A. Maier et al. “CONRAD - A software framework for cone-beam imaging in radiology”. In: *Medical Physics* 40.11 (2013), pp. 111914-1–111914-8.

[12] M. Manhart. *Dynamic Interventional Perfusion Imaging: Reconstruction Algorithms and Clinical Evaluation.* PhD thesis, Friedrich-Alexander-Universität Erlangen-Nürnberg, 2014.

[13] K. Müller. *3-D Imaging of the Heart Chambers with C-arm CT.* PhD thesis, Friedrich-Alexander-Universität Erlangen-Nürnberg, 2014.

[14] Kerstin Müller et al. “Image artefact propagation in motion estimation and reconstruction in interventional cardiac C-arm CT”. In: *Physics in Medicine and Biology* 59.12 (2014), pp. 3121–3138.

[15] Haibo Wu et al. “Spatial-temporal Total Variation Regularization (STTVR) for 4D-CT Reconstruction”. In: *Proceedings of SPIE Medical Imaging 2012.* Ed. by Norbert J. Pelc. Town & Country Resort and Convention Center, San Diego, CA, USA, 2012.

[16] Yan Xia et al. “Towards Clinical Application of a Laplace Operator-based Region of Interest Reconstruction Algorithm in C-arm CT”. In: *IEEE Trans Med Imaging* 33/2014.3 (2014), pp. 593–606. DOI: 10.1109/TMI.2013.2291622.

[17] Y. Xia et al. “Patient-bounded extrapolation using low-dose priors for volume-of-interest imaging in C-arm CT”. In: *Medical Physics* 42.4 (2015), pp. 1787–1796.

[18] Z. Yu et al. “Line plus arc source trajectories and their R-line coverage for long-object cone-beam imaging with a C-arm system”. In: *Physics in Medicine and Biology* 56.12 (2011), pp. 3447–3471.

[19] G. Zeng. *Medical Image Reconstruction: A Conceptual Tutorial.* Springer, 2010. ISBN: 9783642053689.

9

X-Ray Phase-Contrast Imaging

Authors: Johannes Bopp, Lina Felsner, Shiyang Hu,
Sebastian Kaeppler and Christian Riess

9.1 Introduction

Modern medical imaging is achieved with state-of-the-art devices, that use cutting-edge technology from different fields of engineering. Oftentimes, progress is driven by discoveries in a at first sight seemingly unrelated field of research. This enables the construction of new devices that was thought to be impossible before. In this chapter, we introduce a new imaging modality that has the potential to develop into a future medical imaging technology: X-ray phase-contrast imaging. At its current state, its medical use still has to be demonstrated. Yet, several early experimental results indicate that it has some potential for clinical applications.

Conventional X-ray imaging measures the attenuation of X-rays. X-ray attenuation happens due to different interactions between X-ray photons

Geek Box 9.1: Complex Index of Refraction

As stated in Chapter 5, light propagation can be modeled with the index of refraction n. When operating at X-ray energies, the index of refraction is expressed as a complex number,

$$n_{\text{complex}} = 1 - \delta + \mathrm{i}\beta \ , \tag{9.1}$$

where the imaginary coefficient β models attenuation and the real coefficient δ models phase shift. At X-ray energies, n_{complex} is very close to 1, i. e., little attenuation and refraction occurs. For example, for a transition between vacuum and water at a (relatively low) X-ray energy of 20 keV, $\beta = 3.99411 \cdot 10^{-10}$ and $\delta = 5.76149 \cdot 10^{-07}$. Note that for this configuration, δ is by about a factor 1000 larger than β. If we loosely identify β with the quantity measured in traditional X-ray, and δ with the quantity measured in phase-sensitive X-ray, we get an intuition about the vision of early attempts to translate phase-sensitive X-ray into the hospital: shouldn't it be possible with phase-sensitive X-ray systems to obtain a signal that is 1000 times stronger at a radiation dose equal to traditional X-ray? Later research has shown that the necessary compromises in system design to measure phase consume most of this advantage.

and matter (see Chapter 7 for details). However, attenuation does not fully describe X-ray interaction with matter. In the early 1930s, phase contrast microscopy, described in Chapter 5, was introduced. It measures refraction of visible light, which provides an alternative to standard transmission microscopy for mostly translucent objects, such as biological cells. Since visible light and X-ray are both electromagnetic waves, it is theoretically possible to transfer this principle to X-ray imaging. To measure X-ray refraction has two motivations: First, it may allow visualizing materials whose attenuation properties differ only slightly. Second, it was assumed that refraction information would deliver improved contrast over attenuation (see Geek Box 9.1 for details).

However, since the wavelength of X-rays is several orders of magnitude smaller than the wavelength of visible light, it took several decades until manufacturing technologies were developed to realize X-ray phase-contrast imaging.

Several systems have been designed for phase contrast imaging. While all of these approaches are highly interesting from a physics point of view, we limit the presentation in this chapter to the Talbot-Lau Interferometer (TLI). A short description of other approaches can be found in the Geek Box 9.2. Most of these other approaches are more sensitive than TLI, but TLI's relative

Geek Box 9.2: Other Setups

A number of different systems have been proposed to measure the phase of light at X-ray energies. Below is a list of setups that have been regularly mentioned in the recent literature.

- **Propagation-based:** This is probably the simplest phase-sensitive design. Phase is measured via interference: a wavefront that is refracted by a material interferes with itself [19, 22]. To compute the refraction (and hence the phase), it suffices to acquire two or more traditional X-ray images with varying detector distance. On the downside, interference only occurs if the X-ray source has a very small focal spot and the distance between object and detector is large enough. X-ray tubes with a small focal spot currently suffer from low flux, which limits practical applications.
- **Edge illumination:** This setup aims at directly measuring refraction by placing absorption masks in the beam path [14]. Depending on how much the object refracts the beam, a larger or smaller part of a detector pixel is illuminated. This design is conceptually very straightforward, but due to the direct measurement of the angle of refraction, it is less sensitive than other systems.
- **Analyzer-based:** Analyzer-based systems operate on monochromatic X-rays, which allows to precisely measure the refractive angle for a material [6, 4]. The beam is reflected by a crystal (the so-called "analyzer") behind the object. This crystal has the special property that it reflects radiation only at the Bragg angle, i.e., in a very narrow angular interval. Rocking the crystal allows to precisely measure all occurring angles of refraction. While this setup is extremely sensitive to mechanical motion and requires monochromatic X-rays, it is unmatched in its sensitivity and dose efficiency.
- **Speckle tracking:** Another approach to direct phase measurement is to track the refraction of a predefined pattern in the beam path [3]. One can obtain such a pattern by introducing for example a sheet of sandpaper in the beam path. Speckle tracking works best on thin samples and also requires an X-ray source with a small focal spot.

mild system requirements make it currently the most attractive system for implementation in a clinical setup. In particular, it only requires additional gratings to be mounted between a regular medical X-ray tube and detector to be operated. Note that all of the methods presented in this chapter are current research topics and none of them are clinically used at present. However, it is expected that the presented methods will have clinical impact in the future.

We introduce some physical preliminaries, and then the Talbot-Lau interferometer itself. As an outlook, we present potential applications of this modality in medicine and visual inspection.

9.2 Talbot-Lau Interferometer

One of the most promising phase-sensitive setups for medical applications is the so-called Talbot-Lau interferometer (TLI) [5, 15]. It roots in Young's famous double-slit experiment from 1801 to demonstrate interference. Young performed the experiment with visible light, but it can be directly adapted to X-ray. A sketch of this experiment is shown in Fig. 9.1 (left). The light source, in our case an X-ray source, is shown on the left. We assume that X-rays only emerge from a small source point, indicated by the narrow slit on the left. There is a barrier with two narrow slits in the beam path at some distance before an X-ray detector. The observation of the double-slit experiment is that an interference pattern shows at the detector, that is a regular pattern of bright and dark spots. The origin of the interference pattern is illustrated in Fig. 9.1 (right). The interference pattern is determined by the path difference Δd of the two traveling X-ray waves from both slits, namely

$$\Delta d = d\sin(\theta) \ , \tag{9.2}$$

where d is the distance between the two origins. Here, we assume that the distance D between the slits and the screen is large, such that ϑ is close to zero and $\theta \approx \vartheta$. Constructive interference shows as a bright spot. It occurs when the waves arrive "in phase". This is the case if the path difference is zero or an integral multiple of the wavelength,

$$\Delta d = d\sin(\theta) = m\lambda \ , \quad m \in \mathbb{Z} \ . \tag{9.3}$$

Destructive interference appears as a dark spot. It occurs if the path length differs by half the wave length,

$$\Delta d = d\sin(\theta) = (m + \frac{1}{2})\lambda \ , \quad m \in \mathbb{Z} \ . \tag{9.4}$$

Gray spots are observed if the difference of path length is between these two cases.

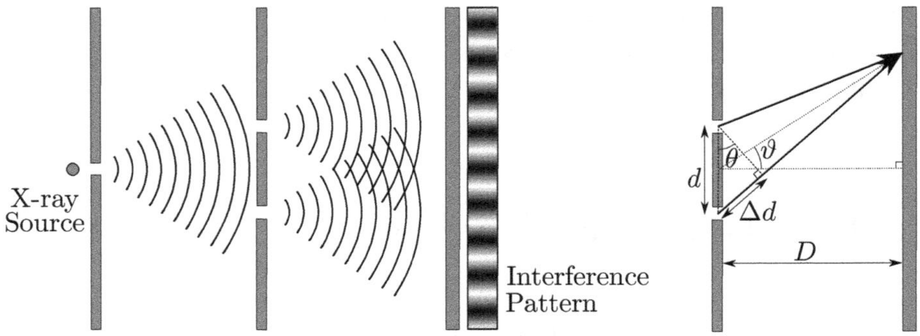

Figure 9.1: Young's Double-Slit Experiment

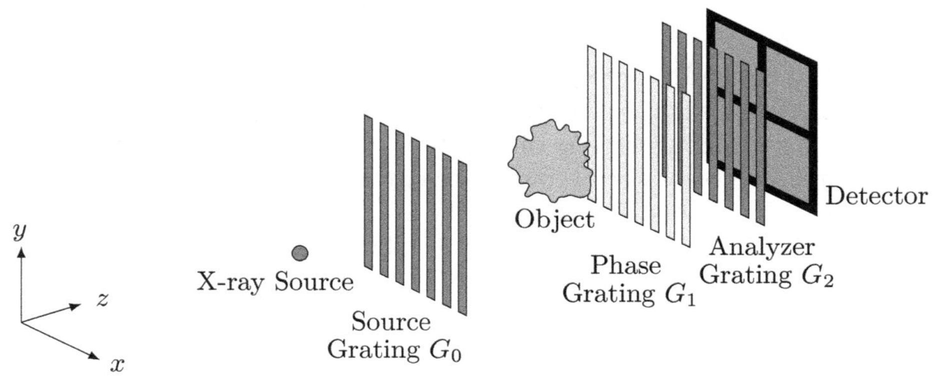

Figure 9.2: Talbot-Lau interferometer. Between X-ray source and detector, the three gratings G_0, G_1, G_2 form an interferometer.

9.2.1 Talbot-Lau Interferometer Setup

The Talbot-Lau interferometer makes use of the interference effect. It consists of a conventional X-ray device with three rectangular gratings G_0, G_1, and G_2 in the beam line (Fig. 9.2). These gratings typically have a period between 1 and 20 µm and a duty cycle of 0.5, i. e., grating bars and slits have the same width. G_1 is a phase grating and constitutes the core of the interferometer. G_0 and G_2 have supporting functions and will be introduced later.

At slits of grating G_1, the wave passes without notable modification. At bars of grating G_1, the phase of the incoming wave is shifted by an additive factor between 0 and 2π. This is a trick to construct from Young's double-slit experiment an actual imaging system. Constructive or destructive interference can now happen between wave sections traveling through two grating slits (as stated above), or between wave sections traveling through a grating slit and a grating bar. In the second case, the path difference Δd between a

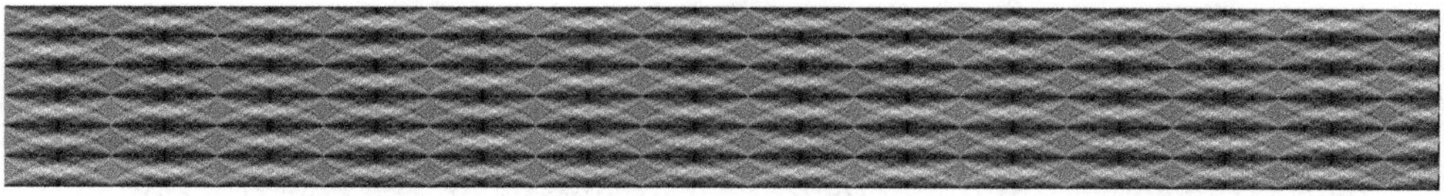

Figure 9.3: Simulated Talbot carpet: interference pattern behind grating G_1 travelling from left to right.

grating bar and a grating slit must now add up to the imprinted phase shift for constructive interference. Due to the Talbot effect, these interference patterns cleanly overlay at the so-called Talbot distances. Fig. 9.3 shows a simulation of the interference pattern behind grating G_1. The wave is assumed to travel from left to right. The detector is placed at a location where constructive and destructive interference form a clearly distinguishable black-and-white pattern. However, the pattern periodically repeats, which is why a system designer can in theory choose from infinitely many positions to place the detector. In practice, however, the pattern quickly washes out, such that the detector has to be located at one of the first replications of the pattern.

Gratings G_0 and G_2 are used to solve several engineering problems such that the interferometer can be built within compact medical X-ray setups. The interference pattern at the detector is normally much smaller than a single detector pixel. To resolve the pattern, the analyzer grating G_2 is used. G_2 is an absorption grating such that only a part of the interference pattern passes through the slits onto the detector. This makes it possible to sample the interference pattern by taking X-ray images while moving G_2 along the pattern (which is further discussed in Sec. 9.2.2).

Grating G_0 addresses another practical problem, namely the size of the focal spot. Interference effects can only be observed on coherent waves. In the sketch on Young's double-slit experiment in Fig. 9.1, coherence is obtained automatically by the small slit behind the X-ray source, which effectively acts as a small focal spot. There exist so-called microfocus X-ray sources that do provide such a small focal spot but they produce only very few X-rays per time. For practical applications, the imaging times are typically much too long. Medical X-ray tubes produce orders of magnitude more X-rays, which allows to take an X-ray image within a fraction of a second. However, such X-ray tubes can only be built with a focal spot that is much larger, typically between half a millimeter and a millimeter. To overcome this issue, grating G_0 is used, which can be seen as a long array of micrometer-sized slits. Each slit acts as a microfocus spot and creates an interference pattern at the detector. The distances between the slits are now chosen in a way that the pattern of each of the slits exactly overlays with the pattern of the other slits. If the setup parameters are chosen correctly (cf. Geek Box 9.3), all these periodic structures at the detector are aligned and add up. This enables imaging using conventional X-ray sources.

Geek Box 9.3: Talbot-Lau Setup Parameters

As described in Section 9.2 the TLI consists of three gratings, a medical X-ray source, and a detector. Many details on the construction of a Talbot-Lau interferometer can be found for example in the Ph.D. thesis by Martin Bech [2].

Optimization of the imaging performance of the whole setup requires to explore a huge parameter space. Each grating design already has multiple degrees of freedom. First of all, the grating material has to be chosen. Typical materials are gold, nickel and aluminum. The choice of the material and the manufacturing technology can constrain the other parameters of the grating, such as the height, period and duty cycle. The duty cycle is the ratio between the width of a grating bar and one grating period. Typical grating periods lie in the rage between 1 µm and 10 µm. Additionally, the grating aspect ratio, which is the grating height divided by the width, is currently limited to about 50. The design of one grating can not be done in isolation. Instead, the whole imaging system has to be considered. For example, The Talbot effect yields a limited set of possible distances between G_1 and G_2 for a specific energy. Another example is the G_0 grating, where the Lau effect can be used to fix either its period or its position.

Due to the huge parameter space, parameters dependencies and the polychromatic spectrum of medical X-ray tubes, optimization of a setup is challenging. In practice, one tries to hold most of the parameters fix. Then, the remaining parameters space is explored by simulating the corresponding interferometer using numerical wave front propagation algorithms.

One quality measure of the TLI can be derived from the system setup directly, the so-called sensitivity s,

$$s = \frac{\mathrm{dist}(\mathrm{G}_1, \mathrm{G}_2)}{2\pi p_2} \quad , \tag{9.5}$$

defined by the distance between G_1 and G_2 and p_2 which is the period of the analyzer grating G_2. The sensitivity can be interpreted as an "amplification factor" of the refractive angle.

9.2.2 Phase Stepping and Reconstruction

Phase stepping denotes the process of shifting one of the gratings (typically G_2) by a fraction of its period to sample the interference pattern. This is

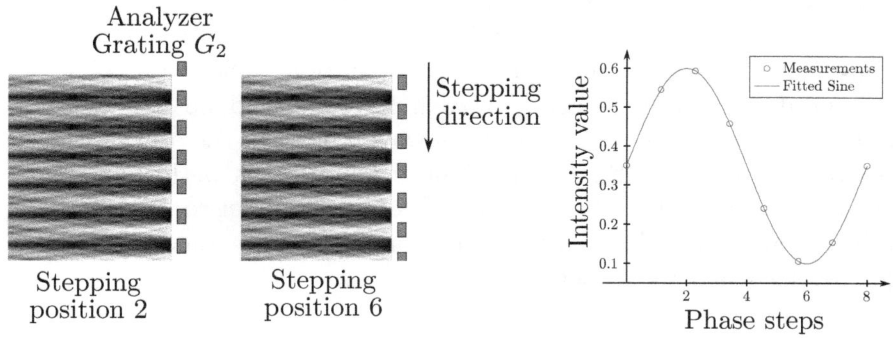

Figure 9.4: Left: phase stepping. The Talbot carpet is sampled at different positions of grating G_2. Right: the intensities at different stepping positions form the sinusoidal phase stepping curve. From this curve, attenuation, differential phase and dark-field can be calculated.

shown in Fig. 9.4 (left): the Talbot carpet forms the interference pattern. At equidistant stepping positions, the detector records an image. The intensity values for a pixel at different stepping positions is called phase stepping curve. This curve can be considered as a convolution of the profile of G_2 with the intensity pattern of the G_1 pattern. Convolution of two rectangular functions of G_1 and G_2 leads ideally to a triangular signal. In reality, blurring from the slits of G_0 leads to a sinusoidal curve that is fitted to the measured steps. These steps are shown in Fig. 9.4 (right). After fitting a sine function to the phase stepping curve, three quantities can be calculated: attenuation, differential phase, and dark-field. Attenuation is the offset of the intensities, which can be computed as the average of all intensities of the phase stepping curve. Differential phase is the phase offset of the sine. Dark-field is one minus the ratio between amplitude of the curve and two times attenuation.

In practice, these three quantities cannot be calculated directly. Instead, it is necessary to acquire two scans: a reference scan and an object scan. The reference scan is acquired without an object in the beam path such that it only shows the background. It captures inhomogeneities in the setup, for example, in the grating bars. The object scan is acquired with an object before or behind G_1. The reference scan is used to normalize the object scan after calculating attenuation, differential phase, and dark-field for both scans. Several works address the further suppression of imaging artifacts in software [9, 8, 11]. More details on the calculation of attenuation, phase, and dark-field can be found in Geek Box 9.4.

A common metric for the quality of an interferometer is visibility. Visibility is a measure of contrast of the intensity modulation and is given by the sine amplitude divided by its offset. Thus, the dark-field signal corresponds to the reduction in interferometer visibility, for example, due to micro scattering.

Geek Box 9.4: Signal Reconstruction

Let us formalize the computation of attenuation, differential phase shift, and dark field information for each pixel. Let R denote the wave profile of the reference scan and O the wave profile of the object scan consisting each of n phase steps. The calculation is performed for each pixel individually which is why we omit the pixel coordinate in the equations below. Attenuation is obtained as the average reference signal over the average object signal by computing

$$\mu = -\ln\left(\frac{\sum_{i=1}^{n} R_i}{\sum_{i=1}^{n} O_i}\right) .$$

The computation of the differential phase shift requires to find parameters for the sinusoidal phase stepping curve. The most robust way to do this is to perform least-squares curve fitting, which gives offset and amplitude of the sine. For the computation of the differential phase, the phase of object and reference wave profiles are subtracted.
The dark-field information ξ is a function of the visibilities of the reference scan V_R and the object scans V_O. V_R is computed as

$$V_R = \frac{\max(R) - \min(R)}{\max(R) + \min(R)} ,$$

where the maximum and minimum operators refer to the maximum and minimum function values of the fitted sine curve on R. The visibility V_O is computed in the same line. Then, the dark-field is defined as

$$D = -\ln\frac{V_R}{V_O} .$$

The visibility of the reference signal is considered an important figure of merit of the interferometer as it determines the noise in the differential phase and dark-field images.

9.3 Applications

An example for the three resulting signals is shown is Fig. 9.5. The shown gummi bears are modified with artificial defects, namely powder, a needle,

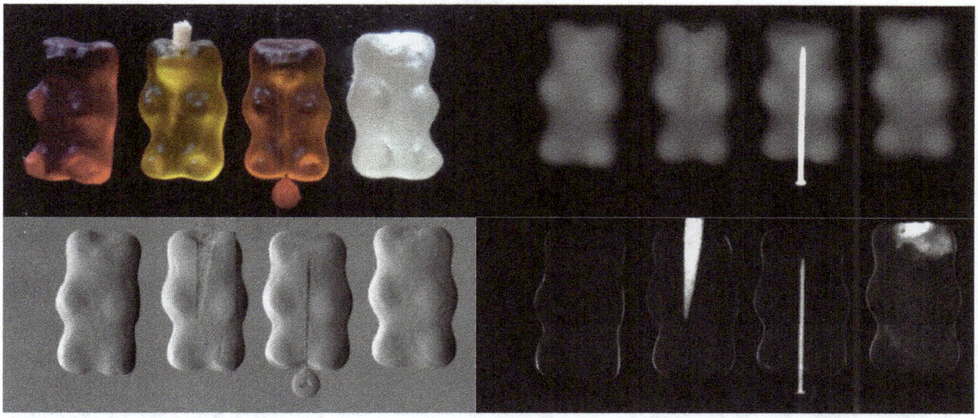

Figure 9.5: Top left: photograph of gummi bears with artificial defects. Attenuation (top right), differential phase (bottom left) and dark-field (bottom right) visualize different modifications in the gummi bears. Differential phase is particularly sensitive to high-frequency variations in the signal. Dark-field is particularly sensitive to micrometer-sized structural variations, such as powders or fibers. Pictures courtesy of ECAP Erlangen.

and a toothpick. In the top right, the absorption image is shown, which clearly shows the metal needle. On the bottom left, the differential phase is shown, which shows a large amount of high-frequency details, including the center of the needle head and the powder structure. In the bottom right, the dark-field signal is shown, which is particularly sensitive to the fine-grained structural variations in the powder and the toothpick.

An example scan on biological data is shown in Fig. 9.6. From left to right, the images show attenuation, differential phase, and dark-field of a female breast [10]. Particularly interesting in this visualization is the dark-field image, which is particularly sensitive to microcalicifications in the breast, a common indication for breast cancer.

Overall, X-ray attenuation visualizes both variations in density and atomic number. Thus, for example, it excels at the visualization of bones. Bones are more dense than the surrounding tissue and also contain a substantial amount of calcium.

Phase information on the other hand is sensitive to variations in electron density. Thus, it is expected to deliver increased contrast over attenuation when there is a similar elemental composition between two structures. One example is imaging of soft tissues. Talbot-Lau interferometers can only obtain differential phase information. Hence, its main advantage is in imaging high frequency details, such as edges that lie perpendicular to the grating bars. Conversely, it is less effective for imaging low-frequencies information.

Dark-field imaging provides two interesting properties that set it apart from absorption and differential phase: First, dark-field is sensitive to den-

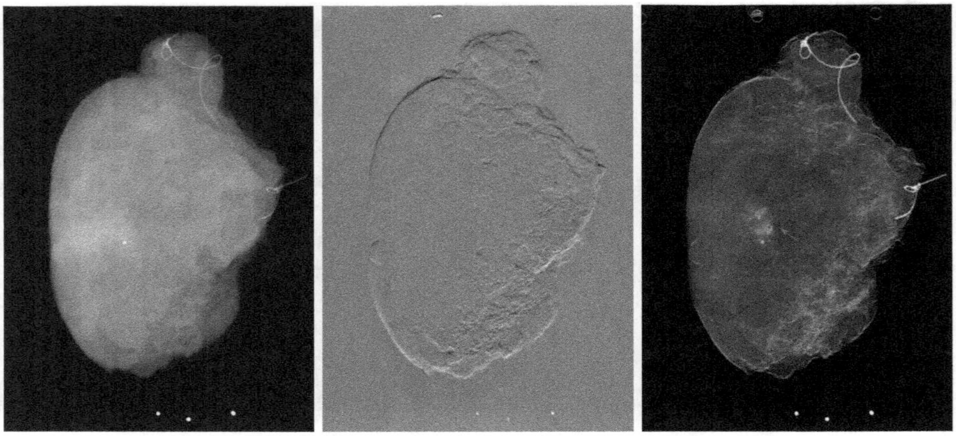

Figure 9.6: Attenuation, differential phase, and dark-field images of a female breast [10]. Microcalcifications in the dark-field signal (red arrows) can indicate cancer.

sity variation at nano- and micrometer scale. This is typically below the resolution of the detector, and as such too small to be resolved in attenuation imaging. Second, when scanning ordered structures such as fibers, the dark-field intensity varies with the angle between the fibers and the gratings. Both properties together can be used to deduce the orientation of fibers below the resolution limit of the detector [7, 12, 1]: when performing tomography on a plane in which micrometer-scaled fibers are located, the dark-field signal oscillates. From this oscillation, the direction of the fibers can be deduced, although the individual fibers are too small to be resolved by the detector. An example is shown in Fig. 9.7. On the left, a wooden block with different layers of wooden fibers is shown. This block is scanned in a tomographic setup, and the fiber orientations are deduced from the signal oscillations [1]. On the right of Fig. 9.7, the reconstructed orientations are shown, in different colors per layer.

Overall, phase-contrast and dark-field signals offer several interesting properties. It depends on the imaging task to decide whether the offerings of phase and dark-field signals or conventional attenuation is advantageous. The list below enumerates applications where Talbot-Lau imaging can potentially offer an advantage over traditional absorption imaging.

- **Mammography.** Mammography relies on imaging soft tissue structures in the breast, as well as on the detection of micro-calcifications. Imaging of soft tissues could benefit from the phase signal since it provides a strong signal to noise ratio at high frequencies. It has also been shown that the dark-field signal can reveal micro-calcifications that are invisible in the attenuation image since their porous structure creates dark-field signals [13].

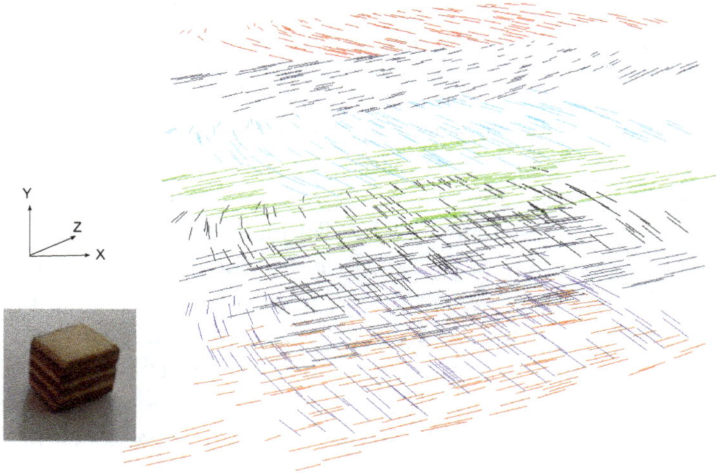

Figure 9.7: Layered wooden block (left) and example dark-field reconstruction of the dominant fiber orientations in each layer (right).

- **Lung imaging.** The human lung relies on millions of small alveoli to perform gas exchange. Lung diseases such as chronic obstructive pulmonary disease (COPD) and pulmonary fibrosis lead to a change in the structure of the alveoli. However, due to their small size, they cannot be resolved individually. The dark-field signal is able to detect abnormalities in the alveoli microstructure and may thus provide a benefit when diagnosing these diseases [23].
- **Bone imaging.** The directionality of the dark-field signal can possibly be used to detect osteoporosis, which can lead to less aligned structures in the bone [21]. Furthermore, the phase signal can visualize low contrast structures such as cartilage and tendons which may not be visible in attenuation imaging.
- **Micro-CT.** CT scanners which provide high resolutions (voxel sizes in the size of micrometers) are called Micro-CT systems. They are used for analyzing small samples and animals. At high resolutions, phase-contrast CT delivers a higher image quality than conventional CT [16]. This can be explained by the fact that the recorded phase signal is differential. A first Talbot-Lau Micro-CT system is commercially available [20].
- **Industrial applications.** Beyond medical imaging, dark-field imaging has been applied to non-destructive testing [18, 17]. For example, it can detect defects in carbon fibers or foreign bodies in food that are undetectable using attenuation imaging.

9.4 Research Challenges

The Talbot-Lau X-ray interferometer is an emerging image modality. Several questions need to be addressed before it can be applied in a clinical environment. Most notable issues are:

- **Grating manufacturing and mechanical setup.** Manufacturing grating structures with a period of a few micrometers and a sufficient grating height (in order to block high energy X-rays) is challenging. Thus, with current technology, the efficiency of the Talbot-Lau interferometer decreases with increasing photon energy. Additionally, the diameter of the gratings is limited to a few centimeters. Stitching procedures, which combine smaller gratings into a big grating, as well as smart scanning approaches that are compatible with smaller gratings are currently under research. Due to the small grating period, system stability in the nanometer range is required during operation. This stability is difficult to achieve in clinical environments.
- **Medical applications and dose.** A Talbot-Lau system is approximately half as dose-effective as a conventional X-ray system since the G_2 grating ideally absorbs half of the radiation. This leads to the question whether the additional information provided by a Talbot-Lau system is worth a reduction in attenuation dose efficiency. Economical aspects also need to be considered: manufacturing the gratings and their support structures adds considerable costs to an X-ray system. Is the benefit of the information provided by the Talbot-Lau system worth this cost?
- **Optimal system design.** Each grating introduces a new set of parameters into the system design (see Geek Box 9.3). Furthermore, the system does not only have to be optimized for attenuation, but also for phase and dark-field imaging performance. Due to this complexity, determining the optimal setup parameters (under the constraints provided by e. g., manufacturing) for a specific imaging task is still an open problem.
- **Image processing algorithms.** Image processing algorithms are needed in many steps of the conventional X-ray imaging pipeline, for example, for artifact correction, denoising, and visualization. Talbot-Lau interferometers suffer from additional issues (e. g. artifacts due to non-exact grating alignment). Also the differential phase and dark-field are affected by similar artifacts as the attenuation image, such as beam hardening. Additionally, the information retrieval from phase stepping data itself requires a reconstruction algorithm. Thus, image processing can be considered as a necessary component of a Talbot-Lau imaging system.
- **Tomographic reconstruction.** The phase information obtained by a Talbot-Lau interferometer can be reconstructed in a similar way to attenuation information by using an appropriate reconstruction filter, the so-called Hilbert filter. However, the dark-field signal (which contains scattering information) is directional and also influenced by signals at the object

edges. This makes its tomographic reconstruction challenging and has led to the development of dedicated algorithms to solve this problem [1].

Further Readings

[1] F. L. Bayer et al. "Reconstruction of scalar and vectorial components in X-ray dark-field tomography". In: *Proceedings of the National Academy of Sciences of the United States of America* 111.35 (Sept. 2014), pp. 12699–12704.

[2] M. Bech. "X-Ray Imaging with a Grating Interferometer". PhD thesis. University of Copenhagen, 2009.

[3] S. Bérujon et al. "Two-Dimensional X-Ray Beam Phase Sensing". In: *Physics Review Letter* 108 (2012), p. 158102.

[4] L. D. Chapman et al. "Diffraction Enhanced X-ray Imaging". In: *Physics in Medicine and Biology* 42.11 (Nov. 1997), pp. 2015–2025.

[5] J. Clauser and M. Reinsch. "New theoretical and experimental results in Fresnel optics with applications to matter-wave and X-ray interferometry". In: *Applied Physics B* 54.5 (1992), pp. 380–395.

[6] T. J. Davis et al. "Phase-contrast Imaging of Weakly Absorbing Materials using Hard X-rays". In: *Nature* 373.6515 (Feb. 1995), pp. 595–598.

[7] T. H. Jensen et al. "Directional x-ray dark-field imaging of strongly ordered systems". In: *Physical Review B* 82.21 (2010), p. 214103.

[8] S. Kaeppler et al. "Improved reconstruction of phase-stepping data for Talbot–Lau x-ray imaging". In: *Journal of Medical Imaging* 4.3 (2017), p. 034005.

[9] S. Kaeppler et al. "Shading Correction for Grating-based Differential Phase Contrast X-ray Imaging". In: *IEEE Nuclear Science Symposium and Medical Imaging Conference (NSS/MIC)*. Nov. 2014.

[10] S. Kaeppler et al. "Signal Decomposition for X-ray Dark-field Imaging". In: *International Conference on Medical Image Computing and Computer-Assisted Intervention (MICCAI)*. Sept. 2014, pp. 170–177.

[11] S. Kaeppler et al. "Talbot-Lau X-ray Phase Contrast for Tiling-based Acquisitions without Reference Scanning". In: *Medical Physics* 44.5 (2017), pp. 1886–1898.

[12] A. Malecki et al. "X-ray tensor tomography". In: *Europhysics Letters* 105.3 (Feb. 2014), p. 38002.

[13] T. Michel et al. "On a dark-field signal generated by micrometer-sized calcifications in phase-contrast mammography". In: *Physics in Medicine & Biology* 58.8 (2013), p. 2713.

[14] A. Olivo and R. Speller. "A coded-aperture technique allowing x-ray phase contrast imaging with conventional sources". In: *Applied Physics Letters* 91 (7 Aug. 2007), p. 074106.

[15] F. Pfeiffer et al. "Phase Retrieval and Differential Phase-contrast Imaging with Low-brilliance X-ray Sources". In: *Nature Physics* 2.4 (Apr. 2006), pp. 258–261.

[16] R. Raupach and T. Flohr. "Analytical Evaluation of the Signal and Noise Propagation in X-ray Differential Phase-Contrast Computed Tomography". In: *Physics in Medicine and Biology* 56.7 (Apr. 2011), pp. 2219–2244.

[17] V. Revol et al. "Laminate fibre structure characterisation by orientation-selective X-ray grating interferometry". In: *Proceedings of the 5th Conference on Industrial Computed Tomography*. Feb. 2014, pp. 45–51.

[18] V. Revol et al. "Sub-pixel Porosity revealed by X-ray Scatter Dark Field Imaging". In: *Journal of Applied Physics* 110 (2011), p. 044912.

[19] A. Snigirev et al. "On the Possibilities of X-ray Phase Contrast Microimaging by Coherent High Energy Synchrotron Radiation". In: *Review of Scientific Instruments* 66.12 (Dec. 1995), pp. 5486–5492. DOI: doi:10.1063/1.1146073.

[20] A. Tapfer et al. "Experimental results from a preclinical X-ray phase-contrast CT scanner". In: *Proceedings of the National Academy of Sciences* 109.39 (2012), pp. 15691–15696.

[21] H. Wen et al. "Fourier X-ray Scattering Radiography Yields Bone Structural Information". In: *Radiology* 251.3 (June 2009), pp. 910–918.

[22] S. W. Wilkins et al. "Phase-contrast Imaging using Polychromatic Hard X-rays". In: *Nature* 384.6607 (Nov. 1996), pp. 335–338. DOI: doi:10.1038/384335a0.

[23] A. Yaroshenko et al. "Pulmonary Emphysema Diagnosis with a Preclinical Small-Animal X-ray Dark-Field Scatter-Contrast Scanner". In: *Radiology* 269.2 (2013), pp. 427–433.

10

Physics and Clinical Applications of Emission Tomography

Author: James Sanders

10.1 Introduction

In contrast to the *structural* imaging used to visualize tissues in the body, *functional* imaging is used to observe biological processes. In the field of nuclear medicine, functional imaging relies on radioisotopes that are tagged to tracers whose biochemical properties cause them to congregate at regions of diagnostic interest in the body. As opposed to transmission tomography with X-ray CT, where the source of imaging radiation is a part of the imaging device, the radiation source in this case is located *within* the patient. For this reason, functional imaging methods in the field of nuclear medicine – also known as molecular imaging – belong to a family of modalities called *emission tomography*, whose differing physical properties make them quite distinct from the transmission case.

The process begins with radioactive decay, which results when an unstable isotope ejects particles from its nucleus while transitioning to a stable state. Although a very complicated process, two modes are of interest to molecular imaging: γ and β. In the former case, gamma rays are ejected directly from the nucleus that can be imaged with a so-called *gamma camera*. 3-D images can then be reconstructed from 2-D projections in a process called SPECT. In the second case, a positron is emitted which travels a small distance until an electron (its antiparticle) is encountered. The ensuing annihilation produces a pair of 511 keV photons traveling in opposite directions that, when detected simultaneously, yield lines of response that can be reconstructed into an image in a process known as positron emission tomography (PET).

Although X-rays produced by bombarding targets with electrons had been in use since their discovery by Röntgen in 1895, the use of naturally decaying radioisotopes for medical imaging did not occur until 1935, when George de Hevesy investigated rats injected with radioactive ^{32}P. Using a Geiger counter, de Hevesy investigated the relative amount of radioactivity in different organs after dissection and found that the skeleton had a disproportionately high level of uptake. In doing so, he not only settled once and for all the ongoing medical question of whether or not bones have an active metabolism (they do, otherwise they would not have taken up the ^{32}P atoms), but he was also the first to use radioisotopes and imaging equipment to investigate the body's biochemistry. Thus, the so-called *tracer principle* was born. For his work in the field of radiotracers, de Hevesy was awarded the Nobel Prize for Chemistry in 1943, and a variant of his original bone-imaging methodology based on phosphates is still in wide use today. In the decades following de Hevesy's discovery, research from the field of radiochemistry and molecular biology have yielded a plethora of tracers with desirable uptake characteristics. Complimentary technical advances have provided imaging devices capable of aiding physicians answer a range of diagnostic questions.

10.2 Physics of Emission Tomography

10.2.1 Photon Emission

Although the properties of γ and β decay are different in many respects, they follow the same basic decay law. Namely, the amount of radioactivity S (expressed in *Bequerel*, or decays per second) in a given sample of radioactive material will decrease until all atoms in the sample reach a stable state. This process follows an exponential curve, and the amount of activity in the sample at a given time t can be expressed as

$$S(t) = S_0 e^{-\ln 2t/t_{1/2}}, \tag{10.1}$$

where S_0 is the initial activity, and $t_{1/2}$ is the isotope's *half-life*, or the time it takes for $S(t)$ to decrease to half of S_0. This process is illustrated in Fig. 10.2, where the blue curve depicts the amount of activity remaining in a sample that initially contained 100 MBq. It can be seen from inspection that the

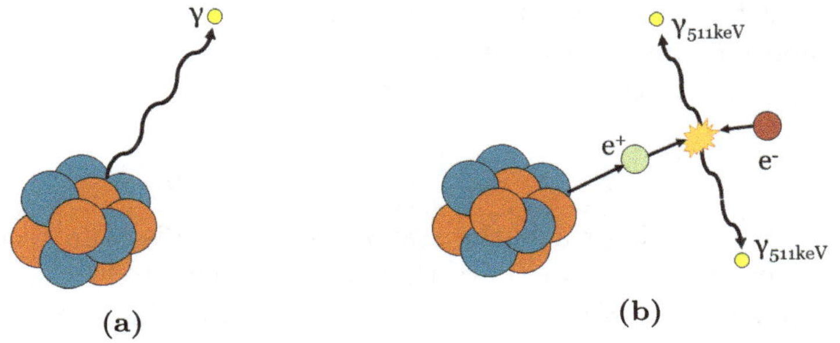

Figure 10.1: Simplified representation of both modes of decay relevant to emission tomography. On the left is a nucleus undergoing γ decay and emitting a single photon directly. On the right is an example of β^+ decay, where a positron is ejected from the nucleus. The positron travels a short distance before coming in contact with an electron. The resulting annihilation produces a pair of 511keV photons traveling in opposite directions.

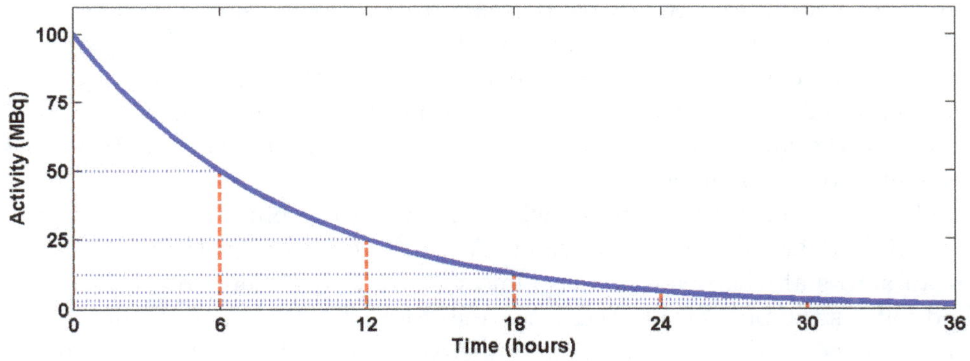

Figure 10.2: Exponential decay curve for a 100 MBq sample of a radioisotope having a half-life of six hours (the same as ^{99m}Tc).

isotope's half-life is six hours, which is the same as that of ^{99m}Tc, the most commonly used isotope for SPECT imaging.

Although Eq. (10.1) represents a sample's aggregate decay properties, the emission of individual photons (or photon pairs for β decay) within a particular time window is a discrete process and follows a Poisson distribution with a mean ν proportional to the amount of radioactivity present. Note that we can assume independence between the voxels and describe an entire image in a vectorized format using for a single voxel and $\boldsymbol{\nu}$ for an entire image. Similarly, the number of photons counted in a particular observation of this process, such as a pixel of a SPECT projection, is a Poisson-distributed random variable as well, provided that the image formation chain is linear.[1] If

[1] In practical scanners, this is not strictly the case, but it is assumed to be here.

we represent the projection pixels and image voxels as vectors, the distribution of photon counts on the detector $\mathcal{D}$ is related to the activity distribution being imaged $\boldsymbol{\nu}$ via the following relation:

$$\mathcal{D} \sim \text{Poisson}\left(\boldsymbol{A\nu}\right), \tag{10.2}$$

where $\boldsymbol{A} \in \mathbb{R}^{M,N}$ is known as the *system matrix* and is composed of elements $a_{m,n}$ representing the probability that a photon emitted from voxel n is detected at pixel m (cf. Geek Box 7.3). M and N are the numbers of detector pixels and image voxels, respectively. Multiplying an image vector $\boldsymbol{\nu}$ by $\boldsymbol{A}$ thus accomplishes a forward projection into the projection space. Acquired projection data $\boldsymbol{d}$ from an emission tomography scan therefore represent a single sample, or observation, drawn from the distribution $\mathcal{D}$.

Eq. (10.2) implies that detected images will always be perturbed by random noise, particularly for small numbers of counts. This effect is shown in Fig. 10.3, where simulated observations are shown for time points $t = 0$, $2t_{1/2}$, $t = 4t_2$, and $t = 6t_{1/2}$. For each simulation, the total activity from the blue curve in Fig. 10.2 corresponding to the time point t was distributed uniformly inside the ellipsoidal object, yielding an amount of activity at each pixel n that corresponds to the mean value of a Poisson process $\boldsymbol{\nu}_n(t)$. A random number was then drawn from the Poisson distribution at each pixel to create the images $\boldsymbol{d}(t)$. This is equivalent to applying Eq. (10.2) with $\boldsymbol{A}$ set equal to the identity matrix.

Central profiles drawn from each image along the blue line on the left of Fig. 10.3(a) are shown at the right. At the aggregate level, the simulated mean across all the pixels $\bar{\boldsymbol{d}}(t)$ is almost exactly equivalent to the true $\bar{\boldsymbol{\nu}}(t)$ and follows the predictable decay curve in Fig. 10.2. However, the noise level in the images and profiles appears to increase with t. This behavior is due to the fact that the mean of a Poisson distribution is equivalent to its variance. But if the variance *decreases* with the mean, then why does the noise appear to *increase*? To answer this, we can define a signal-to-noise ratio SNR within our homogeneous ellipsoid's boundaries to use as a noise measure. In this case, our signal is simply the mean over this object, and the noise is the standard deviation $\sigma_{\boldsymbol{d}}$:

$$SNR = \frac{\bar{\boldsymbol{d}}}{\sigma_{\boldsymbol{d}}} = \frac{\bar{\boldsymbol{d}}}{\sqrt{\bar{\boldsymbol{d}}}} = \sqrt{\bar{\boldsymbol{d}}}. \tag{10.3}$$

The SNR is thus simply the square root of the mean number of photon counts in the object and increases monotonically, albeit with plateauing benefits, with the number of counts in the image.

In X-ray CT imaging, where the radiation source is located outside the body and can be easily controlled by the system, large numbers of photons are easily attainable, as the patient can be irradiated with a high flux for a short period of time. However, in molecular imaging the radioactive source is

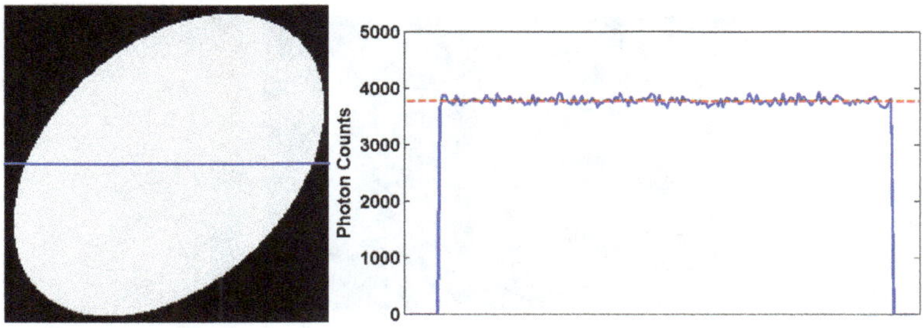

(a) $t = 0$

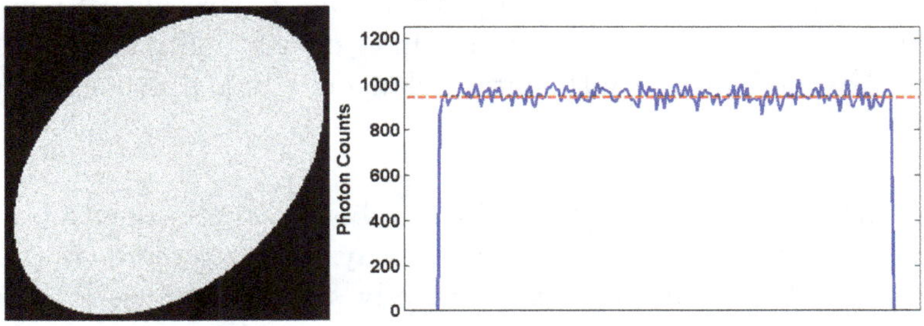

(b) $t = 2t_{1/2}$

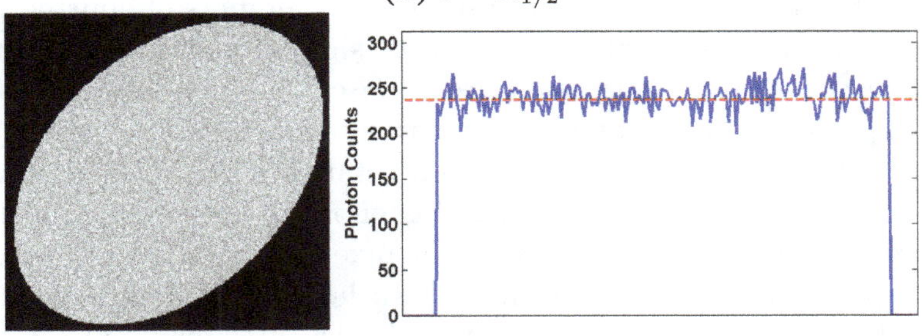

(c) $t = 4t_{1/2}$

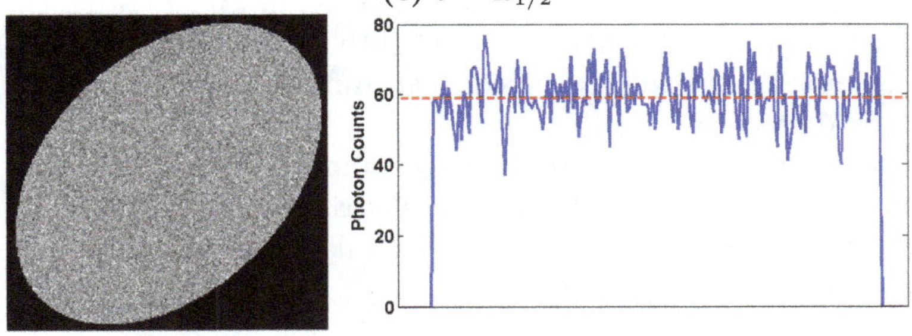

(d) $t = 6t_{1/2}$

Figure 10.3: Simulated images (left) and central horizontal profiles (right) from an object filled with the activity described in Fig. 10.2. The images were simulated after zero, two, four, and six half-lives (a, b, c, and d, respectively). The mean value of the object is shown with a dashed red line through each profile. Note how the images become noisier as the mean decreases.

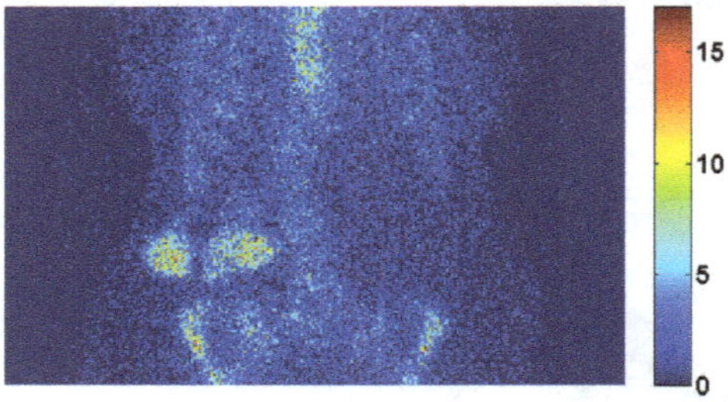

Figure 10.4: Typical 15 second projection from a skeletal SPECT acquisition. Even pixels with the highest counts have only roughly ten photons. Image courtesy of the University Hospital Erlangen, Clinic of Nuclear Medicine.

located within the body and will continue to bombard tissue with potentially harmful ionizing radiation until it either decays or is excreted by the body.

Therefore, to limit patient dose, relatively small amounts of activity are usually injected, typically ranging from 100 to 1,000 MBq. The activity is then distributed throughout the body, leading to low numbers of emitted photons at any given area. The imaging task is thus similar to taking a photograph in a very dark room. A long exposure time can yield a better SNR, but comes with problems of motion blur and patient discomfort. A typical SPECT projection lasts 15 seconds, resulting in a total scan duration of 30 minutes for the usual 120 projections! Despite this effort, projections typically have only about 20 or fewer useful photons per pixel in diagnostically interesting areas. A representative projection from a skeletal SPECT scan in shown in Fig. 10.4. The mean pixel value is a measly 0.6, and maximum is only 17, significantly less than even the noisiest simulation in Fig. 10.3(d). Due higher scanner sensitivities, PET statistics are slightly better, with roughly a factor of 10 more counts per pixel at typical scan durations of 4–6 minutes for an equivalent field of view.

The fundamental challenge in emission tomography is therefore to produce reconstructed images of the activity distribution $\boldsymbol{\nu}$ with acceptable image quality from noisy acquired data. The following sections describe other physical issues encountered as well.

10.2.2 Photon Interactions

Aside from the fundamental problem of noisy data, the second most important physical factor affecting emission tomography is photon attenuation. Photons traveling through a medium may interact with atoms and eventually be absorbed, resulting in a detected flux I less than that originally emitted. In Chapter 8, we learned how to describe this principle using Beer's law and

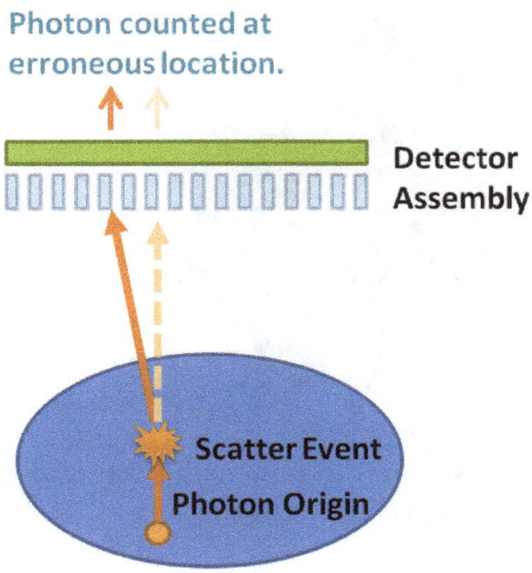

Figure 10.5: A photon is deflected from its original path (vertical) by a scatter event and detected at an erroneous location to the left of its ideal position.

exploit it for imaging. For transmission tomography like X-ray CT, this phenomenon is imaged directly to yield reconstructed images of the medium's (i. e. patient's) structure. This is possible because the location and current of the emitted flux I_0 is known. In emission tomography, however, I_0 is determined by the activity distribution in the body $\boldsymbol{\nu}$, which is unknown. Attenuation is therefore a hindrance that leads to errors if it is not accounted for.

Amongst the photon-matter-interactions, *Compton scatter* is very important for emission tomography (cf. Sec. 7.3). In this interaction, the photon is not absorbed as in attenuation, but merely deflected. The relationship between deflection angle θ and pre- and post-collision energies E_0 and E_{scat} is described by the Klein-Nishina formula:

$$E_{scat} = \frac{E_0}{1 + (\frac{E_0}{511})(1 - \cos\theta)}. \tag{10.4}$$

Scatter is an important component of emission tomography due to its role in the degradation of image quality. Specifically, deflected photons may be erroneously assumed to come from locations in the image volume along their scattered trajectories, rather than their original paths. This process is illustrated in Fig. 10.5, where a photon originating in the image is scattered and counted at a detector pixel corresponding to a trajectory other than its original (vertical) path. This has the effect of reducing resolution, contributing to image noise, and reducing contrast.

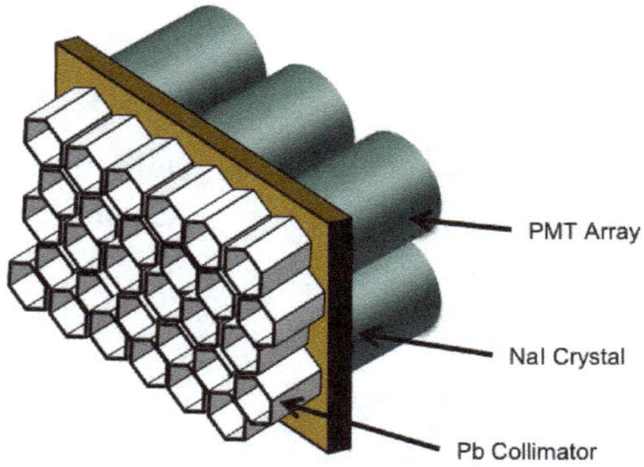

Figure 10.6: Simplified schematic representation of a gamma camera showing three primary components.

10.3 Acquisition Systems

10.3.1 SPECT

Early methods for detecting photons emitted from radiotracers focused on scanning probes (e. g. Geiger counters) over the patient. Scanning a field of view of any reasonable size was therefore a painstaking process, and 3-D reconstruction was out of the question. In 1957, Hal Anger solved this problem with the invention of the gamma camera, shown schematically in Fig. 10.6. A classical gamma camera consists of three components: a collimator, a scintillator, and an array of photomultiplier tubes (PMTs).

The collimator is composed of a lattice of holes separated by septa made of some highly attenuating material (usually lead). Its role is to restrict the angle of acceptance at each point on the detector surface and provide an (ideally) parallel projection of the object being imaged onto the scintillator. In e. g. optical imaging equipment, this is usually accomplished by means of a small aperture known as a pinhole. For this reason, collimators with a parallel-hole geometry consisting of a large array of narrow, parallel bores are the most commonly used type for SPECT imaging..[2]

Ideally, a point source placed in front of the detector would yield a perfect point in the image. However, the bores of a collimator are neither infinitely long nor infinitely narrow, leading to a finite acceptance angle that allows photons traveling from the point to reach the detector via a range of rays about the ideal one (i. e. the shortest path from point to detector). The structure of these alternate paths is described by the collimator's PSF and effectively

[2] Advanced reconstruction algorithms can take advantage of the benefits of non-parallel projection methods, provided they are accomplished by means of multi-hole collimators (fan-beam, convergent, divergent).

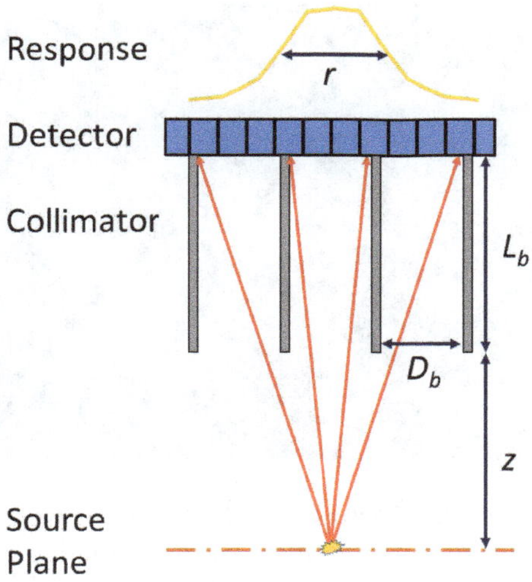

Figure 10.7: Schematic representation of collimator and PSF (yellow). The acceptance angle of a bore is dependent on bore length and width, leading to a widening of the PSF with depth.

blurs more complicated objects being imaged, which can be thought of as collections of many points.

This effect can be seen in Fig. 10.7, which shows a schematic representation of a trio of 1-D parallel collimator bores in front of a detector. A virtual point source placed at the intersection of the red arrows would be able to reach the detector along a number of rays. Photons reaching the detector on direct paths through air are termed geometric, because their PSF is only a function of the detector and collimator geometry. On an infinitely precise detector, the resulting response would be an array of indicator functions, but due to pixelation in the acquired image and other factors, the PSF has a roughly conical shape.

In many applications it is modeled as a Gaussian, and the resolution is characterized by the full width at half maximum (FWHM) r_{PSF}, which may be approximated by the following equation:

$$r_{\mathrm{PSF}} \approx \frac{D_b(L_b + z)}{L_b}, \tag{10.5}$$

where D_b is the bore diameter, L_b its length, and z the distance between the source plane and the face of the collimator. From Eq. (10.5), it can be seen that the resolution is depth-dependent and becomes wider with increasing z for given collimator dimensions.

An image of a point source showing a true PSF is shown in Fig. 10.8. The image is saturated to highlight the complex structure. In the bright central area outlined in red, primarily geometric photons are present. In the

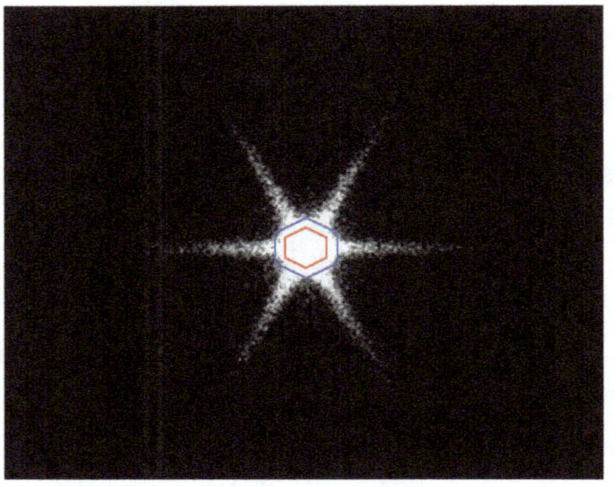

Figure 10.8: Measured PSF from a ^{99m}Tc point source imaged at a distance of 10 cm, shown saturated to emphasize low-intensity regions. The geometric bright geometric is outlined in red, and most extra-geometric counts lie between the red and blue hexagons, where a single partial septal wall is penetrated.

region immediately adjacent to it outlined in blue, photons passing through a portion of a single septum are detected. The long "spider"-like legs are due to septal penetration across multiple walls, which is most probable in a direction perpendicular to the edges of the hexagonal collimator bores. A faint background between these streaks is caused by Compton scattering in the collimator and contaminates the entire function. The magnitude of the spider legs is up to 1.5% of the maximum PSF value, and for ^{99m}Tc up to 10% of photons may be extra-geometric and thus not accounted for by ideal models. Therefore, some in the field have begun to use PSF models based on measured true data rather than ideal calculations.

Issues of resolution and septal penetration are important when designing a collimator. The collimator efficiency ρ is also significant, as it describes the ratio of geometric photons passed through the collimator to the total number emitted towards it. It is ideally constant over z for the parallel hole case and can be approximated as

$$\rho \approx K^2 \left(\frac{D_b}{L_b}\right)^2 \frac{D_b^2}{(D_b + T_s)^2}, \tag{10.6}$$

where T_s is the width of the septal wall and K is a constant based on hole geometry. A typical value of ρ is on the order of 10^{-4}, making it a key, but necessary, limiting factor in the sensitivity of SPECT systems.

In Eq. (10.6), it can be seen that ρ increases as bores are either shortened or widened. However, from Eq. (10.5), we see that these changes decrease resolution. Taking Eq. (10.5) and Eq. (10.6) together, it becomes apparent that the task of collimator design is a compromise between collimator sensitivity and resolution. The former directly impacts the quality of counting statistics, and therefore noise, in an acquired image. The latter is related to the accuracy with which the detector can localize them and properly reproduce small features such as edges. A third consideration appears via the septal thickness which, when increased, limits the star artifacts shown in Fig. 10.8 at the expense of smaller ρ.

Once a photon has passed through the collimator, it impacts the system's scintillator (typically composed of NaI), releasing several lower energy photons in the visible range. These photons then travel to the PMTs, where they initiate an electron avalanche that is detected as a current signal at the PMT output. To determine the 2-D location of a photon, a type of centroid is computed by the output electronics of the PMT array in a process known as Anger Logic, after its inventor. In the 1-D case, the estimated location of the photon detection $\hat{x}$ can be calculated as

$$\hat{x} = \frac{\sum_q x_q G_q}{\sum_q G_q}, \tag{10.7}$$

where G_q and x_q are the signal strength at and location of the q-th PMT. Applied in this fashion directly, images will suffer from nonuniformities and pincushion distortions. These are removed by replacing G_q with some nonlinear function thereof. Even after this correction, the method is not exact, and the resulting finite resolution r_{DET} adds in quadrature with that of the PSF to yield a total system resolution $r_{\mathrm{SYS}} = \sqrt{r_{\mathrm{PSF}}^2 + r_{\mathrm{DET}}^2}$. Another important property of the PMT output is that the value of $\sum_q G_q$ is proportional to the energy of the initial photon. This allows SPECT cameras to be energy resolving as well, allowing the effects of Compton scatter to be mitigated.

10.3.2 PET

As shown in Fig. 10.1, the β decay that forms the basis of PET produces two photons that travel in opposing directions away from each other. This is exploited for imaging purposes by using a ring detector and looking for coincidences in the observed data. This coincidence detection principle is illustrated in Fig. 10.9, where a PET ring composed of many small detector blocks is shown. Extremely high speed electronics monitor each detector's output signal and record a detection event when two impulses are detected simultaneously. The detector blocks themselves are traditionally composed of a scintillator crystal mated to a small PMT array as with the Anger camera. However, no collimator is needed to restrict the scintillator's acceptance angle in this case because the photon's incidence angle is implicitly provided by the detector block at the opposite side of the ring. Nevertheless, inaccuracies in the scintillator blocks and PMTs still induce a finite PSF in PET whose

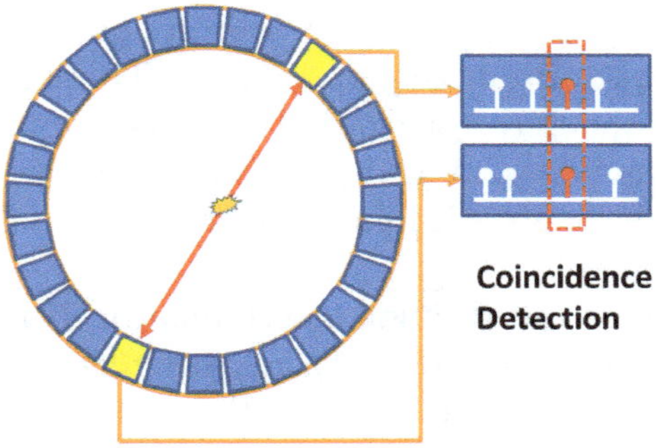

Figure 10.9: PET ring detector and coincidence detection principle. The detector electronics simultaneously monitor signals from each detector block and record counts when an impulse is detected from two blocks at the same time.

geometrical properties vary widely depending on the source's location in the field of view.

The ray connecting the two detection points (red line in Fig. 10.9) is known as the line of response. Integrating along all parallel lines of response at a particular rotation angle will produce a row of a sinogram at that angle that can be used for reconstruction. Early PET systems treated each axial ring of detector blocks as independent slices and thus ignored lines of response with oblique axial angles. This strategy, shown in Fig. 10.10(a), reduces the computational burden on detector electronics (coincidences from fewer blocks must be monitored simultaneously), but sacrifices many counts.

Newer systems utilize a 3-D detection configuration (cf. Fig. 10.10(b)), where lines of response across a finite axial range are observed. This provides an increase in sensitivity due to the fact that, for a given source location, counts can be registered at a greater number of detectors. However, by the same token, it is more probable that false (random) coincidences or pairs of scattered photons will be detected. Also, an extra step of axial rebinning is needed to produce a sinogram. Spatial and Fourier domain strategies exist, but the common goal is to transform the acquired oblique lines of response into approximate virtual lines of response perpendicular to the axial direction.

PET has a number of advantages over SPECT due to more favorable physics. Sensitivity is roughly an order of magnitude higher due to the absence of a collimator, and the ring detector offers better tomographic consistency (i. e. all angles are acquired simultaneously). Furthermore, the reconstruction problem is better defined than with SPECT due to the (ideally) 1-D search space along each line of response. Mathematically, this translates into a system matrix that is better conditioned. By using TOF information derived from slight delays between coincidence detections, the range of possible emission locations can be even further reduced.

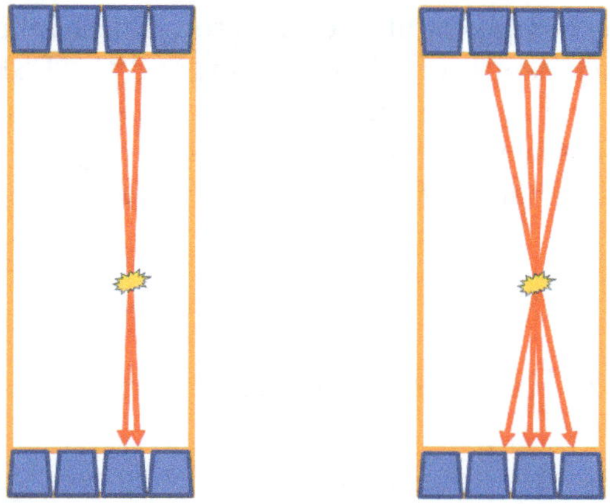

Figure 10.10: 2-D (left) and 3-D (right) detection configurations for PET. The latter offers better sensitivity at the expense of more scatter events.

TOF PET systems with 3-D detection thus typically offer superior resolution and noise characteristics compared to SPECT, but this comes at a price. ^{18}F, the most common isotope used in PET, has a half life of only 110 minutes and is more difficult to produce than ^{99m}Tc, requiring a complex logistical network to minimize the time between production and injection. Furthermore, the higher energy photons imaged in PET require costly exotic scintillator materials. This, combined with highly specialized detector electronics, makes PET systems more expensive to procure and operate than their SPECT counterparts.

10.4 Reconstruction

10.4.1 Filtered Back-Projection

In Chapter 8, we presented the filtered back-projection method of reconstruction in the context of X-ray CT. The advantages of this reconstruction are its speed and simplicity, as well as reconstructed image properties, such as resolution, that are relatively easy to determine. However, while filtered back-projection works quite well for high-count data, it fails to take into account the Poisson statistics outlined in Sec. 10.2.1. This leads to very noisy images in SPECT and PET, where detected counts are several orders of magnitude lower than those seen in CT.

Furthermore, filtered back-projection operates by inverting the Radon transform – the purely geometrical relationship between voxels in the image and their projected pixels at the detector. This ignores all of the other physical factors, such as attenuation, scatter, and the PSF, that play a vital role in the emission tomography image formation chain. This oversight leads to artifacts in reconstructed images that greatly degrade image quality. For these reasons, filtered back-projection is generally no longer used in clinical situations.

10.4.2 Iterative Reconstruction

In order to improve the noise performance of filtered back-projection, we must use the statistical relationship in Eq. (10.2) between the mean activity distribution in each voxel and the observed counts at the detector. Filtered back-projection implicitly assumes a deterministic relationship, but we can take stochastic effects into account by using the definition of the Poisson mass distribution function.

Geek Box 10.1 describes how probable observed detector data are given a set of model parameters, which take the form of a vector of Poisson means $\boldsymbol{\nu}$ for each voxel in our case. Obviously, in emission tomography, these parameters are unknown. However, the likelihood function provides us with a tool to estimate them by searching for the set of $\hat{\boldsymbol{\nu}}^*$ that maximizes $P(\mathcal{D} = \boldsymbol{d})$ and thus yields the *most likely* estimate given our data:

$$\hat{\boldsymbol{\nu}}^* = \underset{\hat{\boldsymbol{\nu}}}{\operatorname{argmax}}\ P(\mathcal{D} = \boldsymbol{d}). \tag{10.8}$$

The relationship described in Geek Box 10.1 is quite complex, and it is not immediately clear how to maximize the likelihood. However, a seminal paper by Shepp and Vardi in 1982 showed that this can be accomplished via the Expectation Maximization (EM) algorithm, whose general framework involves the estimation of the "complete" information, given a set of observations and hidden, "latent", information. Although a detailed description is outside the scope of this text, it is worth outlining that for emission tomography, the complete information is the actual emission distribution $\boldsymbol{\nu}$, and the observations are the counts in the projections $\boldsymbol{d}$. The latent information is comprised of all of the photons originating in the image that escape detection.

As shown by Shepp and Vardi, EM's methodology of alternatingly forming a conditional expectation via marginalization over a particular variable and then maximizing the resulting likelihood provides a convenient framework for attacking Eq. (10.8) as encountered in emission tomography. This expectation/maximization cycle is repeated until a suitable image is obtained, and each one of these repetitions is referred to as one iteration k. The algorithm begins by initializing some estimate of the activity distribution $\hat{\boldsymbol{\nu}}^0$. The process proceeds at each iteration by forward projecting the current estimate $\hat{\boldsymbol{\nu}}^k$, comparing it to the measured data, backprojecting the result, and applying

Geek Box 10.1: Total Likelihood Function

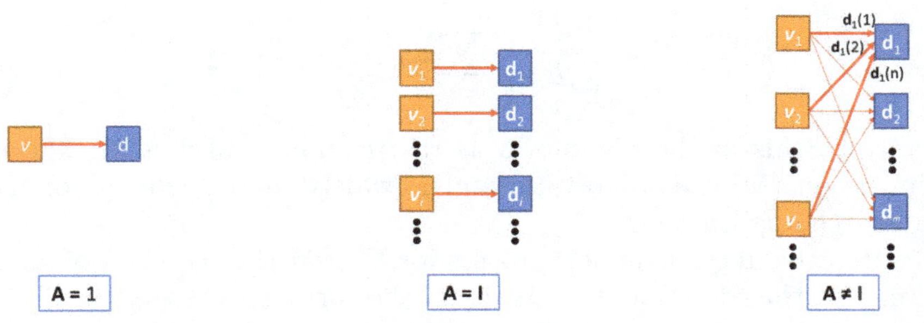

(a) (b) (c)

a) For the simple case of counts from one voxel being emitted directly into a single pixel detector, the probability of a particular observation d given the true mean ν is

$$P(\mathcal{D} = d) = e^{-\nu} \frac{\nu^d}{d!},$$

which is known as the *likelihood* of the observation.

b) Moving one step further, where an array of observations $\boldsymbol{d}$ if formed by photons emitted from a vector of voxels with means $\boldsymbol{\nu}$. This is the same scenario we examined in the example in Fig. 10.3. Here, the system matrix is equivalent to the identity matrix $\boldsymbol{A} = \boldsymbol{I}$, and each voxel contributes to a single detector element. As each observation is independent of the others, we can multiply them together to obtain our likelihood:

$$P(\mathcal{D} = \boldsymbol{d}) = \prod_i \exp(-\nu_i) \frac{\nu_i^{d_i}}{d_i!},$$

where i represents the index of the detector and image elements, which are equivalent in this case.

c) In a true imaging scenario, $\boldsymbol{A} \neq \boldsymbol{I}$, and multiple image voxels contribute to a single detector element. To account for this, we must subdivide the total detected counts in each pixel d_m into contributions from each image voxel: $d_m = \sum_n d_m(n)$. The probabilities contained in the system matrix must also be included. The total likelihood is therefore the sum over each of these possible scenarios:

$$P(\mathcal{D} = \boldsymbol{d}) = \prod_{m,n} \exp(-\nu_m a_{m,n}) \frac{(\nu_m a_{m,n})^{d_m(n)}}{d_m(n)!}$$

The dual product has the effect of incorporating the contribution from each voxel to each pixel.

a weight to the estimate to create a new $\hat{\boldsymbol{\nu}}^{k+1}$.The update mechanism for the algorithm can be expressed using the following equation:

$$\hat{\nu}_n^{k+1} = \frac{\hat{\nu}_n^k}{\sum_{m'} a_{m',n}} \sum_m a_{n,m} \frac{d_m}{\sum_{n'} \hat{\nu}_{n'}^k a_{m,n'}}. \tag{10.9}$$

Collectively, this method is known as the maximum likelihood expectation maximization (MLEM) algorithm and is widely used in many commercial and research applications.

The iterative reconstruction process for MLEM thus consists of an objective function that describes the quality of the current estimate (the likelihood function) and a way of optimizing it (EM). Within the field of image reconstruction, a wide range of objective function/optimizer pairs are available. Another objective function that has found wide use is weighted least squares:

$$\hat{\boldsymbol{\nu}}^* = \underset{\hat{\boldsymbol{\nu}}}{\operatorname{argmin}} \|\boldsymbol{d} - \boldsymbol{A}\hat{\boldsymbol{\nu}}\|_{\boldsymbol{w}}^2 = \underset{\hat{\boldsymbol{\nu}}}{\operatorname{argmin}} \sum_m \boldsymbol{w}_m (\boldsymbol{d}_m - [\boldsymbol{A}\hat{\boldsymbol{\nu}}]_m)^2, \tag{10.10}$$

where $[\boldsymbol{A}\hat{\boldsymbol{\nu}}]_m$ is the m-th pixel of the forward projected estimate and $\boldsymbol{w}$ is a vector of weights. The weights are often used to take noise into account by, for example, setting each element of $\boldsymbol{w}$ equal to an estimate of the variance at the corresponding detector pixel. This has the effect of adjusting each pixel's contribution to the objective function depending on its noise properties. The weighted least squares objective function is convex and can be solved with gradient-based optimization techniques such as the conjugate gradient method.

10.4.3 Quantitative Reconstructions

Although iterative reconstruction is motivated by the underlying statistics of photon emission, another major advantage is its ability to model the physics of the imaging system. This is accomplished via the system matrix. In addition to geometric information, the system matrix can include the effects of attenuation and scatter to allow the reconstruction to correct for them. Furthermore, resolution lost due to PSF blurring may be regained to some extent if this is modeled as well.

Aside from image quality improvements such as contrast enhancement and noise reduction, proper system modeling enables PET and SPECT systems to become *quantitative* as well. In other words, instead of reconstructing images in arbitrary or relative units, absolute units such as activity concentration $\frac{\mathrm{kBq}}{\mathrm{ml}}$ are produced. This important distinction allows scans across different patients, scanners, and time points to be meaningfully compared. This is not only useful for individual patient management, but enables larger, multi-center clinical studies as well.

Assuming an accurate system model is available, the cornerstone of a quantitative imaging system is the calibration. This anchors the counts observed during an acquisition to a physical amount of radioactivity in the detector's field of view. A common way of doing this is to perform an acquisition on a homogeneous phantom with a known activity concentration expressed as $\frac{\text{kBq}}{\text{ml}}$. A volume of interest may then be defined in the reconstructed image, and a count density in units of counts per ml may be determined. Time must then be taken into account by correcting for decay and normalizing by the acquisition duration. After these steps, a volumetric sensitivity factor α_{VOL} may be defined relative to its units as follows:

$$\alpha_{\text{VOL}} = \frac{\frac{\text{counts}}{\text{minute} \cdot \text{ml}}}{\frac{\text{kBq}}{\text{ml}}}. \tag{10.11}$$

With this factor in hand, subsequent acquisitions may be quantified, provided they are acquired with the same isotope and reconstructed in the same way. The procedure for this is straightforward and consists of obtaining the count rate density from a volume of interest in units of $\frac{\text{counts}}{\text{min}\cdot\text{ml}}$ and dividing by α_{VOL}, thus producing the desired absolute units of $\frac{\text{kBq}}{\text{ml}}$.

This solution is not without drawbacks. It requires the filling of a phantom for calibration and is vulnerable to errors and inconsistencies that come from user-defined volumes of interest. A more elegant method is to utilize a planar sensitivity $\alpha_{\text{planar}} = \frac{\text{counts}}{\text{min}\cdot\text{kBq}}$. This value is then incorporated into the system matrix to relate the forward projected counts to absolute activity in the reconstructed volume. The result is a reconstruction that is inherently quantitative and dependent on a calibration factor that can be obtained from less tedious planar acquisitions of a point source.

In the medical community, it is also of interest to normalize for factors such as patient weight and injected dose. The commonly used Standardized Uptake Value (SUV) is an example of this. It is based on the assumptions that a) a tracer in healthy tissue will distribute uniformly throughout the body and b) that the body has a uniform density equal to that of water (i. e. 1 kg/l). Combining these assumptions yields the following relation:

$$\text{SUV} = \frac{\frac{\text{kBq}_{\text{VOI}}}{\text{ml}_{\text{VOI}}}}{\text{MBq}_{\text{INJ}} \cdot \text{kg}}, \tag{10.12}$$

where the subscripts VOI and INJ refer to quantities drawn from a reconstructed volume of interest (e. g. a region surrounding a suspect tumor) and total injected dose, respectively.

Despite the somewhat unintuitive units of $\frac{\text{ml}}{\text{kg}}$, the logic behind the SUV is sound: a value significantly greater than unity indicates a disproportionate

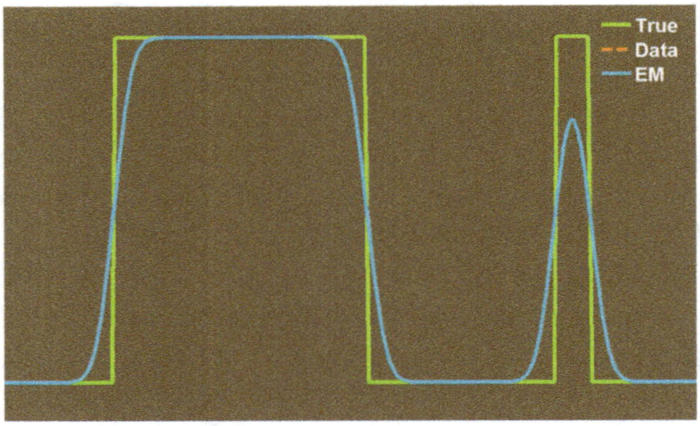

Figure 10.11: 1-D signal (green) convolved with gaussian to yield "observed data" that is reconstructed (i. e. deconvolved) using the MLEM algorithm (blue curve). In this case, the blurring function is not modeled, and the reconstruction cannot improve upon the observed data (the two curves are equal). Figure courtesy of Siemens Molecular Imaging Inc., USA.

amount of uptake and a potential abnormality. This is particularly the case for tracers where assumption (a) from above holds. Furthermore, by normalizing for two factors that vary across acquisitions (injected dose and patient weight), the SUV allows for easier comparison between different patients and time points.

Numerous variations on the SUV exist. One of the most popular is the SUV_{max}, which simply places the maximum activity concentration found in a volume of interest in the numerator of Eq. (10.12) to guard against partial volume effects. Other extensions normalize by lean body mass or body surface area to better account for anatomical variations.

10.4.4 Practical Considerations

Although superior to analytical methods, iterative reconstructions are not without their own complications. Namely, the inclusion of a system model and optimization scheme adds a plethora of parameters that must be tailored to the imaging task at hand. Poor judgment in selecting these values may degrade image quality.

To illustrate this concept, we use a simple 1-D signal with two step functions blurred by a Gaussian. The original signal represents the truth, and its blurred version our observed data. If we initialize a constant function and apply the MLEM algorithm from Eq. (10.9), we can attempt to "reconstruct" the truth from the data. In Fig. 10.11, the results are shown for the case where the blurring function is not modeled (similar to an emission tomography reconstruction without PSF compensation). As expected, the best our

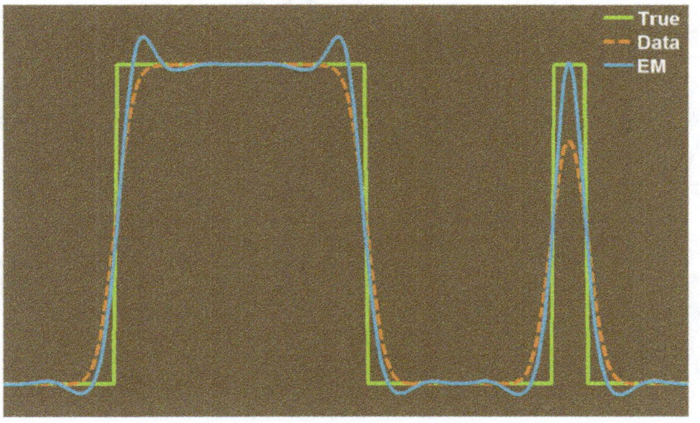

Figure 10.12: Reconstruction after six MLEM iterations where the blurring function is modeled in the system matrix. Edge resolution is improved over Fig. 10.11, but ringing artifacts also become visible. Figure courtesy of Siemens Molecular Imaging Inc, USA.

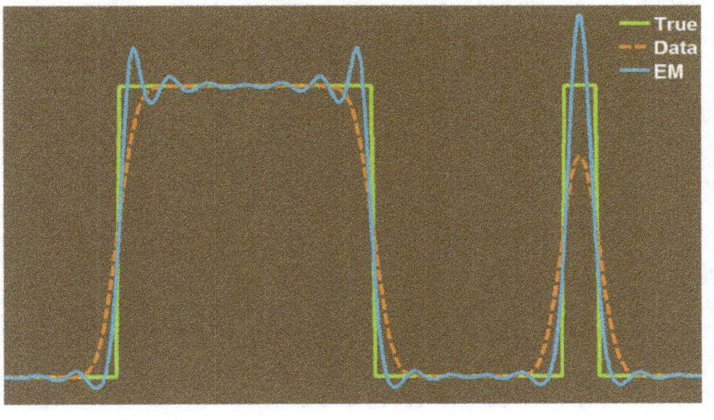

Figure 10.13: MLEM reconstruction after 300 iterations. The edges have become sharper, and artifacts amplified relative to Fig. 10.12. Figure courtesy of Siemens Molecular Imaging Inc., USA.

method can do is to adjust the constant initialization until it matches the blurred observations: the two curves are identical.

Fig. 10.12 shows six MLEM iterations with the blur incorporated into the system matrix. This is equivalent to adding a deconvolution problem to our reconstruction, and we see that the edges have become sharpened as frequencies suppressed by the blur are recovered by the reconstruction. However, ringing artifacts have also become visible due to the fact that the original spectrum is only partially recovered. The results after 300 iterations are shown in Fig. 10.13, where even better edge resolution is achieved, albeit with more severe ringing as well.

If we incorporate Poisson noise into the observed data, we can make our experiment more realistic. How does this change the results? The reconstruction after six iterations shown in Fig. 10.14 indicates that they are broadly

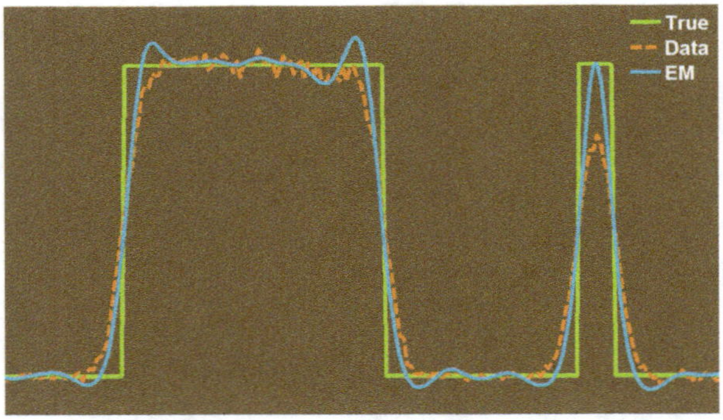

Figure 10.14: Six MLEM iterations with on data perturbed with Poisson noise. The result is slightly irregular but comparable to Fig. 10.12. Figure courtesy of Siemens Molecular Imaging Inc., USA.

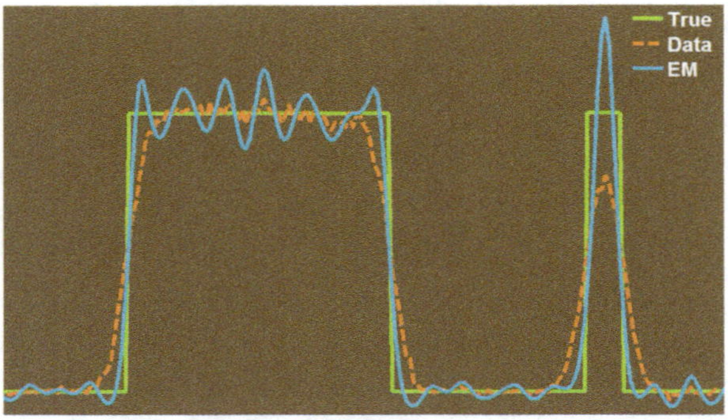

Figure 10.15: 300 MLEM iterations on noisy data. The interior of the large object is highly irregular, and quality is noticably worse than Fig. 10.13. Figure courtesy of Siemens Molecular Imaging Inc., USA.

comparable to the noiseless case in Fig. 10.12, although slight irregularities inside the wide object can be seen. However, the case after 300 iterations shown in Fig. 10.15 is starkly different from its noiseless counterpart, with the interior of the wide object becoming very inhomogeneous.

The noise in the reconstructed signal in Fig. 10.15 is a result of the ill-conditioned nature of the reconstruction problem and can be generalized to the case of emission tomography. During early iterations, low frequencies are recovered that correspond mostly to signal information, such as high-contrast, large objects. However, at higher iterations, the algorithm turns its attention to higher frequencies where the signal and noise energies are comparable. The result is an overfitting of the noise and degradation of image quality.

By iterating further, we can increase resolution and thus reduce quantitative bias due to edge roll-off. However, as seen in Fig. 10.15, this runs the risk of introducing too much noise into the image. The use of image post-smoothing or smoothness regularization can reduce noise while sacrificing some resolution and thus entails making the same type of compromise. In practice, the choice of many reconstruction parameters is therefore another example of the bias/variance trade-off already discussed above with respect to SPECT collimator design.

Another complication for iterative reconstruction in emission tomography is that there are source-dependent factors such as attenuation and scatter in the system matrix. This implies that the properties of the reconstruction will vary from patient to patient, even if the same acquisition and reconstruction parameters are used. Furthermore, depth- and position-dependent PSFs in SPECT and PET lead to shift-variant properties *within* a given image as well. These factors should be taken into account when reconstructing and interpreting images.

10.5 Clinical Applications

Molecular imaging is used in various fields of medicine such as neurology, oncology, cardiology, and orthopedics. Its application areas can be broadly subdivided into two fields: diagnostics and therapy.

10.5.1 Diagnostics

As the most common use for emission tomography, diagnostics is also the most diverse. In the field of neurology, both PET and SPECT offer perfusion tracers that give physicians insight into the amount of blood flow in the brain during the scan, which is proportional to brain activity. An example of a SPECT brain perfusion procedure using ^{99m}Tc-Ethylcysteinat-Dimer (ECD) is shown in Fig. 10.16(a). An epileptic patient is scanned immediately following a seizure and during a neutral state. The reconstructed images are subtracted and fused with an MR of the patient's brain to localize the focus of the seizure. More specialized applications including imaging of amyloid plaques linked to Alzheimer's disease (PET) and dopamine receptor imaging (SPECT) are also available.

For oncology, ^{18}F, the most commonly used PET isotope, may be bonded to a molecule in the glucose family resulting in so-called fludeoxyglucose (FDG). Using these FDG-PET scans, doctors can search for areas with high glucose metabolism – a sign of rapidly growing metastatic tumors. Fig. 10.16(b) shows an FDG-PET scan of a patient with melanoma. Malignant metastases are visible below the liver and beside the heart. A common oncological use for SPECT is skeletal imaging with ^{99m}Tc bonded to phosphorous compounds. High uptake of these tracers is often indicative of secondary lesions from e. g. prostate or breast cancer.

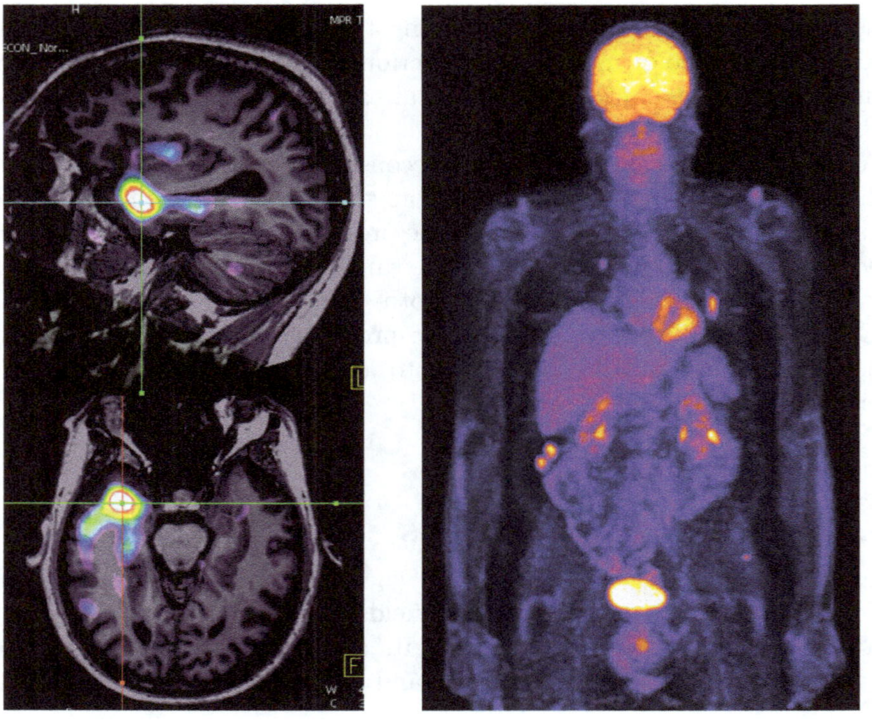

(a) (b)

Figure 10.16: Examples of diagnostic procedures in molecular imaging. a) Differential SPECT scan using ^{99m}Tc-ECD to localize seizure epicenter. b) FDG-PET scan for a patient with melanoma. Several small lesions are visible below liver and beside heart. Images courtesy of the University Hospital Erlangen, Clinic of Nuclear Medicine.

In addition to oncology, bone SPECT is also used in the field of orthopedics to localize and diagnose the source of pain felt by patients with faulty prosthetics, small fractures, or degenerative disease. PET and SPECT also both offer myocardial perfusion tracers, which allow cardiologists to assess the viability of the heart muscle and diagnose various heart diseases.

Using quantitative imaging, physicians are also able to monitor disease over time. By comparing metrics such as SUV at scans taken at different time points, they can track the progression of e. g. metastatic lesions and better assess response to therapy. An example of this is shown in Fig. 10.17, where a breast cancer patient was imaged with ^{99m}Tc-labelled 3,3-diphosphono-1,2-propanodicarboxylic acid (DPD) at three different time points, roughly six months apart. In the first scan (cf. Fig. 10.17(a)), a region was seen in the skull with uptake suspicious of a metastatic bone tumor. In a follow up study, the SUV$_{max}$ was seen to increase, and treatment with bisphosphonates was

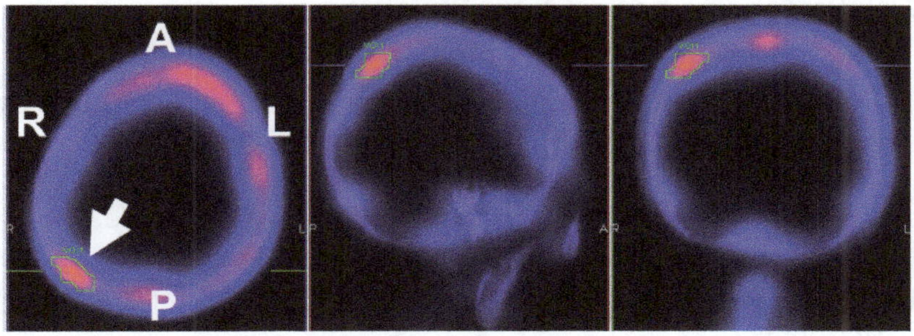

(a) March, 2012; $SUV_{max} = 4.5$

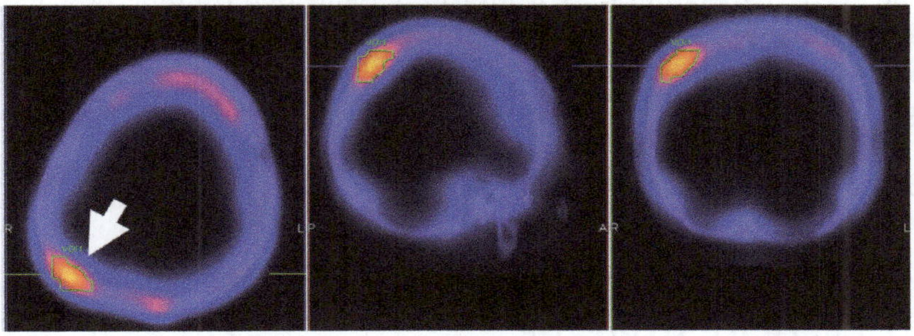

(b) September, 2012; $SUV_{max} = 6.0$

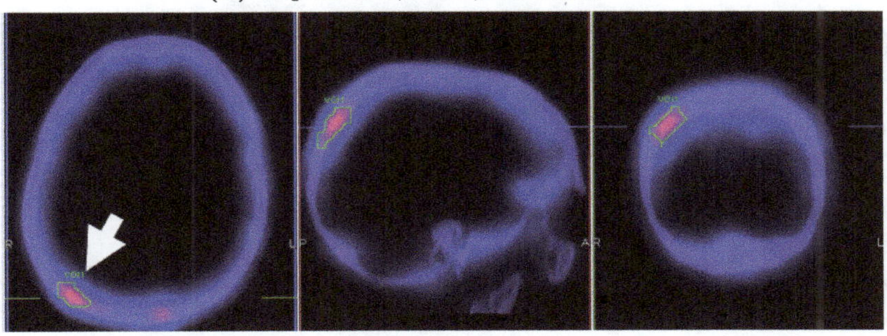

(c) February, 2013; $SUV_{max} = 5.1$

Figure 10.17: Same breast cancer patient imaged on three different dates with ^{99m}Tc-DPD. The calculated SUV_{max} from the volume of interest at the posterior right area of the skull is also shown. A decrease in uptake was noted between the second and third scans, indicating a response to therapy. Images courtesy of the University Hospital Erlangen, Clinic of Nuclear Medicine.

begun. In the final scan shown in Fig. 10.17(c), SUV_{max} decreased, indicating a response to therapy.

10.5.2 Therapy

In addition to purely diagnostic imaging, emission tomography plays an integral role in radioisotope therapy as well. Such procedures utilize the tracer principle to target malignant tissue with radiation. This radiation then eliminates or stems the growth of unwanted cells. However, these positive effects must be weighed against the negative side effects on healthy tissue. To accomplish this, physicians must estimate the dose of a course of therapy on sensitive organs.

This process, known as dosimetry, is quite complex. It relies on quantifying the activity distribution within the patient, determining how long it will remain there, and estimating how much energy will be deposited in healthy tissue. As therapy agents typically involve higher energy emissions and more complicated spectra, the system matrix in such cases becomes more difficult to define. Furthermore, post-processing such as organ segmentation and biological modeling become necessary.

10.6 Hybrid Imaging

10.6.1 Clinical Need

SPECT and PET offer excellent sensitivity for the detection of disease due to the functional information they provide. However, pathological regions of an image may be difficult to localize in the body in the absence of structural information.

Take, for example, a hypothetical surgeon who is planning a biopsy and needs to find the specific Sentinel Lymph Nodes (SLNs) draining a tumor in a breast cancer patient. Prior to surgery, a SPECT scan has clearly shown the presence of an SLN with high uptake in the underarm area, but it is known that there are multiple possible lymph nodes here. This stand-alone SPECT might appear similar to the left pane of Fig. 10.18, where only a single bright spot is visible. How will the surgeon proceed?

Historically, during planar acquisitions, a technologist might trace the outside edge of a patient's body with a radioactive "pen" to provide a rough anatomical point of reference in the image. The advantages of this method are limited, and it is, in any case, not possible for SPECT, where attempts may be made to register a previously acquired CT to the current SLN SPECT study. However, the human anatomy is non-rigid, and shifts in posture and time between scans may lead to errors. Our surgeon would therefore be left with the option to operate in the general area of the suspected SLN and rely on tedious scanning with gamma counting probes to find the exact node.

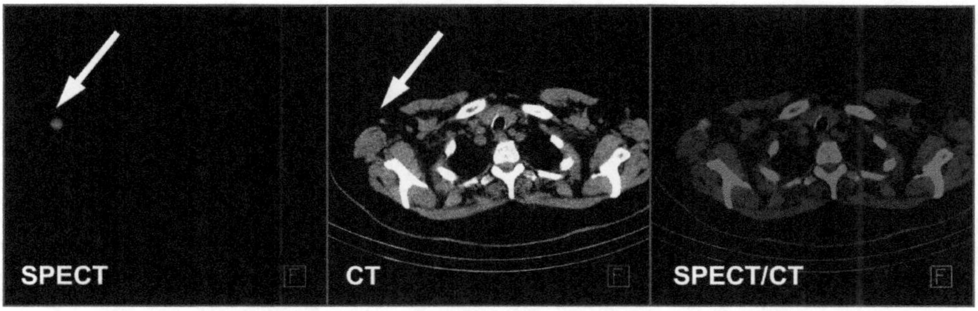

Figure 10.18: SPECT data after labeling of a Sentinel Lymph Node (SLN) with ^{99m}Tc-Nanocoll. The corresponding structural information from a complimentary X-ray CT scan helps provide proper localization of the activity. Images courtesy of the University Hospital Erlangen, Clinic of Nuclear Medicine.

10.6.2 Advent und Acceptance of Hybrid Scanners

In 2000, David Townsend and Ronald Nutt of the University of Geneva, working together with CTI (now a division of Siemens Molecular Imaging), introduced the first hybrid PET/CT scanner. This device offered a PET ring detector and multi-slice spiral CT scanner integrated into the same gantry. Patients could therefore receive PET and CT studies in quick succession without moving, greatly reducing registration errors and providing both structural and functional information in one fell swoop. Six years later, Siemens Molecular Imaging introduced the Symbia SPECT/CT scanner, bringing the same advantages to the field of SPECT. Other manufacturers quickly developed similar hybrid imaging systems as well.

With the advent of hybrid imaging, our hypothetical surgeon can now use the CT acquired with the SPECT study to pinpoint the location of the SLN prior to surgery, reducing both the time needed to perform the operation and the risk of misidentification. This is illustrated in the center and right panes of Fig. 10.18. In the center, a CT acquired immediately after the SPECT to the left is shown, and in the right, the two fused datasets are displayed. As the patient was lying on the same SPECT/CT gantry in the same position during both acquisitions, the surgeon can be sure of the accuracy in the registration between the two datasets.

The integration of PET or SPECT system with an X-ray CT scanner represents a complex engineering task. On the hardware side, care must be taken to ensure that the physical mating of the two systems does not affect their individual performance. On the firm- and software side, separate data transmission protocols, formats, and user interfaces must be unified as well. After the devices are physically complete, system engineers must work with others to develop new calibration and quality control routines. These might, for example, provide the reconstruction software with updated transformations between the SPECT and CT coordinate systems, as these parameters vary over time due to parts wearing down or being replaced.

In addition to the clinical benefits of hybrid imaging, the reconstruction process itself can be improved as well. In Sec. 10.4.3, we briefly discussed the importance of CT attenuation correction for emission tomography. The advent of hybrid devices has made these corrections the standard in most clinics rather than a research topic, reducing attenuation artifacts and paving the way for quantitative imaging.

Hybrid PET and SPECT/CT devices represented a major step forward in medical imaging. However, CT as a structural modality has its own weaknesses. Namely, soft tissue contrast in regions of interest for molecular imaging, such as the liver and brain, is poor. Also, the presence of extra radiation dose from the CT is obviously undesirable. For this reason, MR imaging was proposed as a structural imaging modality for use in hybrid scanners.

Although clinically exciting e. g. for neurology applications due to MR's unparalleled contrast between different brain tissues and PET's array of sensitive neurological tracers, the mating of PET and MR represented a host of new physical challenges. The most important of these was how to eliminate PMTs from the design, which are unusable in MR's strong magnetic fields due to the interference they induce on a PMT's moving electrons. Engineers were able to overcome this by substituting the standard scintillator-PMT setup with semiconductor detectors that convert photons directly to image data. However, another issue is how to derive attenuation maps from the MR data, which does not have the same direct physical meaning that CT's Hounsfield units have and therefore must be processed further to obtain a μ-map. In this case, pattern recognition methods may be used to estimate the density map based on atlas data and segmentation/classification of the patient's tissue.

Having overcome these and other issues to a large extent, beginning in 2011, each of the major manufacturers has released a commercial PET/MR system. Much research is currently being performed to both improve their performance and define new clinical applications.

10.6.3 Further Benefits of Hybrid Imaging

In addition to incorporating the μ-map into the system matrix to improve the physical model of the projection process, CT or MR information may be integrated into the reconstruction in other ways as well. We could assume, for example, that a sharp boundary in an MR brain image should have a correspondingly sharp boundary in the nuclear image because we expect that the radioactivity concentration across two types of tissue (e. g. white and gray matter) will be discontinuous. As the low resolution SPECT or PET reconstructions are not capable of reproducing this high resolution on their

Geek Box 10.2: Maximum a posteriori Estimation

In order to understand the idea of MAP estimation, we have to understand that our model, i. e., the Poisson distribution, introduces conditions on our probability. Thus $P(\mathcal{D} = \boldsymbol{d})$ is actually conditioned by the Poisson means $\boldsymbol{\nu}$. As such, we actually need to denote it as $P(\mathcal{D} = \boldsymbol{d}|\boldsymbol{\nu})$ or $P(\boldsymbol{d}|\boldsymbol{\nu})$ in short. Next, we realize that we are actually interested in $P(\boldsymbol{\nu}|\boldsymbol{d})$, as $\boldsymbol{d}$ is observable in our case and we seek to maximize the probability of $\boldsymbol{\nu}$ given $\boldsymbol{d}$. Fortunately, Bayes' rule applies for conditional probabilities:

$$\hat{\boldsymbol{\nu}}^* = \underset{\hat{\boldsymbol{\nu}}}{\operatorname{argmax}}\, P(\boldsymbol{\nu}|\boldsymbol{d}) = \underset{\hat{\boldsymbol{\nu}}}{\operatorname{argmax}}\, \frac{P(\boldsymbol{d}|\boldsymbol{\nu})P(\boldsymbol{\nu})}{P(\boldsymbol{d})}, \tag{10.13}$$

where $P(\boldsymbol{d}|\boldsymbol{\nu})$ is known from physics, $P(\boldsymbol{d})$ is independent of the optimization and can therefore be neglected, and $P(\boldsymbol{\nu})$ is the prior term. Now $P(\boldsymbol{\nu})$ is independent of the actual observation $\boldsymbol{d}$ and can therefore be used to model any prior knowledge on the distribution of $\boldsymbol{\nu}$. For hybrid applications, $P(\boldsymbol{\nu})$ is chosen based on the CT or MR information. Of course, MAP methods may also be used with purely PET or SPECT data to enforce e. g. smoothness, but their greatest potential benefit is the incorporation of information from other modalities.

own, we could work this prior knowledge from MR into the objective function of an iterative reconstruction algorithm.

The family of maximum a posteriori (MAP) algorithms is capable of doing exactly this by building upon the maximum likelihood method with a term representing some prior information known about the object. As the name implies, the MAP method seeks to maximize the posterior probability of the observed data given the distribution being imaged. We explain this principle in Geek Box 10.2.

Another example of this higher level of integration, although one not relying on the MAP principle, is the xSPECT Bone algorithm from Siemens, which is currently used for reconstructing SPECT skeletal scans. This method works by segmenting the CT into several different tissue classes and forward projecting them separately at each iteration. In addition to voxel-wise image updates, the classes themselves are also allowed to be scaled independently while optimizing the objective function. This scaling allows the SPECT reconstruction to have very sharp edges at the boundaries between tissue classes (e. g. if a cortical bone class has much more uptake than a neighboring lung region), while maintaining a typical SPECT-like resolution within each class.

An example of this method is shown in Fig. 10.19 below. Note how the edges of the vertebrae in the xSPECT image (center) are much sharper than

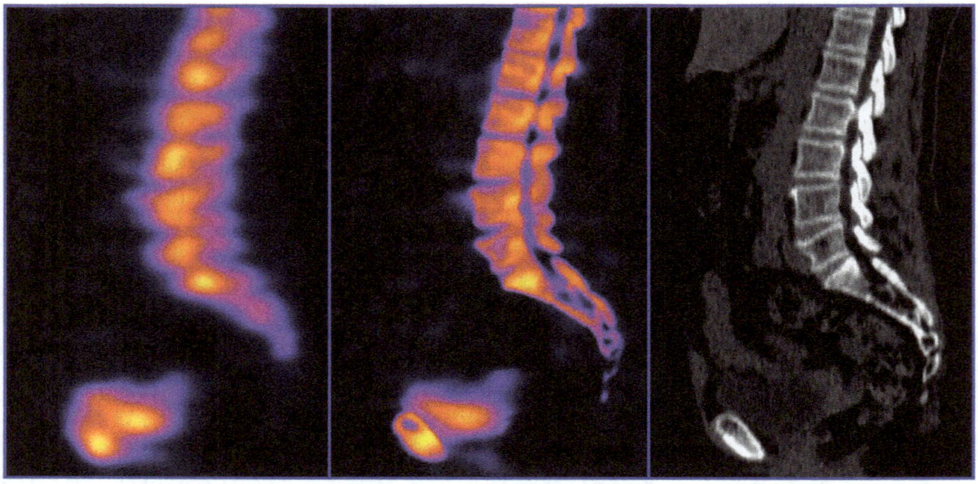

Figure 10.19: MLEM (left) and xSPECT Bone (center) reconstructions. The latter achieves sharper resolution at the edge of tissue classes with the help of extra-modal CT data (right). Images courtesy of the University Hospital Erlangen, Clinic of Nuclear Medicine.

the standard MLEM SPECT reconstruction (left) due to the boundary information provided by the CT (right). However, the bladder appears very similar in the two SPECT reconstructions, as there is little additional CT boundary information here.

Despite the advantages of methods such as MAP and xSPECT Bone, there are risks as well. For example, a MAP method may assume that bone density is always positively correlated to tracer uptake and enforce this behavior to improve quantitative accuracy. This is indeed generally the case, but in the early stages of a bone infarction, there is little or no blood supply to the bone and, hence, no tracer uptake, despite a normal CT. Our example MAP algorithm would then try to allocate activity here during the reconstruction and potentially provide the physician with a false negative. One should therefore be very careful when designing priors, as they are generally based on assumptions about anatomy or biochemistry that may not be true in all cases.

Further Reading

[1] Adam Alessio and Paul Kinahan. "PET Image Reconstruction". In: *Nuclear Medicine* 2 (2006).

[2] Adam Alessio and Paul Kinahan. "Quantitative Accuracy of Clinical 99mTc SPECT/CT Using Ordered-Subset Expectation Maximization

With 3-Dimensional Resolution Recovery, Attenuation, and Scatter Correction". In: *Nuclear Medicine* 2 (2006).

[3] AM Alessio et al. "PET/CT Scanner Instrumentation, Challenges, and Solutions". In: *Radiologic Clinics of North America* 42 (2004), pp. 1017–32.

[4] H.O. Anger. "Scintillation Camera with Multichannel Collimators". In: *Journal of Nuclear Medicine* 5.7 (1964), pp. 515–531.

[5] H.O. Anger. "Scintillation Camera with Multichannel Collimators". In: *Journal of Nuclear Medicine* 5 (1964), pp. 515–531.

[6] H.H. Barrett and K.J. Myers. *Foundations of Image Science.* 1st. Hoboken, NJ, USA: John Wiley & Sons, Inc., 2007.

[7] H.H. Barrett and W. Swindell. *Radiological Imaging: The Theory of Image Formation, Detection, and Processing.* New York, NY, USA: Academic Press, 1981.

[8] S.R. Cherry, J.A. Sorenson, and M.E. Phelps. *Physics in Nuclear Medicine.* Philadelphia, PA, USA: Saunders, 2003.

[9] A.P. Dempster, N.M. Laird, and D.B. Rubin. "Maximum Likelihood from Incomplete Data via the *EM* Algorithm". In: *Journal of the Royal Statistical Society* 39.1 (1977), pp. 1–38.

[10] J.A. Fessler and W.L. Rogers. "Spatial Resolution Properties of Penalized-Likelihood Image Reconstruction: Space-Invariance Tomographs". In: *IEEE Transactions on Image Processing* 5.9 (Sept. 1996), pp. 1346–1358.

[11] R. J. Jaszczak, R. E. Coleman, and C.B. Lim. "SPECT: Single Photon Emission Computed Tomography". In: *IEEE Transactions on Nuclear Science* 27.3 (June 1980), pp. 1137–1153. ISSN: 0018-9499.

[12] Bharath Navalpakkam et al. "Magnetic Resonance-Based Attenuation Correction for PET/MR Hybrid Imaging Using Continuous Valued Attenuation Maps". In: *Investigative Radiology* 48.5 (2013), pp. 323–332.

[13] Hamamatsu Photonics. *Photomultiplier Tube: Principle to Application.* 1st. Hamamatsu City, Japan: Hamamatsu Photonics K.K., Electron Tube Center, 1994.

[14] J. Prekeges. *Nuclear Medicine Implementation.* 2nd. Burlington, MA, USA: Jones & Bartlett Learning, 2013.

[15] Philipp Ritt et al. "Absolute Quantification in SPECT". In: *European Journal of Nuclear Medicine and Molecular Imaging* 38.1 (2011), pp. 69–77.

[16] James Sanders et al. "Fully Automated Data-Driven Respiratory Signal Extraction from SPECT Images Using Laplacian Eigenmaps". In: *IEEE Transactions on Medical Imaging* 35.11 (2016), pp. 2425–2435. DOI: 10.1109/TMI.2016.2576899.

[17] James Sanders et al. "Quantitative SPECT/CT Imaging of (177)Lu with In Vivo Validation in Patients Undergoing Peptide Receptor Radionuclide Therapy". In: *Molecular Imaging and Biology* 17.4 (2015), pp. 585–593. DOI: 10.1007/s11307-014-0806-4.

[18] L. A. Shepp and Y. Vardi. "Maximum Likelihood Reconstruction for Emission Tomography". In: *IEEE Transactions on Medical Imaging* 1.2 (Oct. 1982), pp. 113–122. ISSN: 0278-0062.

[19] B.M.W. Tsui et al. "Comparison Between ML-EM and WLS-CG Algorithms for SPECT Image Reconstruction". In: *IEEE Transactions on Nuclear Science* 38.6 (Dec. 1991), pp. 1766–1772.

[20] M.N. Wernick and J.N. Aarsvold. *Emission Tomography: The Fundamentals of PET and SPECT*. 1st. London, UK: Elsevier Academic Press, 2004.

11

Ultrasound Imaging and its Physics

Authors: Dominik Neumann and Eva Kollorz

11.1 Introduction

Acoustic waves with frequencies ξ between 16 Hz and 20 kHz can be sensed by the human hearing and are thus called audible waves or audible sound. If $\xi > 20$ kHz, one speaks of ultrasound (Tab. 11.1). Some animal species such as bats can perceive ultrasound and use it for echolocation: by measuring the time between sending and receiving (after partial reflection on a surface) ultrasonic waves, the distance of an object (e. g., a wall or prey) to the sender (bat) can be computed accurately, assuming that the sound velocity is known. In the previous century, modern technology started to make use of this technique with applications ranging from marine distance measurement (1920: SONAR) to medicine (1958: first ultrasound device in clinical use). A typical system is shown in Fig. 11.1.

Today, medical ultrasound often is the first-resort clinical imaging modality due to its cost-effectiveness and lack of ionizing radiation. Typical medical ultrasound frequencies are between 2 MHz $< \xi <$ 40 Mhz. Traditionally, medical ultrasound is mainly put to use in diagnostic applications, however, more therapeutic applications are emerging.

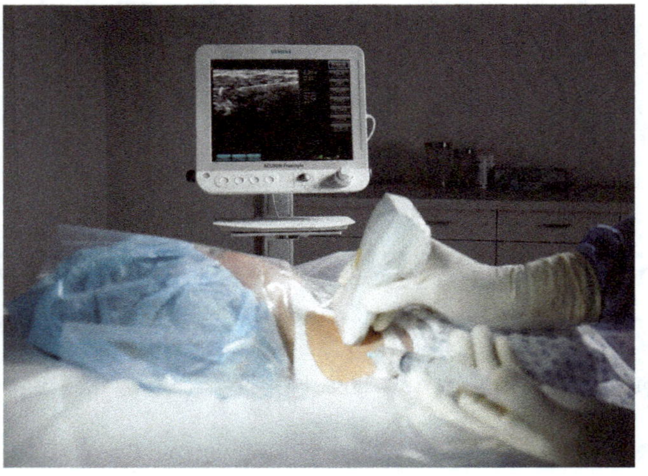

Figure 11.1: Clinical Ultrasound System in action. Image courtesy of Siemens Healthineers AG.

	f	**Examples**
Infrasound	0 ... 16 Hz	Seismic waves
Audible sound	16 Hz ... 20 kHz	Music Human Speech
Ultrasound	$>$ 20 kHz	Bat, Dolphin, and Whale Sounds Acoustic Microscopy Ultrasound Imaging

Table 11.1: Acoustic spectrum.

11.2 Physics of Sound Waves

This section introduces the basic underlying physics of ultrasound imaging.

11.2.1 Sound Waves

Acoustic signals emerge from organized movement of molecules or atoms, which cause local periodic compression of matter (gas, liquids, solid objects). Such spatially propagating, periodically repeating processes are commonly known as waves. Based on the direction of propagation, a distinction between transverse and longitudinal waves is made, where the nature of sound waves is the one of the latter class.

Sound waves are mainly characterized by *frequency*, *velocity*, *wavelength*, and *intensity*. Frequency ξ is measured in Hertz (Hz) and denotes the oscillation count per second. Sound velocity v within a medium, measured in meters

Medium	v [m s^{-1}]	Z [g cm^{-2} s^{-1}]
Air	331	$4.3 \cdot 10^1$
Fat	1470	$1.42 \cdot 10^5$
Water	1492	$1.48 \cdot 10^5$
Brain tissue	1530	$1.56 \cdot 10^5$
Muscles	1568	$1.63 \cdot 10^5$
Bones	3600	$6.12 \cdot 10^5$

Table 11.2: Sound velocity v and impedance Z of various media occurring in the human body.

per second (m s^{-1}), is independent of ξ, but varies with material properties such as elasticity and density. For some prominent examples see Tab. 11.2. The wavelength λ is the distance between two oscillation maxima and measured in meters (m). Recall the *fundamental wave equation* relates wavelength λ with sound velocity c and frequency ξ:

$$\lambda = \frac{c}{\xi} \ . \tag{11.1}$$

Finally, the intensity J of a sound wave is measured in Watts per area (W m^{-2}) and denotes the acoustic power density. Typical values for J in ultrasound diagnostics are between 1 and 10 mW cm^{-2}.

11.2.2 Sound Wave Characteristics at Boundaries

The human body contains various kinds of boundaries between different materials, for instance, at borders between organs and liquids or other tissues. At such boundaries between two media, sound waves are partially reflected and partially transmitted.

11.2.2.1 Reflection

The well known *law of reflection* states that the angle of incidence equals the angle of reflection. This also holds for reflection of sound waves (cf. Fig. 11.2(b)). For perpendicular incidence (cf. Fig. 11.2(a)), the reflection R and transmission T coefficients write:

$$R = \frac{J_r}{J_0} = \left(\frac{Z_2 - Z_1}{Z_2 + Z_1}\right)^2 \tag{11.2}$$

$$T = \frac{J_t}{J_0} = \frac{4Z_1Z_2}{(Z_1 + Z_2)^2} \ , \tag{11.3}$$

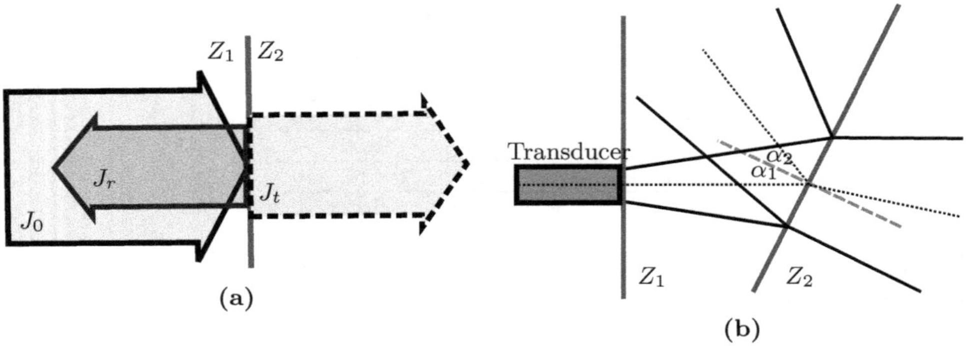

Figure 11.2: (a) Reflected J_r and transmitted J_t wave intensity at border between two different materials with impedance Z_1 and Z_2, respectively. (b) Reflection of sound waves at smooth surfaces ($\alpha_1 = \alpha_2$).

Material 1	Material 2	Reflected
Brain	Skull bone	43.5%
Fat	Muscle	1%
Fat	Kidney	0.6%
Muscle	Blood	0.1%
Soft tissue	Water	0.25%
Soft tissue	Air	99.9%

Table 11.3: Reflectivity at boundaries between two materials.

where J_r, J_t, and J_0 denote the wave intensity of the reflected, transmitted, and incident sound, respectively. Z_1 and Z_2 denote the acoustic impedance of two different media. Acoustic impedance Z, which is measured in $\mathrm{g\,cm^{-2}\,s^{-1}}$, can be computed from the tensile modulus E (elasticity) and the density D of the given medium:

$$Z = \sqrt{(E \cdot D)} \ . \qquad (11.4)$$

For some prominent examples see Tab. 11.2.

From Eq. (11.2), it is interesting to see that for two media with equal impedance $Z_1 = Z_2$, no reflection happens. With similar impedance $Z_1 \approx Z_2$, as often occurring inside the human body at boundaries between similar types of tissue, the reflection coefficient R is rather small, while for $|Z_1 - Z_2| \gg 0$, e.g., at boundaries between air (low impedance) and soft tissue (high impedance), almost the entire wave is reflected (total reflection). The latter immediately leads to the conclusion that organs containing air, such as the lungs, cannot be examined via medical ultrasound. For more details see Tab. 11.3.

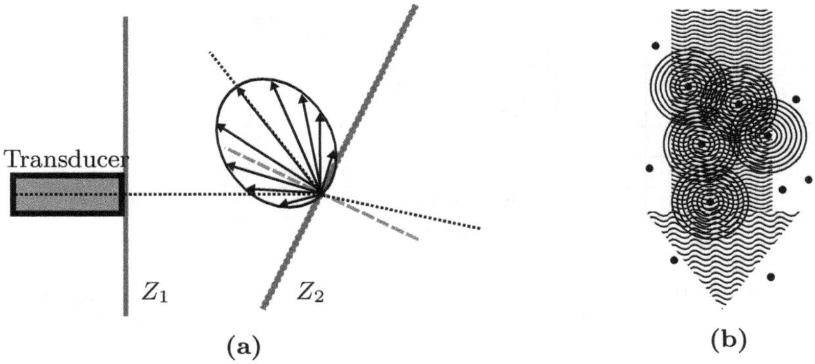

Figure 11.3: Scattering of sound waves at (a) a rough boundary (diffuse reflection) between two different media with impedance Z_1 and Z_2; and scattering at (b) inhomogeneities (depicted as blue dots) in a medium.

11.2.2.2 Scattering

Scattering means diffuse reflection of small portions of a wave in various directions. It should be noted that the law of reflection (see above) holds for each of those portions. Small inhomogeneities in the material cause scattering of sound waves, cf. Fig. 11.3(b). The same holds for boundaries with rough surfaces as shown in Fig. 11.3(a), where the width of the reflection cone increases with decreasing wavelength λ and increasing *roughness* of the surface. Scattering at rough surfaces is highly relevant in medical ultrasound, because in the case of perfectly smooth boundaries, waves are only reflected towards the sender if the direction of the wave is perpendicular to the surface (no diffusion), whereas for rough boundaries, the reflections in various directions enable imaging of tilted boundaries.

11.2.2.3 Diffraction

When sound waves pass barriers, obstacles, or openings on their path, they get diffracted. Diffracion involves a change in direction of the sound wave. Increasing wavelength λ yields an increased amount of diffraction (sharpness of bending), and vice versa. If λ is smaller than the size of the barrier, obstacle, or opening, the occurring diffraction becomes negligible.

11.2.2.4 Refraction

Snell's *law of refraction* known from optics states

ξ [MHz]	$d_{\max}$ [cm]	**Typical Applications**
1.0	50	*n/a*
3.5	15	Fetus, liver, heart, kidney
5.0	10	Brain
7.5	7	Prostate
10	5	Pancreas (intraoperative)
20	1.2	Eye, skin
40	0.6	Intravascular

Table 11.4: Maximum penetration depth $d_{\max}$ for various frequencies f.

$$\frac{v_1}{v_2} = \frac{\sin\alpha_1}{\sin\alpha_2} , \tag{11.5}$$

where α_1 and α_2 denote the angle of refraction in two different media, also applies to sound waves. However, since sound velocities (v_1, v_2) in human soft tissue differ only marginally (see Tab. 11.2), the little effects of refraction in medical ultrasound are negligible and therefore not considered further in this chapter.

11.2.3 Attenuation

Attenuation is the reduction in sound wave intensity J that occurs when a wave penetrates a medium. It follows the well-known *exponential law of attenuation*:

$$J(x) = J_0 \exp\left(-\mu x\right) , \tag{11.6}$$

where J_0 denotes the initial intensity. The attenuation coefficient μ denotes the attenuation that occurs with each cm the sound wave travels inside a medium. It depends on material (tissue type) and ultrasound frequency ξ and is measured in decibel (dB). The attenuation coefficient mainly consists of two additive components $\mu = \mu_a + \mu_s$, namely absorption μ_a and scattering μ_s (see above). Absorption μ_a causes tissue to heat.

From Eq. (11.6), it can be easily seen that the acoustic intensity J decreases with increasing penetration depth x. For a high maximum penetration depth, low frequencies are necessary as shown in Tab. 11.4. However, the resolution of the acquired images decreases with decreasing frequency (cf. Sec. 11.3.3). Thus, the deeper the tissue penetration, the lower the spatial resolution.

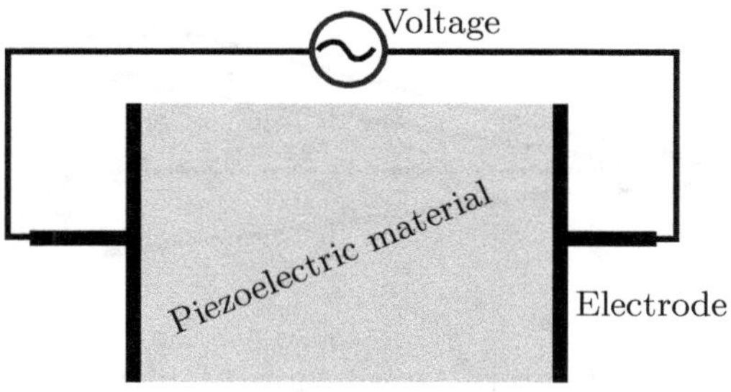

Figure 11.4: Piezoelectric effect.

11.3 Image Acquisition for Diagnostics

11.3.1 Transducers

An ultrasound transducer functions as both: a generator and a detector of ultrasonic waves. It converts mechanical energy into electrical energy and vice versa. When the transducer is pressed against the skin, it directs high-frequency sound waves into the body. Since sound waves produced by the transducer can barely penetrate air (cf. Tab. 11.3), gel is applied to the skin to help to minimize the amount of air between the transducer and the skin. As the waves penetrate the body, sound echoes are generated from the body's fluids and tissues due to (diffuse) reflection and scattering. The strength and character of these sound echoes are recorded by the transducer and, depending on the type of transducer, can be transformed into 1-D, 2-D or 3-D images, which can be rendered and viewed to the user.

11.3.2 Piezoelectric Effect

In order to generate and detect ultrasonic waves, transducers rely on the so-called *piezoelectric effect*. It describes the conversion of electrical energy into mechanical energy and vice versa in piezoelectric materials. On the one hand, mechanical pressure (pressure translates to "piezo" (gr.)) is converted to electric polarization, which generates electric voltage. The electric voltage can be measured using two electrodes, as shown in Fig. 11.4. On the other hand, electrical fields cause contraction or stretching of the piezoelectric material. This contraction and stretching can be used to generate ultrasound waves by applying a high frequency alternating voltage.

Typical piezoelectric materials used in medical ultrasound transducers are barium titanate ($BaTiO_3$) and lead zirconium titanate (PZT).

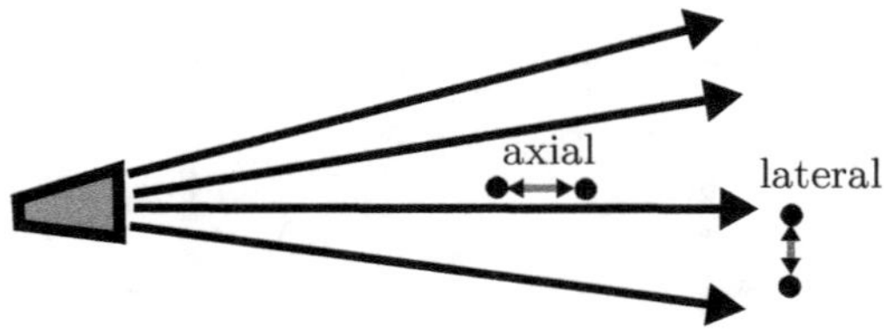

Figure 11.5: Axial and lateral resolution of ultrasound devices. Minimal distance between two structures (blue dots) in axial/lateral direction that allows for distinguishing between them in the ultrasound image.

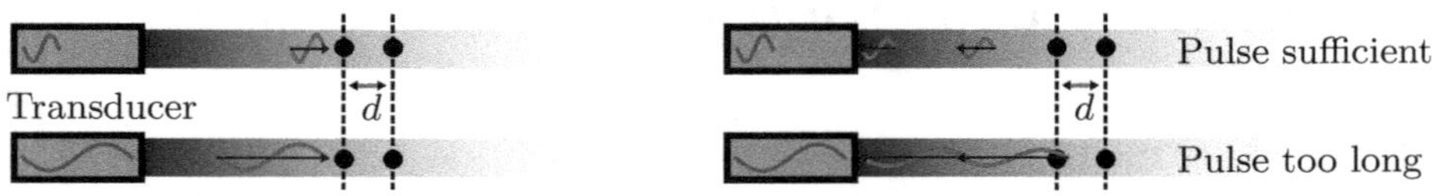

Figure 11.6: Axial resolution: illustration of dependence on wave frequency f. Left and right shows two different timesteps, where d denotes the distance between two structures (blue dots). The high frequency (top) wave allows for distinguishing between the two structures, as clearly separated echoes are sent back to the sender. Using the low frequency wave, the echoes cannot be separated (echoes are merged).

11.3.3 Spatial Resolution

In ultrasound imaging, a distinction is made between two different kinds of spatial resolutions, in particular axial and lateral resolution (cf. Fig. 11.5).

11.3.3.1 Axial Resolution

Axial resolution concerns structures lying behind each other w. r. t. the direction of the ultrasound waves. The better the axial resolution, the smaller the distance between two structures can be such that they can be distinguished by the transducer. Axial resolution is highly dependent on the ultrasound wave frequency f. The illustration in Fig. 11.6 explains that dependency based on a simple example, where an ultrasonic pulse generated by the transducer consists in a single wave only (shortest possible pulse). The distance d between the structures needs to be $d \geq \lambda/2$ in order to be able distinguish between them.

11.3.3.2 Lateral Resolution

Lateral resolution concerns the distinguishability of structures located next to each other in the same lateral distance to the transducer (same penetration depth). Lateral resolution is always inferior to axial resolution.

11.3.3.3 Frequency Trade-off

As described above, axial and lateral transducer resolution depend on the ultrasound frequency ξ, and thus on the wavelength λ. As a rule of thumb:

$$\text{axial:} \quad \Delta z \geq \lambda/2, \tag{11.7}$$

$$\text{lateral:} \quad \Delta x \sim 3 \cdot \lambda \ , \tag{11.8}$$

where Δz and Δx denote the minimum distance between to structures in axial/lateral direction such that the ultrasound echo is distinguishable. Hence, high ξ yields high resolution, whereas low ξ yields low resolution. However, the frequency is also directly related to attenuation (cf. Sec. 11.2.3), where high ξ yields high attenuation and vice versa. Thus, with high frequency f, the penetration depth is low but the images will have high resolution. At low ξ, deeper penetration is possible, but the resolution will be lower. Depending on the application, a trade-off between the desired properties (deep penetration versus high resolution) needs to be found, and the transducer frequency be adjusted accordingly.

11.3.4 Imaging Modes

Ultrasound offers a large variety of different imaging modes. The most common ones include A-mode, B-mode, and M-mode. A- and M-mode generate one-dimensional (1-D) images (signals), whereas B-mode can be used to acquire 2-D or even 3-D images (cf. Geek Box 11.1). Doppler (cf. Geek Box 11.2) can be acquired in 1-D and 2-D, and with the most recent generations of transducers also in 3-D.

11.3.4.1 A-Mode (Amplitude Mode)

A-mode is the simplest scanning mode. The height of the amplitude of the reflected ultrasound is displayed over the sonic runtime in the sonic ray direction. Extractable measurements are: frequency, modulated frequency, height of the impulse/amplitude, runtime, wave phase, phase shift, and attenuation.

However, the major disadvantage is that only very localized information (one single line through the body) is acquired.

The backward scattered ultrasound intensity along a single ray is called *A-mode*. From a continuously running high-frequency generator, a wave packet is cut out with a "gate" and is passed to the transducer. The returning echo is given through a duplexer to a time-dependent amplifier (Time Gain Compensation). Later arriving echoes, which are weaker because of the absorption, are more amplified than the signals from the surface. Signals of high depth (15 cm) are raised up to 120 dB. The signal height of an interface reflected signal is independent of the penetration depth from which the echo comes. The signal-to-noise ratio becomes worse with increasing depth. The next sonic impulse will be emitted if all echoes of the preliminary sonic impulse are decayed. The repeat rate depends on the penetration depth and therewith on the used frequency.

11.3.4.2 B-Mode (Brightness Mode)

B-mode is the most common ultrasound mode. B-mode images are generated by systematically combining a multitude of A-mode (1-D) scans into a single 2-D image, where the intensity of a pixel is defined by the amplitude of the corresponding ultrasonic ray. In brief, in order to acquire 2-D images of the inner body, the ultrasound device has to sample not only on a 1-D ray (as in A-mode), but on a 2-D plane in 3-D space. Hence, various rays are sent in different directions. To achieve this, two techniques are commonly used: the mechanical and the electronic method.

Mechanical scanners The transducer librates in front of the patient, without any external movement of the gaging head. Thus, a slice of the human body is represented in the form of a circle segment. The intensity of the echo is transformed into gray scales and is inserted into an image matrix (*B-Mode*). An image consists of a fan of typically 100 lines.

Electronic scanners (linear/curved arrays) Here, many (60 to 100) and very small (0.5 mm to 1 mm) transducers are used, which are arranged in a row ("array"). A group of transducers is activated simultaneously. For scanning, the whole group of elements is shifted. With a curved arrangement of transducers, an image detail can be represented as a circle segment.

Electronic scanners (phased arrays) Every transducer element of an array can be accessed for both sending and receiving with an individual adjustable delay.

Geek Box 11.1: 3-D Ultrasound

In 3-D ultrasound imaging, several 2-D images (B-mode) at different angles (w. r. t. axial direction) are combined into one 3-D volume. Real-time processing and visualization (rendering) of 3-D ultrasound images (volumes) requires high computational power, where graphics processing units can be used. Arbitrary section planes and "virtual travels through the body" are possible. The first 3-D ultrasound system was reported by Kazunori Baba in 1984. Slowly but steadily, 3-D ultrasound is becoming the standard of care in various medical fields (e. g., echocardiography), where 2-D imaging was traditionally used. One common application is to show their children to parents even before birth. An example is found right below this text.

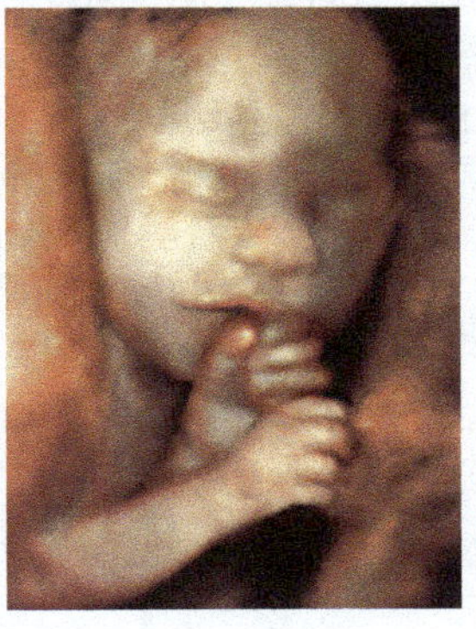

11.3.4.3 M-Mode (Motion Mode)

In motion mode, ultrasonic pulses are emitted from the transducer in quick succession without movement of the transducer. Either an A-mode or a B-mode image is acquired each time. This allows for time-dependent measurement of organ movement relative to the probe. Thus, the velocity of specific organ structures can be obtained. This can be useful, for instance, when the movement of the cardiac wall (myocardium) is to be analyzed (echocardiography).

11.4 Safety Aspects

Ultrasound imaging offers many benefits over other imaging techniques, including:

- Non-invasiveness (no injections or needles in most cases) and mostly painless.

Geek Box 11.2: 3-D Ultrasound

Medical Doppler ultrasonography enables the measuring and visualization of blood flow (blood velocities). Two modes are frequently used: continuous wave (CW) Doppler and pulsed wave (PW) Doppler. In CW Doppler, half of the transducer array emits, and the other half detects pulses. It has the advantage that it allows for continuous imaging due to simultaneous emission and detection. However, no distance information can be measured. In PW Doppler, which is pulse-based, distance information can be obtained using time-gating. However, no continuous imaging is possible.
Doppler ultrasonography exploits the well-known *Doppler effect*. The Doppler effect is named after its discoverer Christian Johann Doppler (1803–1853) and can be observed in various situations, for instance, the noise of the siren of the ambulance when an ambulance passes at high speed. Other examples can be found in astronomy: the astronomical red-shift. Most relevant to medical Doppler ultrasonography, however, is blood flow, i. e., Doppler ultrasonography can visualize blood velocities. The Doppler effect describes the change in wave frequency by a relative movement between *source* and *observer*. A characteristic frequency shift appears, which is proportional to the relative velocity. Doppler ultrasonography aims at measuring the shift in frequency to estimate velocities (e. g., of blood in vessels).

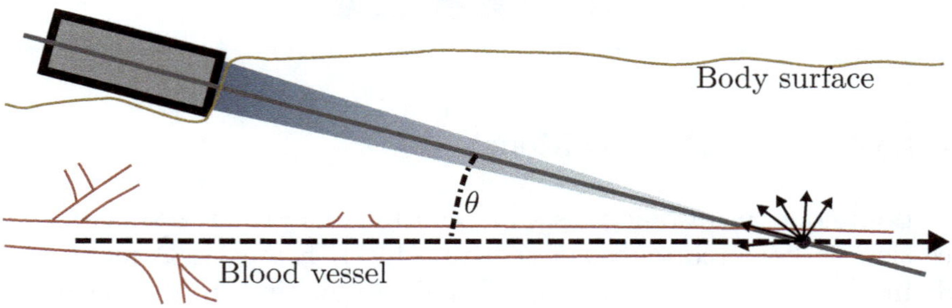

In Doppler blood flow imaging, the *source* are the moving blood cells, at which the waves scatter. The *observer* is the ultrasound transducer. The smaller the angle between the direction of blood flow in the vessel and the ultrasound wave direction, the better the Doppler effect can be exploited.

- Image acquisition is fast and relatively easy to learn.
- No ionizing radiation (contrary to X-ray/CT).
- Large number of potential applications: ultrasound can visualize structure, movement, and function of the body's organs and blood vessels.

However, ultrasound waves can harm the body:

- through heating, proportional to absorbed acoustic intensity, or
- through *cavitation*, which means gas bubbles that emerge in the low pressure phases of sound waves and collapse at high pressure phases.

Since acoustic intensities for medical diagnostics are rather low, the potentially harmful effects described above have proven to be harmless. Medical ultrasound is considered one of the least harmful imaging techniques available today and is even used during pregnancy.

Therapeutical use of ultrasound can be found in gallstone and kidney stone therapies, where high intensity localized ultrasound is used to break up the stones. The heating effect of ultrasound waves can further be used to destroy diseased or cancerous tissue.

Further Reading

[1] Olaf Dössel. *Bildgebende Verfahren in der Medizin: Von der Technik zur medizinischen Anwendung.* Springer, 1999. ISBN: 978-3-540-66014-9.

[2] G Goretzki. *Medizinische Strahlenkunde: physikalisch-technische Grundlagen.* Elsevier, Urban und Fischer, 2004. ISBN: 978-3-437-47200-8.

[3] Paul Suetens. *Fundamentals of Medical Imaging.* Cambridge University Press, 2009. ISBN: 978-0-521-51915-1.

12

OCT and its Principles

Authors: Lennart Husvogt, Stefan Ploner and Andreas Maier

OCT is an interferometry based three-dimensional imaging modality that can be used on scattering media, including several types of body tissues. It provides physicians with in-situ image data in micrometer resolution within seconds. OCT's working principle is similar to ultrasound but uses light instead of sound waves and is also free of potentially harmful ionizing radiation while being non-invasive.

OCT in ophthalmology (the branch of medicine concerned with the eyes) has been pioneered by David Huang, Eric Swanson, and James G. Fujimoto and has since become a standard modality and is widely used by clinicians on a daily basis. Since then, OCT has been continuously developed further, providing significant increases in imaging speed and resolution.

12.1 Working Principle of OCT

OCT uses low-coherence interferometry to determine depth and reflectivity within scattering tissues. In order to understand this process, we recall some basic properties of light and waves from the previous chapters.

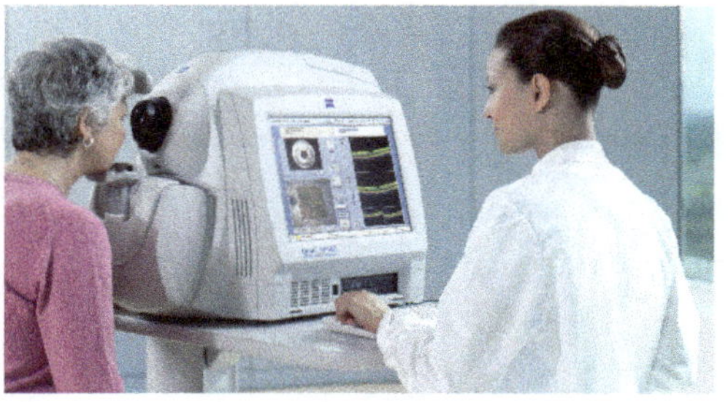

Figure 12.1: Patient being imaged with a commercial OCT device. Image courtesy of Carl Zeiss Meditec AG.

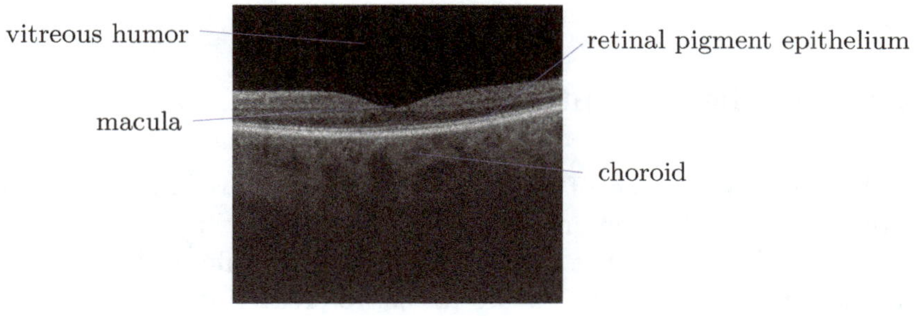

Figure 12.2: OCT B-scan of the retina. Brighter pixels indicate tissue which reflects more light. The upper portion of the figure shows the vitreous humor which has very low reflectivity. The small pit in the center is the macula, the center of vision with the highest resolution. The lowest horizontal bright band corresponds to the retinal pigment epithelium and the cloud-like structure below depicts the choroid, a blood vessel network supplying the retina with nutrients and oxygen.

- Light exhibits properties of particles and waves of which only the latter are relevant for this chapter. Light's electromagnetic wave properties form the basis for OCT.
- Coherence: two waves (or their sources) are described as being coherent with each other, when they have matching wavelengths and the same shift in phase.
- Interference: coherent waves superpose with each other (superposition principle) and can cancel each other out (destructive interference) or reinforce each other (constructive interference).
- Bandwidth describes the width of the spectrum that a light source emits. In contrast, a light source which is monochromatic, only emits light with one wavelength. Such a light source has a bandwidth of 0.

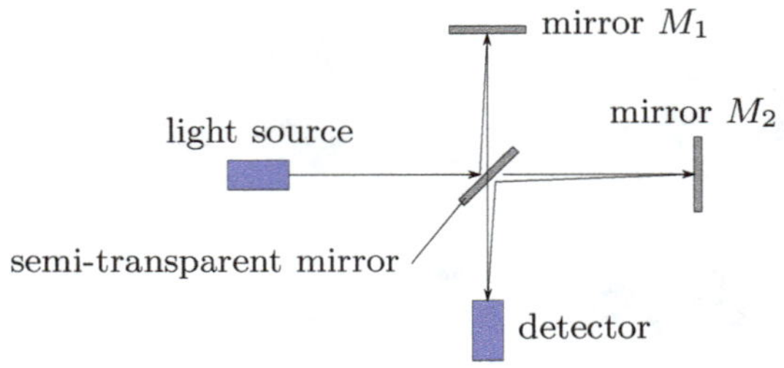

Figure 12.3: Michelson interferometer. Half of the light from the light source travels to mirrors M_1 and M_2 each, before arriving at the detector. Differences in path lengths lead to interference.

12.1.1 Michelson Interferometer

To observe interference of light, interferometers are used. Fig. 12.3 shows a Michelson interferometer. It splits light, coming from a source, into two different paths, where the light can be treated differently, and merges the light, coming back from these two paths, to create interference. Light is split at the semi-transparent mirror in the center and half of it is reflected towards mirror M_1 while the other half passes through the semi-transparent mirror towards mirror M_2. Mirror M_1 reflects the light back towards the semi-transparent mirror where half of the light passes through to a detector. Half of the light coming from mirror M_2 is reflected by the semi-transparent mirror and also travels to the detector. Interference occurs along the distance between the central semi-transparent mirror and the detector. The distance that light travels is called path length and the two paths that the light takes are called arms. If the distances between the semi-transparent mirror and the mirrors M_1 and M_2 are equal, the path lengths are equal and constructive interference will occur.

The detector does not directly detect the waves that form the electromagnetic field, but it detects the intensity of the light, averaged over a small time span, with the detected intensity I being the square of the electromagnetic field E

$$I = E^2. \tag{12.1}$$

12.1.2 Coherence Length

In practice, interference is limited by the coherence length. The coherence length describes how big the difference in path lengths can be for interference to occur. Is the difference in path lengths greater than the coherence length, no interference can be observed. Coherence length is inversely proportional

Geek Box 12.1: Coherence Length

The coherence length l_c of a light source is calculated by

$$l_c = \frac{2\ln 2}{\pi}\frac{\lambda_0^2}{\Delta\lambda} \tag{12.2}$$

with λ_0 being the central wavelength of the light source and $\Delta\lambda$ its bandwidth. As can be seen, a higher bandwidth leads to a smaller coherence length.

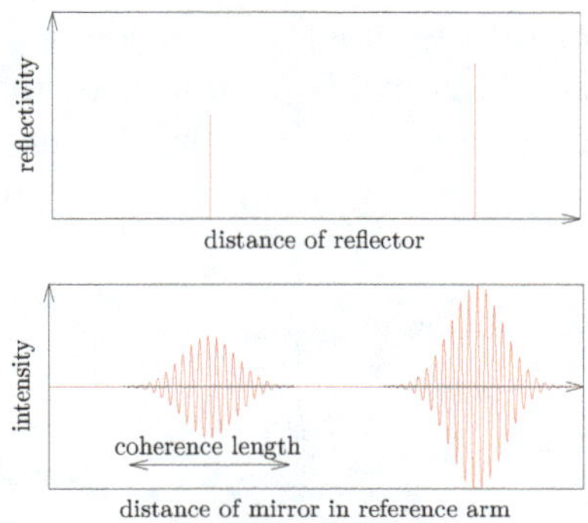

The upper half of the plot shows two reflectors with different reflectivities at different distances (as Dirac impulses). If the reference mirror is moved to match the path length of the reflectors, the measured intensity becomes maximal. Lower coherence lengths also increase resolution.

to the bandwidth (see Geek Box 12.1 for more details on coherence length). Now, if the Michelson interferometer uses a low-coherence light source (a light source which emits a spectrum), the coherence length can be used to determine the distance of a reflector in one of the interferometer's arms by gradually moving the mirror in the other arm. Fig. 12.4 illustrates this, where by moving mirror M_1 to match the distances z_{M_1} and z_{M_2}, will generate an intensity peak in the detector. The plot in Geek Box 12.1 shows how the intensity peaks when z_{M_1} and z_{M_2} are matched.

12.2 Time Domain OCT

The principle of low-coherence interferometry is used by OCT to image scattering samples. The Michelson interferometer is adapted replacing one mirror (M_2 in this case) with a sample (e. g. a patient's eye) to be imaged (cf.

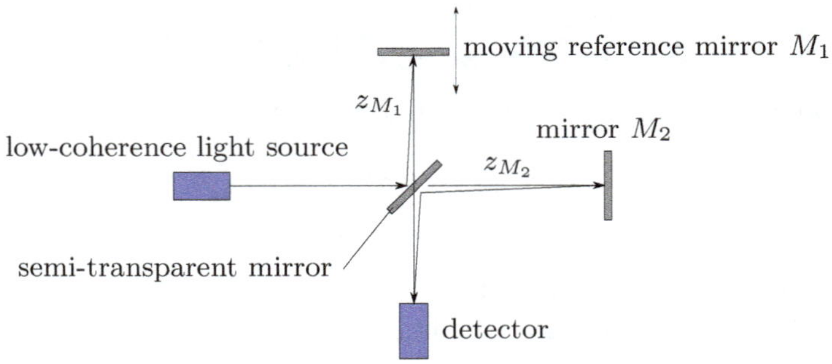

Figure 12.4: Michelson interferometer with low-coherence light source to measure the distance z_{M_2}. Mirror M_1 is moved to match the distances z_{M_1} and z_{M_2} which will generate an intensity peak in the detector.

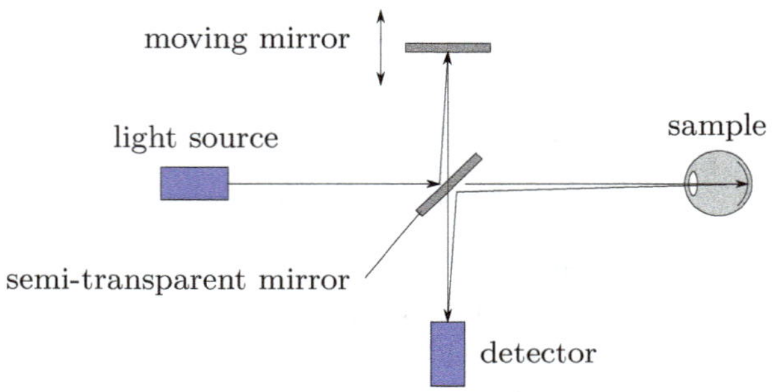

Figure 12.5: Setup of a time-domain OCT system, one mirror has been replaced with a sample. The other mirror can move to acquire an A-scan. The mirror is located in the reference arm, the sample in the sample arm.

Fig. 12.5). The remaining mirror M_1 forms part of the reference arm, whereas the sample becomes part of the sample arm. The sample has to be translucent enough to permit light to travel through it and to reflect back from different layers. Thus, movement of the mirror over time results in a depth profile of intensities of reflection at one position of the sample. This is called an A-scan. Directing the beam along a line across the sample, while acquiring A-scans at regular intervals, yields a two-dimensional image which is called a B-scan. Creating a raster scan of B-scans yields a volume. Every pixel column in Fig. 12.2 is an A-scan. The moving mirror is a disadvantage though, since it limits the maximum sampling speed of the OCT device.

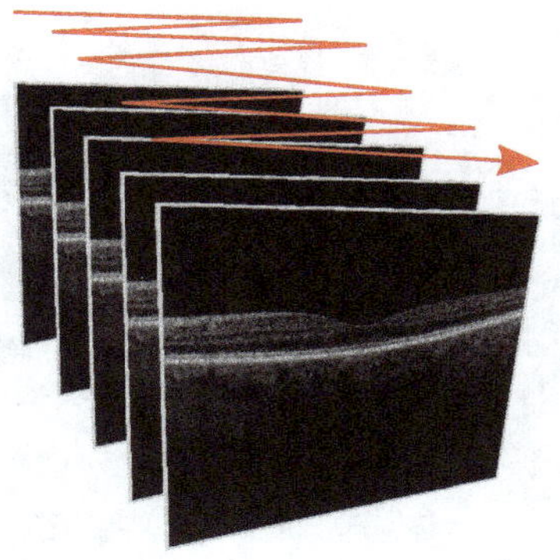

Figure 12.6: The OCT beam raster-scans the surface of the retina. Moving the beam along a line results in a B-scan (2-D image). Every column in a B-scan image is an A-scan. After each B-scan, the beam travels to the beginning of the next one.

12.3 Fourier Domain OCT

Modern Fourier domain OCT systems work differently. The spectrum of the A-scan can be acquired simultaneously and the moving mirror in the reference arm becomes unnecessary. Since we acquire the spectrum of the A-scan, we can apply an inverse Fourier-transform which yields the respective A-scan. This enables significantly higher acquisition speeds since the OCT device does not contain moving parts anymore.

Fourier domain OCT can be grouped into two variants. The first one is Spectral-domain OCT, where a spectrometer acquires the spectrum. The speed is limited by how fast the spectrometer can acquire the spectrum. Currently, resolutions of 3 µm with a scanning speed of up to 312.500 A-scans per second can be achieved.

The second one is swept-source OCT, where the light source sweeps across a spectrum and a detector samples the spectrum over time. The speed limit is set by how fast the light source can sweep across the spectrum, but the speed is generally higher than the speed of spectrometers used for Spectral-domain OCT. Resolutions of 5 µm while scanning 800.000 to 3.350.000 A-scans per second are currently possible in research systems.

12.4 OCT Angiography

OCT devices operate in the infrared light regime with wavelengths in the micrometer regime. Blood cells have diameters that lie in a similar range, i. e., white blood cells have diameters of 10–12 µm, red blood cells of 6–8 µm,

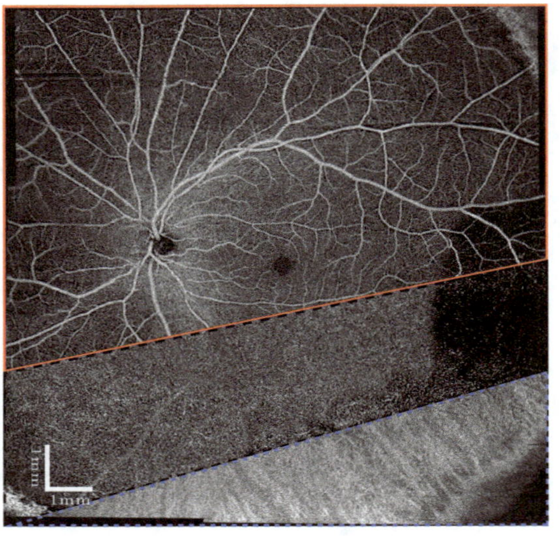

Figure 12.7: 3-D OCT angiography results in a layered reconstruction of the vessels for each retinal layer. Here we show a wide 12 mm × 12 mm field of view of the superficial and deep retina as well as the choroid (from top to bottom). Image data courtesy of New England Eye Center, USA.

and platelets of 2–3 µm. This size is just about right to induce high speckle noise in the image. In OCT angiography, this effect is exploited to create a visualization of vessels without the need of contrast agent. The idea is to scan the same area of the retina multiple times to generate a map of variance. This map will have a high response in areas that contain vessels. Using the structural OCT image (cf. Fig. 12.2), the retinal layers are then segmented and used to create projections of each layer. Fig. 12.7 shows such projections for the superficial and deep vascular plexi as well as the choroid. In Geek Box 12.2, we detail measures for OCT angiography reconstruction. Note that comparison of scans that were acquired in rapid sequence also allows for the estimation of blood flow speed. This topic is scope of current OCT research.

12.5 Applications

OCT is predominantly used for imaging the eye. However, its application is also quite common in other body regions. In the following, we summarize shortly OCT's fields of application.

- Ophthalmic Imaging: Retinal imaging is currently the major application for OCT. Both the retina and anterior eye can be imaged for diagnostic purposes completely non-invasively in 3-D. Furthermore, as described above, the vessel structure can also be investigated in 3-D without the use

Geek Box 12.2: OCT Angiography Signal Generation

In order to quantify the variance in OCT images, several measures have been proposed. *Speckle variance* assumes a normal distribution to compute the signal variance

$$\sigma_{\mathrm{SV}}^2 = \frac{1}{N} \sum_{n=0}^{N-1} (I_n - \bar{I})^2 \tag{12.3}$$

where I_n are the individual structural measurements and $\bar{I}$ their corresponding mean value.
In order to accommodate the acquisition sequence, above concept can be expanded to only compare neighboring acquisitions. The resulting method is called *inter-frame variance*

$$\sigma_{\mathrm{IF}}^2 = \frac{1}{N-1} \sum_{i=1}^{N-1} (I_{n-1} - I_n)^2 \tag{12.4}$$

Note that this measure again uses a normal distribution as underlying assumption. This time, however, we assume that the inter-frame differences are normally distributed and their mean is 0.
Another extension to this is the so-called *amplitude decorrelation* in which we introduce additional scaling to the variance computation.

$$\sigma_{\mathrm{AD}}^2 = \frac{1}{N-1} \sum_{n=1}^{N-1} \frac{(I_{n-1} - I_n)^2}{I_{n-1}^2 + I_n^2}. \tag{12.5}$$

This concept is very similar to inter-frame variance, however, a local scaling of $\sqrt{I_{n-1}^2 + I_n^2}$ is introduced for every amplitude difference. Doing so, amplitude decorrelation is always scaled between 0 and 1 and therefore can be interpreted as an "inverse correlation" where 0 is obtained for correlated observations and 1 for independent measurements.

of contrast agent. As such, OCT has become the standard of care for the diagnosis of eye diseases. Fig. 12.8 shows a volume of the anterior eye and part of the retina.

- Cardiovascular Imaging: OCT can be used to diagnose cardiovascular diseases. In order to do so, optical fibers are embedded into a catheter that is inserted minimally invasively into the vessel system. Doing so, the vessel wall can be imaged and areas of concern can be investigated. These are typically calcifications and plaques that are attached to the vessel wall.

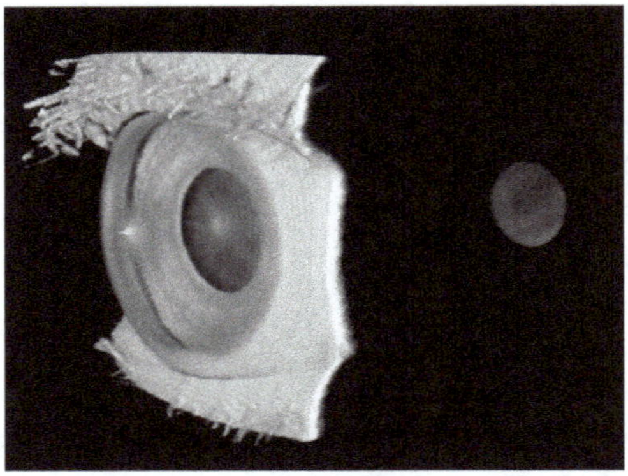

Figure 12.8: OCT volume showing the structure of the cornea, lens, and iris of the anterior eye. The disc in the background is part of the retina which is visible through the lens. These volumes are used in the visualization and diagnosis of corneal pathologies and glaucoma.

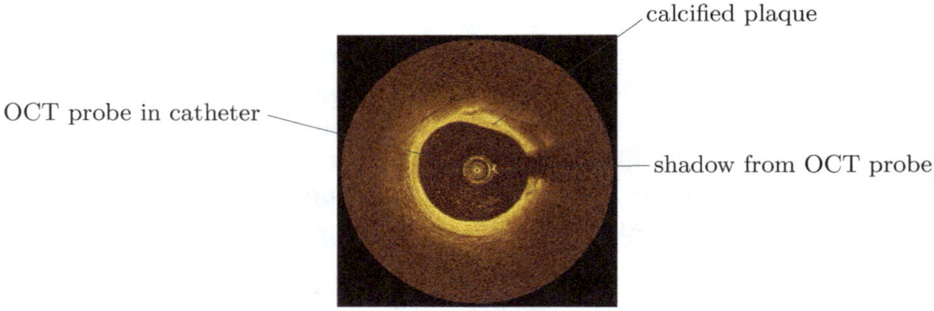

Figure 12.9: B-scan from a blood vessel. The small circle in the middle is the OCT probe within the dark lumen. The bright ring around the lumen is the vessel's endothelium (inner surface). The gap on the right side is caused by constructional properties of the probe. A calcified plaque is visible in the top right quadrant of the endothelium.

Fig. 12.9 shows a cross section of a blood vessel. A rotating mirror is mounted at the tip of the catheter and deflects the OCT beam into the tissue around the probe. OCT offers higher resolution when compared to intravascular ultrasound.

- Gastrointestinal Imaging: OCT is also used in gastrointestinal imaging, where it might have the potential to enable earlier detection and prevention of cancer. Current research investigates application in the esophagus and the colon.
- Dermatology: OCT angiography is investigated to detect skin cancer which has increased blood flow due to rapid growth of cancerous cells. Again, the combination of structural and functional imaging potentially can enable new ways of treatment. This topic is scope of current research.

Further Reading

[1] Bernhard Baumann et al. "Total retinal blood flow measurement with ultrahigh speed swept source/Fourier domain OCT". In: *Biomedical Optics Express* 2.6 (2011), pp. 1539–1552. DOI: 10.1364/BOE.2.001539.

[2] Mark E Brezinski. *Optical coherence tomography: principles and applications*. Academic press, 2006.

[3] Emily Cole et al. "The definition, rationale, and effects of thresholding in OCT angiography". In: *Ophthalmology Retina* 1/2017.5 (2017), pp. 435–447. DOI: 10.1016/j.oret.2017.01.019.

[4] Wolfgang Drexler and James G. Fujimoto. *Optical coherence tomography: technology and applications*. Springer, 2008.

[5] David Huang et al. "Optical Coherence Tomography". In: *Science* 254.5035 (Nov. 1991), pp. 1178–1181. DOI: 10.1126/science.1957169.

[6] Martin Kraus et al. "Quantitative 3D-OCT motion correction with tilt and illumination correction, robust similarity measure and regularization". In: *Biomedical Optics Express* 5.8 (2014), pp. 2591–2613.

[7] Jonathan J. Liu et al. "In vivo imaging of the rodent eye with swept source/Fourier domain OCT". In: *Biomedical Optics Express* 4.2 (2013), pp. 351–363. DOI: 10.1364/BOE.4.000351.

[8] Markus Mayer et al. "Retinal Nerve Fiber Layer Segmentation on FD-OCT Scans of Normal Subjects and Glaucoma Patients". In: *Biomedical Optics Express* 1.5 (2010), pp. 1358–1383.

[9] Stefan Ploner et al. "A Joint Probabilistic Model for Speckle Variance, Amplitude Decorrelation and Interframe Variance (IFV) Optical Coherence Tomography Angiography". In: *Bildverarbeitung für die Medizin 2018*. Ed. by Andreas Maier et al. Informatik aktuell. Erlangen, 2018, pp. 98–102. ISBN: 3662565374. DOI: 10.1007/978-3-662-56537-7.

[10] Stefan Ploner et al. "Toward Quantitative Optical Coherence Tomography Angiography: Visualizing Blood Flow Speeds in Ocular Pathology Using Variable Interscan Time Analysis". In: *Retina* 32 (2016). DOI: 10.1097/IAE.0000000000001328.

[11] Carl Rebhun et al. "Analyzing relative blood flow speeds in choroidal neovascularization using variable interscan time analysis OCT angiography". In: *Ophthalmology Retina* 2.4 (2018), pp. 306–319. DOI: 10.1016/j.oret.2017.08.013.

[12] Franziska Schirrmacher et al. "QuaSI: Quantile Sparse Image Prior for Spatio-Temporal Denoising of Retinal OCT Data". In: *Medical Image Computing and Computer-Assisted Intervention - MICCAI 2017, Proceedings, Part II*. Ed. by Maxime Descoteaux et al. Quebec City, QC, Canada, 2017, pp. 83–91.

Permissions

All chapters in this book were first published by Springer; hereby published with permission under the Creative Commons Attribution License or equivalent. Every chapter published in this book has been scrutinized by our experts. Their significance has been extensively debated. The topics covered herein carry significant information for a comprehensive understanding. They may even be implemented as practical applications or may be referred to as a beginning point for further studies.

The contributors of this book come from diverse backgrounds, making this book a truly international effort. We would like to thank all the contributing authors for lending their expertise to make the book truly unique. They have played a crucial role in the development of this book. Without their invaluable contributions this book wouldn't have been possible. They have made vital efforts to compile up to date information on the varied aspects of this subject to make this book a valuable addition to the collection of many professionals and students.

This book was conceptualized with the vision of imparting up-to-date and integrated information in this field. To ensure the same, a matchless editorial board was set up. Every individual on the board went through rigorous rounds of assessment to prove their worth. After which they invested a large part of their time researching and compiling the most relevant data for our readers.

The editorial board has been involved in producing this book since its inception. They have spent rigorous hours researching and exploring the diverse topics which have resulted in the successful publishing of this book. They have passed on their knowledge of decades through this book. To expedite this challenging task, the publisher supported the team at every step. A small team of assistant editors was also appointed to further simplify the editing procedure and attain best results for the readers.

Apart from the editorial board, the designing team has also invested a significant amount of their time in understanding the subject and creating the most relevant covers. They scrutinized every image to scout for the most suitable representation of the subject and create an appropriate cover for the book.

The publishing team has been an ardent support to the editorial, designing and production team. Their endless efforts to recruit the best for this project, has resulted in the accomplishment of this book. They are a veteran in the field of academics and their pool of knowledge is as vast as their experience in printing. Their expertise and guidance has proved useful at every step. Their uncompromising quality standards have made this book an exceptional effort. Their encouragement from time to time has been an inspiration for everyone.

The publisher and the editorial board hope that this book will prove to be a valuable piece of knowledge for students, practitioners and scholars across the globe.

Index

www.ingramcontent.com/pod-product-compliance
Lightning Source LLC
LaVergne TN
LVHW062229200926
848484LV00006B/1507